The Appraisal of *Nursing Facilities*

Steve:
Thanks for your support over the years. Your voice was heard in the writing of this book.
Jim

by James K. Tellatin, MAI

Readers of this text may be interested in the following publications from the Appraisal Institute:

- *The Appraisal of Real Estate*, 13th edition
- *Capitalization Theory and Techniques Study Guide*, 3d edition
- *The Dictionary of Real Estate Appraisal*, 4th edition
- *Market Analysis for Real Estate: Concepts and Applications in Valuation and Highest and Best Use*
- *Real Estate Damages: Applied Economics and Detrimental Conditions*, 2d edition
- *Shopping Center Appraisal and Analysis*, 2d edition
- *Subdivision Valuation*

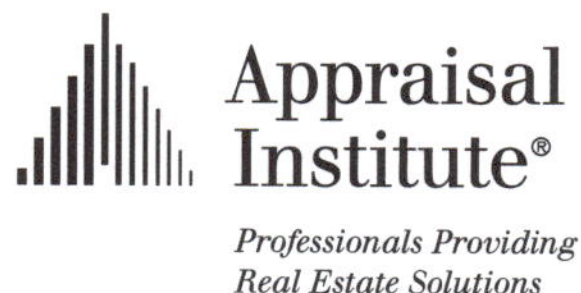

The Appraisal of *Nursing Facilities*

by James K. Tellatin, MAI

Appraisal Institute • 550 West Van Buren • Chicago, IL 60607 • www.appraisalinstitute.org

The Appraisal Institute advances global standards, methodologies, and practices through the professional development of property economics worldwide.

Reviewers: Mark R. Linne, MAI
Michael S. MaRous, MAI, SRA
Jeanne J. McNairy, MAI, SRA

Chief Executive Officer: Frederick H. Grubbe
Director, Communications, Marketing & Member Resources: Hope Atuel
Senior Manager, Publications: Stephanie Shea-Joyce
Manager, Book Design/Production: Michael Landis
Book Production Specialist: Sandra Williams
Senior Book Coordinator: Colette Nicolay

For Educational Purposes Only

The materials presented in this book represent the opinions and views of the author. Although these materials may have been reviewed by members of the Appraisal Institute, the views and opinions expressed herein are not endorsed or approved by the Appraisal Institute as policy unless adopted by the Board of Directors pursuant to the Bylaws of the Appraisal Institute. While substantial care has been taken to provide accurate and current data and information, the Appraisal Institute does not warrant the accuracy or timeliness of the data and information contained herein. Further, any principles and conclusions presented in this publication are subject to court decisions and to local, state and federal laws and regulations and any revisions of such laws and regulations.

This textbook is sold for educational and informational purposes only with the understanding that the Appraisal Institute is not engaged in rendering legal, accounting or other professional advice or services. Nothing in these materials is to be construed as the offering of such advice or services. If expert advice or services are required, readers are responsible for obtaining such advice or services from appropriate professionals.

Nondiscrimination Policy

The Appraisal Institute advocates equal opportunity and nondiscrimination in the appraisal profession and conducts its activities in accordance with applicable federal, state, and local laws.

Printed in the United States of America

Library of Congress Cataloging-in-Publication Data

Tellatin, James K.
The appraisal of nursing facilities / James K. Tellatin.
p. cm.
ISBN 978-1-935328-03-2
1. Nursing homes–Valuation–United States. I. Title
RA977.T45 2009
362.16–dc22

2009015996

Table of Contents

About the Author

James K. Tellatin, MAI, began his career in the appraisal business in 1976, after earning a degree in geography from Missouri State University. While his early career was spent appraising a wide variety of commercial real estate and farmland, his focus turned to health care property in the early 1980s. Since then Mr. Tellatin has appraised several thousand nursing facilities and various types of senior housing and hospital properties in nearly every state in the United States.

Mr. Tellatin has contributed two articles to *The Appraisal Journal* on nursing facility valuation topics and developed The Appraisal of Nursing Facilities seminar for the Appraisal Institute. He has also lectured and instructed governmental, financial, and professional association groups on healthcare valuation issues throughout the nation. He has spoken at national conferences for the National Investment Center for Long Term Care Financing (NIC), Robert Morris Associates (RMA), the International Association of Assessing Officers (IAAO), and the World Research Group. Mr. Tellatin has also been instrumental in the development of appraisal guidelines for healthcare properties for the U.S. Department of Housing and Urban Development (HUD). He is the founding partner in Tellatin, Short & Hansen, Inc.

Acknowledgments

My thanks go out to a great number of clients, appraisers, lenders, and healthcare facility operators who have provided me with more than 25 years of experience in appraising nursing facilities and the download of information contained in this book. Special thanks to Melanie Kosich, for assistance in reviewing the lengthy case study, and to my appraisal partners, Sterling Short, MAI, and C. Mark Hansen, for their support on this project.

There are a number of members of the Appraisal Institute and others who have been an influence in my appraisal career: Charles Pilmer, MAI, Thomas J. O'Toole, MAI, Tae-Sung Song, MAI, Robert Pratt, Grace Guderjahn, Michael Coufalik, Paul Neidenberg, James F. Olsen, MAI, Richard C. Sorenson, MAI, and Debra Cafaro. Their confidence in my professionalism helped inspire the writing of this manuscript.

A very special thanks to Stephanie (Tep) Shea-Joyce, the Appraisal Institute's senior manager of Publications and the Publicatons staff.

I'm very grateful to my friends, my family, and my wife, Janet, for their support.

Foreword

An aging population and soaring healthcare costs make housing for the elderly a fascinating topic and a growing concern for all Americans. As the federal government and individual states struggle to regulate and fund long-term care, increased knowledge and expertise is required of appraisers, developers, investors, lenders, and other real estate professionals. To address this need, the Appraisal Institute is proud to introduce *The Appraisal of Nursing Facilities*, which provides readers with a rare opportunity to look at a complex and growing industry from an insider's perspective, to understand its operation, and to learn to value its assets.

In this book, healthcare property valuation expert James K. Tellatin, MAI, explores long-term care facilities from both a physical and an economic perspective. The text follows the development of the industry over the past 50 years and identifies the various types of facilities that now serve the elderly population. The discussion focuses on skilled nursing facilities and the services and amenities required to serve this particular market segment and compete with other care options such as assisted living facilities and acute-care hospitals. The intricacies of Medicare and Medicaid funding are explained in depth as reimbursements from federal and state programs are crucial to the operation of both for-profit and non-profit nursing facilities. Location, site, and improvement characteristics are analyzed as are trends in new development. The supply and demand factors at work in the competitive market for skilled nursing facilities are investigated as they affect occupancy, patient mix, revenue, income, and expenses.

In addition to a large quantity of current demographic and operational data, *The Appraisal of Nursing Facilities* provides a wealth of practical examples. Readers will learn how to use Medicare and Medicaid cost reports, market surveys, interviews, sales, and data from other sources to calculate reimbursements, develop competitive market analyses, and forecast occupancy, census, payor mix, income, and expenses. All three approaches to value are discussed and illustrated, step-by-step, through the use of detailed, real-world examples. With a single case study developed throughout the text, readers are exposed to numerous techniques and tools that can be applied to address different valuation scenarios. The allocation of business assets is also explored and suggested methodology is presented to address this and other valuation challenges.

In short, *The Appraisal of Nursing Facilities* is a welcome addition to the Appraisal Institute's library of publications, which teach appraisers about new opportunities and new ways to demonstrate and expand their skills.

Jim Amorin, MAI, SRA
2009 President
Appraisal Institute

Chapter 1

Introduction and Overview

The purpose of this book is to familiarize those interested in nursing home valuation issues with the forces that affect earnings and valuation and to provide the specific tools and techniques needed to perform comprehensive valuations to assist in acquisition, lending, investing, developing, and assessing nursing facilities. Readers will include lenders, nursing home operators and developers, industry analysts, assessors, attorneys, and others, but the focus here is appraisal. The text presents a comprehensive treatment of Medicare and Medicaid programs, which have a unique and profound impact on value. Other critical topics include tools and techniques for developing well-supported occupancy, payor mix, revenue and operating expense forecasts and approaches to collecting and analyzing market sales data to extract clear and consistent price indicators.

A single case study is developed throughout the text to demonstrate the concepts and techniques. The case study begins in Chapter 10, with forecasting occupancy, and then proceeds through the remaining chapters to provide a practical application for payor mix, revenue, and expense forecasting. The case study is also used in later chapters to demonstrate the income capitalization, sales comparison, and cost approaches, the final reconciliation of value, and the allocation of the various assets of the business or going concern.

The terms *business value*, *going-concern value*, and *value of the total assets of the business* will be used interchangeably throughout the text since the appraisal community has not settled on a single term. The primary focus of the book is the valuation of the total assets of the business or going concern assuming fee simple interest in the real estate. Valuation of partial interests and components of the total assets of the business is examined in the final chapter.

To set the stage for the discussions that follow, each chapter of the book is summarized below.

Chapter 2. Types of Long-Term Care and Health Care Facilities

Nursing facilities are one segment of the health care industry and represent approximately 8% of the nation's total spending on health care. They offer both short- and long-term services. On one end of the health care spectrum offering a residential component are senior housing facilities that provide slight to moderate levels of personal care to residents, usually on a permanent, residential basis. On the other end are hospitals, providing intense medical care, usually on a short-term basis. This work does not delve into other types of health care and senior housing properties. However, appraisal principles are universal and many of the specific analyses, techniques, and information presented here are applicable to other, related property types.

Chapter 3. History of the Nursing Home Industry

The nursing home industry, like so many other businesses, has evolved over time from small, local proprietors into large businesses with substantial capital needs. The interplay of changing social, governmental, economic, and medical technology forces have profoundly affected the attitudes, approaches, and funding of long-term care. Medical treatments (surgery and medications) have lengthened the fragile final stages of life. Life style and family changes have left many of the elderly dependent on commercial or institutional care. Enactment of the Social Security Act in the 1930s, followed by the Medicare and Medicaid programs in the 1960s, have launched an industry that provides skilled nursing care to nearly 1.5 million Americans and employs another 1.5 million. Nearly every aspect of the industry is changing, including patient acuity levels, specialized care, competition from alternatives, government regulations, and program reimbursements. Residents in a nursing facility are referred to as *patients* or *residents*; however there is a growing preference to use the term *resident.*

Chapter 4. Assets of the Going Concern, Interest Appraised, and Ownership Structure

Because nursing facilities are business enterprises or going concerns, an appraiser will typically value the total assets of the business or going concern. The assets of a nursing facility include real estate, tangible personal property or furniture, fixtures, and equipment, and intangible personal property, which usually includes assembled work forces, licenses, certifications, approvals, patient records, goodwill, and management know-how.

The ownership of a nursing facility enterprise is often fragmented, with an operating entity controlling the license(s) and operations while a separate, and sometimes unrelated, party holds title to the real estate. In this legally complex and litigious business environment, the division of control and ownership can minimize some types of liability. The appraiser must properly identify the interest appraised and identify the entities or entity that control that interest.

Note that most appraisal engagements and sales transactions exclude current assets (working capital, cash, accounts receivable, etc.) from the purchase price consideration. Similarly, seller liabilities stay with the seller, and the buyer or successor in the business typically gains indemnity for the seller's liabilities. It is important for appraisers to confirm what current assets and liabilities, if any, are included in the consideration specified in a sale transaction.

Chapter 5. Medicare Program and Reimbursement for Skilled Nursing Facilities

Medicare plays a very significant role in the operations and value of nursing facilities. It is essential that the Medicare census forecasting be treated in a comprehensive manner within the competitive market analysis, as slight variations will impact earnings and value. Competition is most intense for patients receiving Medicare because this component is highly profitable.

Medicare is a federal entitlement program that provides medical insurance coverage for U.S. citizens aged 65 and older. While Medicare has four benefit components (Parts A, B, C and D), nursing facilities focus on Medicare Part A. Part A provides short-term coverage for those who require skilled nursing or rehabilitative care after a qualified discharge from a hospital. It pays the operator for restorative care, i.e. physical, speech, and occupational therapies, and for pharmacy and medical supply expenses, which collectively are referred to as *ancillary services.* This federal program is administrated by the Centers for Medicare & Medicaid Services (CMS) and a single reimbursement method is applied nationally. Part B is optional coverage that requires an individual to pay a monthly premium to receive some coverage for physician, outpatient, diagnostic, therapeutic, and nursing services and for some durable medical equipment. Part C is known as Medicare Advantage and it gives Medicare beneficiaries the option to receive their Medicare benefits through private health insurance plans, instead of through the original Medicare plan (Parts A and B). Part D is the recently created prescription drug plan, which offers Medicare recipients limited drug insurance coverage.

Medicare pays nursing facilities for Part A services using a Prospective Payment System (PPS). The Part A portion is a flat-rate case-mix, prospective system with adjustments for differences in regional labor costs and a patient's medical classification. There are four components to PPS rates: nursing, therapy, therapy–non-case mix, and non-case mix. The details of rate calculation are addressed in the discussion of this topic and should provide the reader with all the necessary tools to develop a very well-supported Medicare revenue forecast.

Chapter 6. Medicaid Program and Reimbursement for Skilled Nursing Facilities

Medicaid patients constitute the largest portion of a nursing facility's patient census and are generally the least profitable. Medicaid is the payor of last resort and pays the portion of the nursing home bill that the patient is unable to cover with his or her Social Security and pension income. To qualify for Medicaid, a person must have a medical need and have spent down nearly all of their personal assets. The program is a federal-state partnership administered at the state level. The program is very costly to states, which fund their share of the program through various tax revenues. There are as many different Medicaid programs as there are states. Most states reimburse nursing facilities for their actual, allowable operating expenses, provided those costs remain below prescribed limits. Reimbursement for interest, depreciation, and return on equity is also limited, often to the original cost basis before inflation. A growing number of states are abandoning the traditional, facility-specific, cost-based system and instead pay all operators the same reimbursement. It is beyond the scope of this book to delve into specific state reimbursement rules. However, the general principles are covered and issues that affect short- and long-run earnings are stressed.

Chapter 7. Regional and Neighborhood Influences

Regional and neighborhood physical, social, political and economic forces have a different effect on nursing facilities than they have on most residential and commercial real estate. The current and future elderly population requires scrutiny as these demographics drive demand. Household income levels are correlated to private-pay/Medicaid demand. Housing characteristics, including the percentage of home ownership, the average house value, and the age of the housing stock, are also correlated to private-pay/Medicaid demand. The size of the current and future labor pool and wage and unemployment levels are important factors to be analyzed as labor represents more than half of the operating expenses for most nursing facilities.

Neighborhoods tend to experience life cycles, and the economic performance of a nursing facility is inextricably tied into this cycle. Nursing facilities located near major medical centers may be more influenced by the hospital than the cycles in the surrounding neighborhoods.

Chapter 8. Site and Improvement Data and Analysis

A nursing home site must adapt to the environment. The sizes of sites differ in urban, suburban, and rural settings. Besides the building, the site should accommodate employee and visitor parking, deliveries, strolling areas for patients and guests, and water drainage. Other environmental issues may also need to be addressed.

Nursing facilities are generally designed and built for that specific use and must comply with many state and federal standards, over and above local codes. Designs have evolved to keep up with continued growth in economic wealth and medical and technological advances. There are four functional areas of nursing facilities: patient rooms, nursing and therapy areas, common areas shared by the patients, and support areas. Patient rooms are typically designed for double occupancy and either have a private wash closet or one shared with an adjoining room. Older facilities tend to have smaller patient rooms, shared wash closets, and sometimes even patient rooms with three or more beds. Newer facilities tend to incorporate a greater percentage of private patient rooms to compete more effectively for profitable Medicare and private-pay patients. In the early 1990s nursing homes began incorporating greater areas for therapy services to match the growing demand for these services. (Prior to 1989, Medicare only provided very limited coverage for skilled nursing care.) Common areas for patients include living, activity, and dining areas. Support areas include administrative offices, which are typically situated near the front entrance and laundry, kitchen, maintenance, and other functional space clustered together, often at the rear or on one side of the building.

Nursing home construction varies in structural type and quality. Nursing facilities are heavily used structures. They are open for business every hour of every day of every week. As a result, the building finishes and mechanical systems may deteriorate more rapidly than similar items in residential or commercial buildings. Because of changes in market preferences, increasing patient acuity levels, and continual code upgrading, nursing facilities experience obsolescence from many causes. In states where there are certificate of need policies limiting the development of new facilities, older facilities may be able to remain competitive because supply is tightly regulated.

Chapter 9. Competitive Market Analysis—Supply and Demand

Market analysis sets the stage for the development of occupancy, payor mix, absorption, and private-pay rate forecasting. The ultimate target of a nursing facility is the patient, yet it is often the family or the medical community that has the largest voice in selecting a facility. Market analysis of a nursing facility addresses the following topics.

- Market delineation–primary and secondary
- Certificate of need and its impact on supply and demand
- Identification of existing, under-development, and proposed supply and tools used to obtain accurate factual information
- Analysis of factors that drive and measure demand.
- Data sources that will help the analyst inventory existing and proposed supply, develop an accurate assessment of existing demand, identify new supply and demand, and collect objective data for rating and comparing the subject and competitive facilities.

Chapter 10. Projecting Occupancy

Supply and demand analysis proceeds through the forecasting of occupancy levels and absorption rates. The appraiser must adopt sound approaches to compare the facilities in the market, calculate market share and penetration rates, and develop an occupancy forecast. There are several techniques for estimating absorption. One technique that is not often applied, but proves to be highly reliable, is the bed turnover process, which essentially redistributes the admissions and discharges in the market to include the new facility. An example illustrating this technique is included in Chapter 10.

Chapter 11. Payor Census Mix Analysis

The four major sources of payment for skilled nursing care are Medicaid, Medicare, private insurance (managed care), and private-pay or self-pay. Profitability levels vary between these three groups, with Medicare generally being the most profitable and Medicaid the least profitable. The mix of these payment types significantly affects earnings and value. The location, physical plant, and quality of care greatly influence payor mix.

Chapter 12. Revenue Forecasting

Nursing facilities achieve revenue through routine and ancillary services. Routine services include payments for shelter, food, nursing and personal care, social services, and activities. These services constitute the primary sources of revenue. Ancillary revenues are derived from therapies, medical supplies, prescription medications, and charges for other services. Routine revenue forecasting involves applying the occupancy and payor mix (patient days by payor) to daily rates for each payment source.

The discussions of Medicaid and Medicare in Chapters 5 and 6 address principles of reimbursement. The specific development of these reimbursements is demonstrated through the case study. Appraisers must understand how to interpret historical revenue line items in a standard operating statement because many companies in the nursing home industry report revenues in a complicated set of accounts.

In most cases, the only rates that are set by competitive market forces are private-pay and, to a lesser degree, private insurance rates. Private-pay rates for routine services vary depending on the type of room (private, semi-private, etc.) and the level of care within a facility. Private-pay rate forecasting involves comparisons between competitive facilities, the same type of comparisons performed in analyzing occupancy and patient mix. Private insurance rates are typically the result of negotiations between an insurance company and the facility.

The vast majority of ancillary revenue is reimbursed through Medicare Parts A and B and from managed care and other private insurance. These revenues are also discussed in Chapter 12.

Chapter 13. Operating Expense Analysis

A standardized process for classifying, comparing, analyzing, and forecasting operating expenses is presented. The appraiser begins by classifying expenses by function (usually in alignment with Medicaid reimbursement categories) and identifying the best units of comparisons. Next, forecasts are made based on historical results and expense levels for comparable facilities, adjusted for reimbursement ceilings and changes in occupancy and patient acuity mix. Nearly every state's Medicaid reimbursement system requires individual nursing facilities to file annual cost reports. These highly detailed statements require each facility to report census, revenue, and expenses in a consistent, standardized accounting system. The data is available to anyone who requests it under the Freedom of Information Act. Most states provide the data promptly and often in electronic form. The data is extremely useful for comparing operating expenses, mining information for comparable sales and occupancy statistics, and developing a competitive market analysis.

A facility's expense forecast and Medicaid and Medicare reimbursements are interdependent. Many Medicaid reimbursement systems base reimbursement on the actual operating expenses of the facility, and thus the Medicaid revenue is expense-driven. Medicare reimbursement is not based on the specific costs of the facility, but it is sensitive to patient acuity and the amount of therapy that each patient is required to receive. The primary unit of comparison for operating expenses is per-patient day. Some property expenses can be analyzed on a square-foot basis; management expenses are typically reflected as a percentage of net revenue. Other units of comparison can also be applied to gain additional perspective.

Chapter 14. Highest and Best Use Issues

The appraiser analyzes the highest and best use of the property as vacant and as improved by applying the four tests of legal permissibility, physical possibility, financial feasibility, and maximum productivity. The analysis of the highest and best use as though vacant of a nursing facility is complicated by the consideration of obsolescence, leases, and intangible assets. The analysis of the highest and best use of the property as improved must include consideration of the business and operational aspects of the facility.

Chapter 15. Income Capitalization and Discounted Cash Flow Analysis

After census, revenue, and operating expense forecasts are developed, the three approaches to value can be applied. Since nursing facilities are primarily viewed as businesses, the income capitalization approach typically receives greater emphasis than the sales comparison and cost approaches.

As in commercial real estate appraising, overall capitalization rates derived from comparable sales data can be conclusive evidence for estimating value. The technique is most effective when the net operating income is expected to be fairly stable through the forecast period. However, irregularities in the cash flow can occur as a result of changes in competitive market conditions, reimbursements, or operations. In these cases, a discounted cash flow (DCF) analysis may prove more reliable than direct capitalization.

Overall capitalization employs a simple equation that states: value equals income divided by rate. To solve for rate, income is divided by price. The primary technique used in the development of an overall capitalization rate involves extracting rates from comparable sales and surveys. For consistency, the net operating income figures developed from comparable sales should reflect the same factors found in the subject facility. The net operating income of the sales must reflect forecasted census, revenue, and operating expenses if the net operating income being capitalized for the subject is based on forecasted figures. It is inconsistent and misleading to develop capitalization rates using trailing or past revenue and expense figures for the comparables if the rates developed from these analyses are applied to forecasted earnings for the subject. Other issues of consistency include use of a management expense, reserves for replacement, and fee simple interest sales. Portfolio sale transaction capitalization rates have the advantage of averaging out highs and lows, but they can reflect pricing discounts or premiums that may not be appropriate for a single property. Medicaid rate rebasing due to changes in ownership should be considered in the development of capitalization rates from comparable sales.

Overall capitalization rates are also developed through other techniques. The band of investments technique considers market levels of mortgage and equity ratios and rates. Residual techniques, which isolate rates for the different assets in the going concern, can be applied, but they generally require the use of a number of assumptions that are difficult to support. The simple debt coverage ratio can be applied but, rather than applying the lender's advertised ratio, the appraiser should develop the debt coverage ratio from actual transactions. Lenders will often underwrite based on conservative, trailing figures.

Discounted cash flow analysis is especially applicable in situations where there is a reasonable expectation that the earnings in the forecast will be irregular, but predictable. Internal rates of return or yield rates used in the development of the DCF can be supported using traditional methods including surveying investors, developing formulas using market capitalization rates and forecasted changes in value and NOI, and abstracting implied yield rates from comparable sale data.

Chapter 16. Sales Comparison Approach

The sales comparison approach can produce a sound value indication when well-discerned adjustments for the appropriate elements of comparison are applied to a small group of comparable nursing facility sales. Although a myriad of issues can complicate the development and application of the sales comparison approach, collecting and confirming sale data is made easier because changes in ownership are typically registered at state licensing agencies, and Medicaid cost reports can be used to extract considerable operating and financial information.

Nursing facilities are typically priced on a per-bed basis, and the sales comparison approach should address this unit of comparison first. Other sales analyses, often applied as tests of reasonableness, may include the use of net revenue multipliers, prices per square foot, and implied overall capitalization rates. The process of applying price adjustments to nursing facility sales is the same as that followed for other property types. Some unique elements of comparison that pertain to nursing facilities include conveyances of property rights and economic factors that center around payor mix and Medicaid capital reimbursement.

Chapter 17. Cost Approach

The cost approach is the least applicable technique in the valuation of the going concern of a nursing facility. Its greatest use may be in allocating the going concern to real estate and to the tangible and intangible personal property assets. Relevant development costs include the price of the land and the costs of obtaining use entitlements, and hard costs associated with constructing and equipping the facility. The array of soft development costs include architect and engineering fees, financing and other third-party fees, the cost of obtaining approvals such as a certificate of need, developer fees, incentives and profit, and the cost of operating deficits before the facility achieves economic stability.

Depreciation estimates for nursing home improvements are developed using the same principles applied to any type of commercial real estate. Special attention is given to functional and external obsolescence. Depreciation methods include economic age-life methods and methods that break down depreciation by specific causes. Extracting depreciation rates from market sales data is problematic since the sales will often involve a significant and unidentified intangible component.

Chapter 18. Reconciliation of Value Indications and Allocation of the Going Concern Value

The appropriateness of each approach and the quality, quantity, and the accuracy of the data and adjustments weigh into the final reconciliation. Generally, the income capitalization approach is favored over the sales comparison approach, and the sales comparison approach is favored over the cost approach. However, the sales comparison approach may provide more insights into value if there are a number of comparable sales that required little adjusting and are priced within a tight range. Moreover, the sales comparison approach can step to the forefront when the estimated net operating income is based on a number of uncertainties.

The methods for allocating the going concern of a health care facility are the subject of an on-going debate. There is no sure, single technique to separate the real estate value from the value of the business enterprise. The cost approach may be the best indicator of the value of the tangible assets. This is especially true when the facility is newer. However, the cost approach is ineffective when the total value of the business or going concern is less than the value indicated from the cost approach.

Another often-used technique is to capitalize an entrepreneurial or proprietary profit to arrive at an indication of intangible value. This method requires the appraiser to allocate earnings between the various assets. Parsing the operating revenues and expenses between the various assets involves considerable subjectivity since market evidence is not available.

Some market participants suggest that the percentage difference between the net operating income and the market rate rent represents the proprietor's profit, and the capitalized profit represents a significant proportion of the value of the intangible assets. An argument can be made that long-term, absolute net leases are based largely on real estate value and, therefore, recently leased properties with rents and other conditions set at market levels are proxies for real estate value. Certain components of intangible value, such as the value of the certificate of need, may be demonstrated by analyzing prices from actual market transactions. For facilities that rely primarily on Medicaid, the tangible asset value could be tethered to the allowable property cost basis of the facility as recognized in the Medicaid reimbursement rules.

A less-favored technique for arriving at a real estate value indication involves comparing sales of similarly constructed and located real estate designed and used for different purposes. Residential and medical office buildings often have location and construction qualities similar to nursing facilities. The sale prices of these properties may require adjustments to reflect differences in cost and depreciation. Other techniques should not be ruled out. The key to the use of any allocation method is reasonableness.

Chapter 19. Valuation of Partial Interests

Many nursing home ownerships are structured so that separate, unrelated parties own the property and operate the facility and a lease agreement binds the two. The value of the leased fee interest is the right to receive rents over the expected term, plus the residual value of the property at the termination of the lease. The income capitalization approach is generally applied to the valuation of the leased fee interest, and both direct capitalization and discounted cash flow methods are very useful. To assess the landlord's risk, the net operating income and contract rent are compared. Most lease rents are set at a level that allows the operators to earn some profit for their efforts, skills, and invested capital. Leased fee capitalization and discount rates are fairly easy to obtain from sale transactions and market surveys. The value of the leasehold interest is developed by capitalizing or discounting the tenant's profit. Because the lease term is finite, discounting the anticipated profits to a present value is considered more reliable than capitalizing a single year's profit. The difference between the value of the hypothetical fee simple interest and the leased fee interest, or the fee simple and leasehold interests, does not necessarily represent the market value of the partial interest.

Case Study

A case study is used to examine salient issues presented in the chapters. Case study discussions are presented immediately after a concept is discussed or the end of the chapter.

Chapter 2

Types of Long-Term Care and Health Care Facilities

A large array of building types are designed and constructed to serve general health care and senior housing. The subsequent chapters of this book will focus on nursing facilities and, more specifically, skilled nursing facilities. Nursing facilities are one segment of the health care industry. They offer short- to long-term services falling between senior housing facilities, which provide little to moderate levels of personal care to residents (usually on a permanent, residential basis) and various types of hospitals, which provide intense medical care (usually on a short-term basis). Non-residential care for the elderly is available through adult day care centers and geriatric outpatient clinics. The general categories of senior housing and health care facilities include:

- Independent living facilities (ILFs)
- Assisted living facilities (ALFs)
- Intermediate and skilled care nursing facilities (ICFs/SNFs)
- Hospitals

Most long-term care facilities fall into one of these categories, but multiple levels of service and facilities are common and are frequently referred to as "continuum of care" retirement communities.

Independent Living Facilities (ILFs)

Independent living facilities, also known as *adult congregate living facilities*, *catered living*, or *senior service apartments*, may include one or more of the following property types.

Active adult communities. Active adult communities primarily contain for-sale, single-family homes, townhomes, cluster homes, mobile homes, and/or condominiums with no specialized services. These communities are typically restricted or targeted to adults at least 55 years of age. Residents generally have independent lifestyles. Communities may include amenities such as a clubhouse, golf course, recreational spaces, and houses of worship.

Independent living facilities. Independent living facilities are age-restricted multifamily properties with central dining facilities that provide residents with access to meals and other services such as housekeeping, linen service, transportation, and social and recreational activities. The physical plant and operating characteristics of ILFs are similar in many ways to apartment and hotel properties.

Independent living facilities are for residents who can live without significant healthcare support, but choose a lifestyle that offers freedom from property responsibilities and a package of housekeeping, security, meals, and social services. Most ILFs provide full apartment rental units plus an array of public areas. The apartments range from studios to expansive three-bedroom units. In addition, many facilities also have detached housing units, generally referred to as *villas* or *cottages.* Newer developments typically include wider doors and accessibility hardware; grab bars in bathrooms; and hard-wired emergency call devices in the bedrooms and bathrooms of each unit. Washers and dryers are often provided in shared areas of the residential wings. Larger facilities can offer more common area amenities. Basic common areas include dining, social, and activity spaces. Other common areas may include educational areas such as expanded libraries with computers, multi-purpose auditoriums that can function as lecture halls, live performance centers, or theaters, and fitness centers with indoor pools and exercise equipment. The facilities also include administrative offices and areas for back-of-the house functions.

Assisted Living Facilities (ALFs)

Assisted living facilities are typically state-regulated rental properties that have the same services as independent living facilities, but also provide supportive care from trained employees to residents who require assistance with activities of daily living such as medication, bathing, dressing, toileting, walking, and eating. Because states have different ways of licensing and reimbursing assisted living, there are various names for assisted living, including *residential care, sheltered care, supervisory care home, supportive care home, personal care boarding home, rest home, domiciliary home,* and *home for the aged.* Alzheimer's/

dementia care facilities are a subset of ALFs that specialize in caring for those afflicted with Alzheimer's disease and similar forms of dementia or memory loss.

The licensing of assisted living facilities varies greatly from state to state; the physical facilities and scope of services vary too. Services generally include:

- 24-hour, on-site supervision
- Three meals and snacks each day
- Activities, social services, and transportation
- Personal care and assistance with activities of daily living, including personalized care plans
- Light housekeeping, laundry, and linen service
- Landlord-paid utilities (except telephone, cable TV, and internet access) and building maintenance

States are increasingly developing Medicaid waiver programs to shift lower-acuity nursing facility patients to lower-cost assisted living environments. Medicare will not pay for assisted living services. An excellent Web site for information on the assisted living industry is www.alfa.org.

Assisted living facilities share many design and construction features with independent living facilities. In fact, many independent living facilities have converted entire residential wings into assisted living areas without incurring substantial capital expense. The residential units of assisted living facilities are typically smaller and, because the resident requires more personal care services, designs include more accessibility features. Typically, assisted living facilities will offer semi-private, studio, one-bedroom, and two-bedroom units and shared suites. Smaller kitchens are typical since residents are provided with three daily meals and may have cognitive impairments that prohibit them from safely preparing meals on their own. Bathrooms are typically designed with larger shower areas and low thresholds for improved accessibility. Corridor lengths are typically shorter than in independent living facilities because assisted living residents are less mobile. Common and support areas are similar to independent living facilities but usually not on the same scale since assisted living facilities tend to have fewer living units.

As mentioned, one subset of assisted living is a separate type of facility that provides specialized care for residents with memory loss caused by Alzheimer's and other diseases that cause dementia. Estimates show that more than four million persons in the United States suffer from various forms of dementia. These diseases generally progress through stages that destroy memory, reason, judgment, speech, and eventually control of muscles. Memory care can be offered in licensed nursing and assisted living settings. In an assisted living setting, memory care units are residential in character. (Evidence shows that residents function better in a home-like setting rather than an institutional setting.)

In memory care units, resident units may include a Dutch door arrangement that allows the bottom half of the door to remain closed while the top half is open or of see-through glass. Making the corridor visible improves the residents' visual orientation and connection. Resident bathrooms typically include three fixtures or separate bathing facilities. Ideally, the toilet should be directly visible from the bed as a visual reminder to reduce incontinence. Kitchens are reduced to a few cabinets, a small refrigerator, and a sink. Most memory care facilities contain fewer units than traditional assisted living facilities and common areas are smaller and fewer. Communal dining is typically designed to include a large home-like kitchen and dining area. Memory care units have secured-perimeter outdoor areas; facilities must always be on guard for residents who may attempt to leave the facility unaccompanied.

Nursing Facilities

Nursing facilities provide various levels of health care service on a 24-hour basis in addition to shelter, dietary, housekeeping, laundry, and social needs. Nursing facilities include intermediate, skilled, and subacute care. The California Office of Statewide Health Planning and Development defines these levels of nursing care as follows:

- *Intermediate care* A level of nursing care services that provides care for patients who are ambulatory or semi-ambulatory and have a recurring need for skilled nursing supervision and supportive care but who do not require continuous skilled nursing care.
- *Skilled care* A level of nursing and supportive care provided by licensed nurses to patients who need 24-hour nursing services on an extended basis.
- *Sub-acute care* A level of nursing and supportive care services for patients who have a fragile medical condition, requiring intensive therapy, nursing, and/or medical treatment. Such care is more intensive than skilled nursing care, but less intensive than the usual medical, surgical, and pediatric acute care requirements. Staffing requires specially trained, licensed nursing personnel and therapists (physical, speech, occupational). Sub-acute care can be found as a freestanding facility or as a unit within a nursing facility or hospital.

These are typically smaller units (less bed capacity). Many sub-acute units specialize in specific treatments, e.g. head injury rehabilitation or ventilator dependent care.

Some nursing facilities are either specifically designed or have evolved into specialty care units that may receive additional or different licensure and certification as facilities for Alzheimer's, mental health, developmental disabilities, hospice and palliative care, or traumatic brain injury. While the focus of this book is on general types of nursing facilities, these specialty care facilities may have very similar descriptions, reimbursement programs, and competitive market conditions and the valuation methodologies presented here may apply to them as well.

Nursing facilities are typically licensed by agencies with the state health department, and most states regulate the supply of nursing homes via a certificate of need program. This program maintains an equilibrium between supply and demand, which should result in lower costs. A facility's certifications, licenses, and other approvals are components of intangible value.

The physical layout of nursing facilities differs from other elderly housing in that most patient rooms are semi-private with restrooms often shared between rooms; bathing facilities are communal; corridors and doorways are wider; and nurses' stations are positioned to view down all patient corridors. Further information on building features of nursing facilities are covered later in this text.

The largest association for for-profit nursing homes is the American Health Care Association (http://www.ahca.org).

Continuing Care Retirement Communities (CCRCs)

Continuing care retirement communities (CCRCs) can include a combination of detached homes, an independent living facility, an assisted living facility, and/or a skilled nursing facility on one campus. These communities are often very large, and they provide residents with all their residential needs and much of their non-hospital and non-physician health care for the remainder of their lives. CCRC payment plans include:

- Entry fees–substantial up-front fees with reduced monthly service fees
- Condominium purchases with monthly fees for services
- Straight rental or monthly fees

Valuations of CCRCs are difficult because the appraiser must analyze the competitive market for independent living (rent-only and entry fee structures), assisted living, and skilled nursing facilities. The analysis of entry fee revenues is akin to a lease-by-lease analysis of a regional mall or office building with hundreds of tenants since each resident has a different life expectancy and entry fee refund liability. CCRCs are substantially similar in design and construction features to independent living, assisted living, and skilled nursing facilities. CCRCs include separate, freestanding housing around portions of the site perimeter.

Hospitals

There are four major categories of hospitals:

- Acute care hospitals are traditional medical centers that provide a wide range of inpatient and outpatient services, including, but not limited to, surgery, emergency room treatment, rehabilitation, therapy, and clinical laboratories. In recent years, specialty acute care hospitals have been developed to focus on heart, orthopedic, neurological, and oncology treatment. Nursing facilities receive a number of patients discharged from acute care hospitals. Many small, rural hospitals have a special designation as *critical access hospitals*, which allows them to receive additional reimbursement from Medicare in order to make health care services available and economically viable in rural areas.
- Long-term acute care hospitals (LTACHs) serve medically complex, chronically ill patients who require a high level of monitoring and specialized care, but whose conditions do not necessitate the continued services of an intensive care unit. LTACHs have the capability to treat patients who suffer from multiple systemic failures or conditions such as neurological disorders, head injuries, brain stem and spinal cord trauma, cerebral vascular accidents, chemical brain injuries, central nervous system disorders, developmental anomalies, and cardiopulmonary disorders. Chronic patients are often dependent on technology such as ventilators, total parenteral nutrition, respiration or cardiac monitors, and dialysis machines for continued life support. Due to their severe medical conditions, these patients generally are not clinically appropriate for admission to a nursing facility or rehabilitation hospital. The average length of stay in an LTACH exceeds 25 days.
- Rehabilitation hospitals (inpatient rehabilitation facilities–IRFs) are specially licensed and certified hospitals that provide services to patients who require intensive inpatient rehabilitative care. Inpatient rehabilitation patients typically experience significant physical disabilities due to conditions

such as head injury, spinal cord injury, stroke, certain orthopedic problems, and neuromuscular disease. IRFs provide medical, nursing, therapy, and ancillary services, but not surgical procedures.
- Inpatient psychiatric hospitals specialize in the treatment of persons with mental illness. Some acute care hospitals contain psychiatric units within the larger hospital complex.

An excellent site for free and fee-based hospital data is the American Hospital Directory (www.ahd.com).

Some hospitals offer more than one of the general categories of service described here and Medicare reimbursements differ for each hospital type. Some hospitals will include a skilled nursing unit within the building complex or in a freestanding unit on the campus. Generally, when a hospital has its own skilled nursing facility, it focuses on providing rehabilitation and skilled nursing care on a short-term basis for patients needing a transition step between the hospital and home. These units represent significant competition for freestanding nursing facilities.

Summary

Healthcare enterprises occupy a wide range of general and special-purpose buildings, including retail, office, residential, industrial, and institutional properties in many settings. In contrast, nursing facilities are purpose-built structures that take on residential, commercial and institutional locations and structural characteristics. In the continuum of care, nursing facilities fall between hospitals and senior housing. Senior housing properties include independent and assisted living facilities, which are normally contained in purpose-built structures configured for one or more levels of service. Developments that combine independent living, assisted living, and skilled nursing are generally referred to continuing care retirement centers (CCRCs). While there are four general hospital categories–acute care, psychiatric, long-term acute care, and inpatient rehabilitation–many nursing facility patients come from acute care hospital discharges.

Most nursing homes are freestanding facilities; the buildings are not shared by hospital, senior housing, or other functions. However, nursing facilities can be combined into buildings that contain space for other purposes. There are three general categories of nursing facilities: intermediate, skilled and subacute care. Intermediate care facilities are falling by the wayside as the market has pressured the facilities to either upgrade (physically and/or by license) to skilled care to meet growing demand, or fall prey to growing competition from lower-cost, more attractive assisted living facility and home healthcare alternatives. A growing proportion of nursing facilities are offering intense levels of nursing and rehabilitation services to patients being discharged earlier from hospitals. Such facilities are often refered to as subacute facilities. These adjustments in the market necessitate physical and operational changes for nursing facilities. Nursing facility beds or units are sometimes contained within hospital and senior housing settings. The combination of different levels of care within a property adds considerable complexity to an appraisal.

Chapter 3

History of the Nursing Home Industry

Nursing home care in the United States has evolved in response to changing social, governmental, economic, and technological forces. The average life expectancy of a white female increased from 48.7 years in 1900 to 80.1 years in 2000[1]. Medical treatments (surgical and medications) have lengthened the fragile final stages of life, necessitating closer medical supervision and professional care giving. Life style and family changes have left many elderly widowed or geographically separated from their children. Younger family members, who once made room for their aging parents in their homes, have moved away to live and work in distant communities. Government insurance programs, beginning with the Social Security Act in the 1930s, subsequent amendments to the act in the 1950s, and Medicare and Medicaid programs signed into law in the 1960s, have combined with social and economic trends to enrich the nursing home industry. Change in the industry is constant. Acuity levels within nursing homes continue to increase and specialization in long-term care to treat diseases that affect large numbers of the elderly is becoming more common.

This chapter will examine important historical events that have impacted this changing and highly regulated industry.

Early 20th Century

During the early 1900s, federal assistance for the elderly was simply not available. Nursing home care depended on the patient's personal resources and was provided by family, local and state government, and religious and other private non-profit

1. National Center for Health Statistics, *Health, United States, 2006, with Chartbook on Trends in the Health of Americans*, Hyattsville, MD: 2006

Table 3.1 Timeline of Important Events Affecting the Nursing Home Industry

Decade	Business Trends	Average Life Expectancy*	Government Policies
1930s	Largely non-profit and government operated	52.0 years	Social Security enacted
1950s	Largely non-profit and government operated	68.2 years	Amendments to SS act, still no federal payments for nursing home care
1960s	Rapid development of the industry	69.7 years	Medicare/Medicaid established, states begin to receive federal moneys for nursing homes
1970s	For-profit operators grow and consolidate	70.8 years	States fine-tune their newly created Medicaid programs
1980s	Hospitals discharge patients earlier	73.7 years	Medicare pays flat fees for hospital stays; Medicare expands nursing home benefits
1990s	Increased offering of higher-acuity care and rehabilitation services	75.4 years	Medicare reimbursements change from facility-specific, cost-based to a flat-rate structure
2000s		77.0 years	Growing use of Medicaid waivers by states to shift nursing home patients into assisted living

* From http://www.cdc.gov/nchs/data/hus06.pdf#027

organizations. Many impoverished frail and elderly persons were placed in "poor farms" or "almshouses," which were often administered by local governmental agencies that were poorly funded. These facilities were often found in dilapidated buildings and provided inadequate care. These conditions gradually improved through the first half of the century. In 1900, the average life expectancy at birth was 47.3 years and the major causes of death were pneumonia (all forms) and influenza, tuberculosis, diarrhea, enteritis, and ulceration of the intestines, and diseases of the heart.

The 1930s and 1940s: Roosevelt and Truman Administrations

Franklin D. Roosevelt's New Deal introduced the idea that elderly citizens should receive federal benefits on the basis of need. The Social Security Act was enacted by President Roosevelt on August 14, 1935. The act provided matching grants to each state for Old Age Assistance (OAA) provided to retired workers. To discourage almshouse living, people living in public institutions were not eligible for the payments. That paved the way for the opening of a variety of private old-age homes where elderly people could live in a care facility and still collect the Old Age Assistance payments.

The Depression and World War II restricted the growth of the nation's health care services, and little improvement was observed in the fragmented and loosely regulated nursing home industry in this period. The optimism that followed the war provided the impetus for The Hospital Survey and Construction Act, known as the Hill-Burton Act, in 1946 during the early part of the Truman administration. The Hill-Burton Act provided funding for the constructing of state-of-the-art hospitals that satisfied an enormous backlog of need and incorporated new medical treatments. In 1945 President Truman asked Congress to develop a government-sponsored national health care insurance program. By the end of his administration, Truman backed away from his proposed universal health insurance program and instead supported a plan that would focus on providing health insurance aid to those with Social Security benefits. This plan would percolate through two more administrations before becoming law.

The 1950s: Eisenhower Administration

During the 1950s there were significant amendments to the Social Security Act, including a requirement that states establish some form of nursing home licensure. The amendments also eliminated a ban on providing funding to residents of public facilities and health service providers. The Social Security amendments transformed nursing homes from part of the welfare system to part of the health care system. A change in federal law in 1954 provided hospitals with federal grants for nursing home construction "in conjunction with a hospital" to improve the quality of care. With this grant, nursing home designs and construction began to change and be modeled after hospitals.[2] By 1950 the average life expectancy at birth had increased to 68.2 years[3] and the leading causes of death were heart diseases, various forms of cancer, vascular lesions affecting the central nervous system–i.e., strokes, and accidents. Influenza, pneumonia, and tuberculosis were being brought under control with new medicines.

The 1960s: Kennedy and Johnson Administrations

The 1960s was the most formative decade in the nursing home industry as the federal government implemented the Medicare and Medicaid programs through Title XVIII and Title XIX of the

2. *The Online NewsHour with Jim Lehrer,* Henry J. Kaiser Family Foundation/Harvard School of Public Health National Survey on Nursing Homes—http://www.pbs.org/newshour/health/nursinghomes/timeline.html
3. National Center for Health Statistics, *Health, United States, 2006, with Chartbook on Trends in the Health of Americans*, Hyattsville, MD.

Social Security Act. President Lyndon Johnson signed the law on July 30, 1965, in the presence of Harry Truman at his home in Independence, Missouri. Truman became the first Medicare enrollee and, at the signing ceremony, President Johnson said:

> Thirty years ago, the American people made a basic decision that the later years of life should not be years of despondency and drift. The result was enactment of our Social Security program... Compassion and reason dictate that this logical extension of our proven Social Security system will supply the prudent, feasible, and dignified way to free the aged from the fear of financial hardship in the event of illness.

As will be discussed in detail in Chapters 5 and 6, Medicare, which is strictly a federal program funded by a distinct federal payroll tax, focuses on hospital, physician, and therapy services for those that qualify for Social Security benefits. Initially, the program included moderate benefits for nursing home care. In contrast, Medicaid is essentially a joint venture between each state and the federal government and is funded through general tax revenues. It is one of a number of aid programs and provides nursing home coverage to qualifying indigent persons.

The enactment of the Medicare and Medicaid programs triggered an enormous expansion in nursing home services and widespread development in ensuing years. In many rural states that have experienced limited population or economic growth since the 1960s, much of the existing nursing home bed supply was developed in the wave of development between 1966 and 1975.

The 1970s

The rollout of Medicare brought rapid and unexpected use of program benefits for nursing home care. Then, in 1969, the Department of Health and Human Services, the federal agency responsible for administrating the Title XVIII and XIX programs, issued Intermediary Letter 371, which substantially reduced nursing home coverage through Medicare. The letter was effective immediately and the sudden policy change required thousands of recipients and their families to pay nursing home bills with private funds. Many of these bills would never be paid, causing financial strain on the nursing home industry.

With the new Medicaid and Medicare programs came higher government standards for care and physical plants, with which most facilities were unable to comply. By 1971, six years after the enactment of Medicare and Medicaid, the U.S. Congress passed the Miller Amendment, which allowed states to offer a lower-acuity licensure for facilities known as *intermediate care facilities.* Intermediate care facilities (ICFs) were allowed to provide fewer skilled nursing resources and operate in buildings with inferior standards. Because these facilities were also eligible for Medicaid reimbursements, ICF licensure was less costly for states and the federal government. Some argue that these ICFs were the precursors to today's assisted living facilities.

During the early years of the Medicaid program, billing fraud and patient abuse were rampant. Most states used relatively arbitrary fee schedules to compensate nursing home operators. In 1972 the federal government passed reforms to improve patient care and compensate owners through a reasonable cost-based system. In other words, nursing home operators were to be reimbursed according to their actual operating expenses, subject to limitations typically set by comparing costs at comparable facilities. Unfortunately, these changes were not enough to substantially eliminate poor patient care and provider fraud.

The 1980s: Reagan and Bush Administrations

During the 1970s, Medicaid expenditures were growing rapidly and were one of the largest costs in state budgets. Many states attempted to limit the expense by developing payment systems that did not adequately cover reasonable nursing home costs. In 1981 the Boren Amendment was enacted, requiring states to provide for "reasonable and adequate" reimbursements. This forced many states to increase payments to nursing homes, creating state budget difficulties. Governors were unsuccessful in their legal attempts to rescind the Boren Amendment and many state nursing home associations effectively employed the Boren Amendment to leverage higher compensation from states, often through the use of lawsuits. It should be noted that most states have constitutions that prohibit deficits spending, while the federal government has increased the federal deficit nearly every year since 1956.[4]

In 1983 Medicare switched from paying inpatient hospital services using a cost-based structure to a flat fee system known as *diagnostically related groupings*, or DRGs. This system pays a hospital a flat amount, regardless of the actual costs or length of stay for a specific DRG. This gave hospitals an incentive to discharge patients earlier, often into nursing homes, which elevated acuity levels at nursing facilities. Hospitals pressured Medicare to increase nursing home benefits to patients being discharged from hospitals earlier under the DRG system. This made sense to the government as these patients could receive

4. U.S. Department of the Treasury, Web site: www.treasurydirect.gov/govt/reports/pd/histdebt/histdebt_histo5.htm

similar care in a lower-cost, nursing home environment. However, it was not until 1989 that Medicare increased benefits for skilled nursing care through the Medicare Catastrophic Protection Act. This program, which was introduced along with a number of improved benefits, provided for up to 150 days of Medicare coverage at a nursing home after a qualified hospital stay. To fund the expanded Medicare benefits, many elderly were required to pay a surtax on their regular income taxes. This tax was extremely unpopular and the program was discontinued after just one year.

One benefit that remained in place, although in a somewhat reduced form, was the nursing home component. The program is still in effect today. It allows Medicare patients who are discharged from hospitals after a stay of three days or more, but require qualified rehabilitation or medical treatments, to receive a nursing home benefit of up to 100 covered days in a skilled nursing facility. In the late 1980s, many nursing facilities ramped up their levels of service to provide rehabilitation and other sub-acute care and take advantage of this growing, and profitable, patient segment. As nursing homes were facing tighter operating margins due to declining numbers of higher-paying private-pay patients and compressed Medicaid reimbursement, the expanded Medicare program, which employed an actual-cost-plus payment system, largely carried the industry out of a very lean period and into a generally prosperous new decade.

In 1987 President Ronald Reagan signed into law the first major revision of the federal standards for nursing home care since Medicare and Medicaid were created. The Omnibus Budget Reconciliation Act of 1987, or OBRA 87, effectively mandated that nursing facilities provide enough services so that each patient can "attain and maintain his or her highest practicable physical, mental, and psycho-social well-being." (Congress usually wraps up much of its budgetary and substantive work in one large bill, which is referred to as an "Omnibus Budget Reconciliation Act.")

According to the National Long Term Care Ombudsman Resource Center, the significant OBRA 87 provisions include:[5]

- Emphasis on a resident's quality of life and care
- A goal to maintain or improve each patient's ability to perform activities of daily living, absent medical reasons
- Development of an individualized care plan for each patient

5. The National Long Term Care Ombudsman Resource Center *www.ltcombudsman.org/ombpublic/49_346_1023.cfm*, Developed by Hollis Turnham, Esq.

- Increased staff training
- A serious push to transfer patients with developmental disabilities to smaller, de-institutionalized, residential settings (the Olmstead act)
- Substantial elimination of inappropriate physical and chemical restraints for patients who respond well to restraint solutions
- Uniform standards for Medicare and Medicaid certification
- Facilities are prohibited from requesting or receiving compensation from families or others for patients using Medicare and Medicaid
- State inspectors expanded their scope from reliance on staff interviews and facility records to include interviews with residents and families and observation of dining and medication administration.

The 1990s: Clinton Administration

During the 1990s the industry saw acuity levels increase as facilities took on an increasing proportion of Medicare patients, who were sicker and coming directly from hospitals, and decreasing proportions of lower-acuity, private-pay patients. These patients were being siphoned off by the rapidly growing assisted living industry. Patients and their families generally prefer assisted living facilities because they offer apartment-like living units, have a newer, fresher appearance, and serve a healthier population. The assisted living industry began moving into the old IFC (intermediate care facility) territory, and the private-pay market welcomed this new alternative.

The 1997 Balance Budget Agreement (BBA) introduced sweeping changes to Medicare reimbursement for nursing homes by phasing out facility-specific, cost-based reimbursement in favor of a "managed care" approach. Managed care pays a single rate to all operators for a specific care level, with the rate adjusted for regional wage differences. This new Medicare system, known as a *prospective payment system*, or *PPS*, was designed to reduce Medicare spending and motivate operators to reduce costs.

Under the prior reimbursement system, Medicare paid nursing homes for their actual, allowable costs, subject to certain limits or ceilings. The cost of this program was increasing at a rate well beyond the general inflation rate. To counter this trend, the PPS was implemented. Like the DRG structure under which hospitals were paid for inpatient services, the new PPS called for nursing homes to receive pre-set reimbursements based on a patient's medical classification, or resource utilization grouping (RUG). The reimbursement for each of the original

44 RUG classifications was the same for all nursing facilities, regardless of individual cost experiences and ownership structures, but subject to regional wage indexing adjustments. This reimbursement scheme is still in effect and will be discussed in detail in Chapter 5.

The switch from a facility-specific, cost-based system to the current prospective payment system caused considerable financial hardship for large, highly leveraged providers who were unable to change their business models quickly. Several of the nation's largest publicly traded nursing home companies (Vencor-Kindred, Integrated, Mariner, Genesis, and Sun Healthcare) went bankrupt in the late 1990s within a few years after the roll out of PPS and attributed their bankruptcies to PPS. Actually, most of these companies leveraged up prior to 1997 to acquire and expand into other types of healthcare services, including home health, pharmacy, and therapy businesses. These services experienced substantial reductions in Medicare payments due to the 1997 Balanced Budget Act. In contrast, those nursing home companies that have learned how to provide quality rehabilitation services at low costs have benefited under PPS. It is quite possible for a typical nursing facility to derive more than half of its earnings from Medicare reimbursements even though the Medicare patients represent less than 20% of the total census.

The 21st Century

Moving into the first decade of the 21st century, nursing facilities have continued to experience the following trends:

- Increasing reimbursement pressures from Medicaid and Medicare
- Further attrition of low-acuity patients to assisted living and home healthcare alternatives
- Increasing pressure from states using Medicaid waivers to shift some low-acuity Medicaid patients to assisted living environments
- Increased competition from new facilities designed to target higher profit service areas such as rehabilitation and high-end private-pay clientele

Continued change is expected in this mature and heavily regulated industry. Considerable pressure will be exerted by

- Growing federal and state budget concerns
- Increasing demand from aging baby boomers
- An inventory of aging and deteriorating physical plants

- A consumer market seeking more desirable alternatives for long-term care.

Future changes will be greatly affected by societal choices and physical needs and largely directed by governmental and economic forces.

Demographic Trends

The most significant issues for the industry are the growth of an aging society and its ability to pay for health care in general and long-term care specifically. Some facts and trends warrant examination from the outset.

Life expectancy from birth increased substantially between 1900 and 1950 as the three leading causes of death in 1900 (pneumonia, tuberculosis, and intestinal diseases) were substantially reduced through medical discoveries (see Table 3.2).[6]

Table 3.2 **Life Expectancy in Years at Birth for the United States**

Year	Total	Male	Female
1900	47.3	46.3	48.3
1940	62.9	60.8	65.2
1950	68.2	65.6	71.1
1960	69.7	66.6	73.1
1970	70.8	67.1	74.7
1980	73.7	70.0	77.4
1990	75.4	71.8	78.8
2000	77.0	74.3	79.7
2004	77.8	75.2	80.4

Source: National Center for Health Statistics, *Health, United States, 2006, with Chartbook on Trends in the Health of Americans*, Hyattsville, MD.

Increases in life expectancy since the 1950s have been less remarkable, but steady. When Social Security was enacted, the average life expectancy at birth was less than 65, the qualifying age for benefits. Thus, less than half of the nation's population could ever expect to receive any Social Security benefits

As shown in Figure 3.1, the average life expectancy for all Americans over the age of 65 in 1950 was 78.9 years (13.9 addition years), and that average increased 4.8 years to 83.7 years in 2000.[7] Much of this increase is attributed to healthier lifestyles and improved diagnostics and medical treatments (surgical and pharmaceutical).

As the number of Medicaid and Medicare beneficiaries increases as a percentage of the working-age, or contributing,

6. Centers for Disease Control and Prevention, *Leading Causes of Death, 1900-1998*
7. National Center for Health Statistics, *Health, United States, 2006, with Chartbook on Trends in the Health of Americans*, Hyattsville, MD: 2006

Figure 3.1 **Total Life Expectancy at Age 65 by Sex, United States, Selected Decades, 1950 to 2000, Plus 2004**

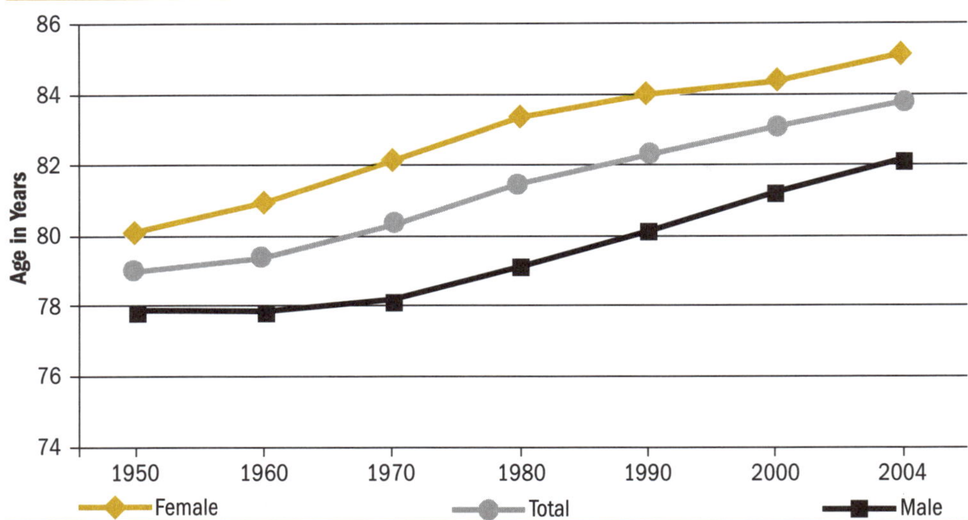

Source: National Center for Health Statistics, *Health, United States, 2006, with Chartbook on Trends in the Health of Americans*, Hyattsville, MD.

population, a greater fiscal strain will be exerted on government programs and the private economy. Baby boomers will be migrating through the later stages of their demographic cycle in the coming decades, significantly increasing the nation's retirement and old-aged dependency ratios and creating enormous pressure on Social Security, Medicare, and Medicaid. These massive federal programs were developed prior to the 1960s and 1970s, when family size began to steadily shrink due to the development and acceptance of birth control methods and other lifestyle changes. As shown in Table 3.3 and Figure 3.2, the old-age dependency ratio is expected to increase from 10.0% in 2000 to 17.0% in 2030. In total population, the 75-plus age cohort will essentially double between 2000 and 2030, while the "economically productive" age cohort will increase only 18.7% over the same 30-year period.

The demographic pressures are enormous and, without significant tax increases and/or reductions in benefits, dire consequences cannot be avoided. Reduced benefits such as lower dollar coverage

Table 3.3 **Dependency Population and Ratios for the U.S. Population—2000 and 2030**

	2000	2030
Age 0 to 19	80,473,265	95,103,878
Age 20 to 64	165,956,888	197,027,086
Age 65+	34,991,753	71,453,471
Retirement-aged dependency ratio*	21.1%	36.3%
75+	16,600,767	33,505,538
Old-age dependency ratio†	10.0%	17.0%
Total dependency ratio‡	69.6%	84.5%

* Retirement-age dependency ratio = Age 65 and over / Age 20 to 64

† Old-age dependency ratio = Age 65 and over / Age 20 to 64

‡ Dependency ratio = (Age under 20 + Age 65 and over) / (Age 20 to 64)

Source: U.S. Census Bureau, Population Division, *Interim State Population Projections, 2005.* Internet release date: April 21, 2005.

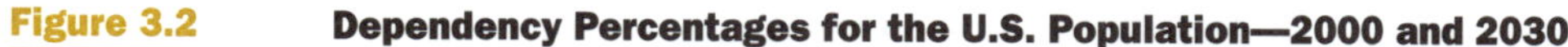

Figure 3.2 **Dependency Percentages for the U.S. Population—2000 and 2030**

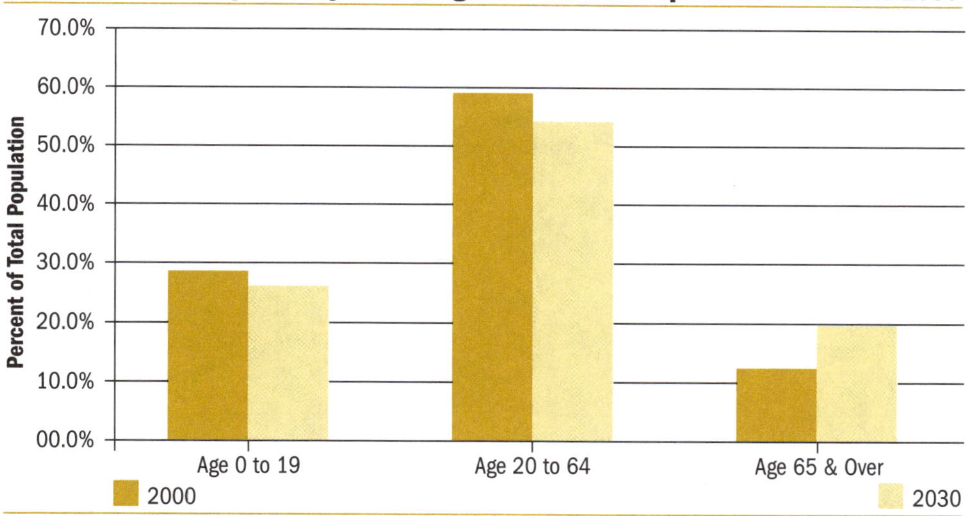

Source: *Interim State Population Projections, 2005.*

and payments, higher deductibles and co-pays, higher age eligibility, and limits to lifetime benefits have been suggested.

Comparing U.S. spending on health care to spending in other nations suggests that substantial reductions could be achieved (see Table 3.4). In 2003 the United States spent 15.0% of its gross domestic product (GDP) on health care.[8] No other major, first-world economy comes close to this level of spending, either in total dollars or as a percentage of GDP. Yet, when comparing healthcare spending to life expectancy, the United States falls below a number of countries that spend far less. The arguments for life expectancy and healthcare spending variances are multiple and continue to be debated.

Now, focusing in on where healthcare spending occurs in the United States, nursing facilities consumed 8.4% of total healthcare spending in 2000. That amounted to an expenditure of $95.0 billion in 2000 which, when divided by the total U.S. population aged 75 and over, indicates an average annual cost of $5,738 for this age cohort (developed from figures in the two previous tables). Prior to the enactment of Medicare and Medicaid, nursing facilities captured only 3.4% of total U.S. healthcare spending.

In 1960, before the creation of Medicare and Medicaid, out-of-pocket (private-pay) spending on health care represented 55.2% of the nation's total healthcare expenditures. By 1980 out-of-pocket spending was reduced to 27.2%, and in 2000 it declined to just 16.9%. Private health insurance has picked up

8. The Organization for Economic Cooperation and Development, *Health Data File 2005*, incorporating revisions to the annual update. Available from: www.oecd.org/els/health.

Table 3.4 **Total Health Expenditures as a Percent of Gross Domestic Product and Per Capita Health Expenditures in Dollars, By Selected Countries: Selected Years 1960-2000**

	Per Capita Income (rounded to nearest $100)		Per Capita Health Expenditures*		Health Expenditures as a Percentage of GDP		Life Expectancy in 2000
Country†	**1980**	**2000**	**1980**	**2000**	**1980**	**2000**	
Australia	$9,900	$24,700	$691	$2,220	7.0%	9.0%	79.8
Canada	11,000	28,100	783	2,503	7.1%	8.9%	79.4
Czech Republic	–	14,600	–	962	–	6.6%	74.8
Denmark	10,500	28,400	955	2,382	9.1%	8.4%	76.7
France	10,000	26,400	711	2,456	7.1%	9.3%	78.8
Germany	11,100	25,200	965	2,671	8.7%	10.6%	78.1
Hungary	–	12,100	–	857	–	7.1%	71.4
Italy	–	25,300	–	2,049	–	8.1%	79.1
Japan	8,900	25,900	580	1,971	6.5%	7.6%	81.1
South Korea	–	16,400	–	771	–	4.7%	75.6
Mexico	–	8,900	–	499	–	5.6%	73.9
Poland	–	10,300	–	587	–	5.7%	73.8
Switzerland	14,000	30,600	1,033	3,182	7.4%	10.4%	79.7
Turkey	2,300	6,800	75	452	3.3%	6.6%	71.0
United Kingdom	8,600	25,100	482	1,833	5.6%	7.3%	77.8
United States	12,100	34,600	1,055	4,539	8.7%	13.1%	76.6

* Per capita health expenditures for each country have been adjusted to U.S. dollars using gross domestic product purchasing power parities (PPP) for each year.

† The Organization for Economic Cooperation and Development (OECD) estimates

Source: For selected years 1960-2000: The Organization for Economic Cooperation and Development, *Health Data File 2005*, incorporating revisions to the annual update. Available from: *www.oecd.org/els/health*. For average life expectancy: U.S. Census Bureau Web site: http://www.census.gov/cgi-bin/ipc/agggen

much of the decline in private spending between 1980 and 2000, increasing from 28.4% to 35.3% over the 20-year period. Total government spending on health care increased from 21.4% to 40.0% between 1960 and 1980, with much of the increase coming through the Medicare and Medicaid programs.

Hospitals gained a greater share of the total healthcare spending between 1960 and 1980 with the advent of the Medicare program. The change in hospital inpatient reimbursement, from a cost-based system that encouraged inpatient services to the prospective payment system using fixed prices for each DGR, motivates hospitals to discharge patients more quickly. Since Medicare's use of DRG payments begin in 1984, total healthcare spending within hospitals declined to 36.6% by 2000 (see Table 3.5). Hospitals have also seen their market share erode through expansion of independent, freestanding outpatient clinics and surgical and diagnostic facilities.

As shown in Table 3.6, private-pay sources funded 83.6% of total nursing facility expenditures in 1960, declining to

Table 3.5 **Personal Health Care Expenditures, by Source of Funds and Type of Expenditure: United States, 1960, 1980, and 2000**

Classification of Health Care Service	1960	1980	2000
Hospital care expenditures	39.5%	46.9%	36.6%
Physician and clinical services expenditures	23.2%	21.9%	25.3%
Prescription drug expenditures	11.6%	5.6%	10.6%
All other personal health care expenditures*	22.7%	16.8%	19.1%
Nursing home expenditures	**3.4%**	**8.8%**	**8.4%**
Totals (may not add due to rounding)	100.0%	100.0%	100.0%
Sources of Funds for All U.S. Health Care			
Out-of-pocket payments	55.2%	27.2%	16.9%
Private health insurance	21.4%	28.4%	35.3%
Other private funds	2.0%	4.3%	5.0%
Government	21.4%	40.0%	42.8%
Medicaid	8.7%	28.9%	32.6%
Medicare	12.7%	11.1%	10.2%
All sources of funds	100.0%	100.0%	100.0%

* Includes dental services, home health care, durable and non-durable medical equipment and products, other professional services, other personal health care, public health activities, and structures and equipment.

Source: Centers for Medicare & Medicaid Services, Office of the Actuary, National Health Statistics Group, National Health Accounts, National Health Expenditures, 2004. Available from: www.cms.hhs.gov/NationalHealthExpendData/.

Table 3.6 **Nursing Facility Expenditures, by Source of Funds: United States, 1960, 1980, and 2000**

Total Nursing Facility Spending (in millions)	1960	1980	2000
Private funds	$678	$7,541	$41,120
Federal spending			
Medicare	–	307	10,112
Federal share of Medicaid (Title XIX)	–	5,713	24,385
All other federal programs	67	363	1,884
Total federal funds	67	6,383	36,381
State spending			
State's share of Medicaid (Title XIX)	–	4,529	17,610
All other state programs	66	21	151
State and local funds	66	4,550	17,761
Public funds	$133	$10,934	$54,142
Total spending	$811	$18,475	$95,262
Segment Spending as a Percent of Total			
Private funds	83.6%	40.8%	43.2%
Federal spending			
Medicare	0.0%	1.7%	10.6%
Federal share of Medicaid (Title XIX)	0.0%	30.9%	25.6%
All other federal programs	8.3%	2.0%	2.0%
Total federal funds	8.3%	34.5%	38.2%
State spending			
State's share of Medicaid (Title XIX)	0.0%	24.5%	18.5%
All other state programs	8.1%	0.1%	0.2%
State and local funds	8.1%	24.6%	18.6%
Public funds	16.4%	59.2%	56.8%
Total spending	100.0%	100.0%	100.0%

Source: Centers for Medicare & Medicaid Services

40.8% in 1980 after the Medicaid and Medicare programs were firmly established. Medicare's contribution to nursing facilities' revenues increased from 1.7% in 1980, prior to the expanded benefits covering skilled nursing and rehabilitation, to 10.6% in 2000. Since 1980 the federal share of expenditures has increased while the state share has declined.

Funding Nursing Facilities in the Future

With the aging U.S. population, costs for health care in general and long-term care in particular will probably continue to increase at rates that exceed the national GDP. The current trends of rising demand, higher-acuity patients, inflation, nursing shortages, and market demands for improved staffing levels and care will further challenge the nursing home industry.

As long as nursing facility operators find higher-acuity patients such as Medicare patients more profitable, the industry will expand further into that sector and lose the lower-acuity patient market share to assisted living and community-based alternatives. The continuation of this trend is expected to favor building designs that have more private patient rooms, greater amounts of therapy space, and more amenities desired by short-stay patients. Nursing facilities will continue to serve as a step in patients' rehabilitation programs before they return to their homes. As mentioned earlier, government funding in the 1950s encouraged nursing homes to model "institutional" hospital designs. Today, a push towards home-like environments is picking up momentum in markets where there is deep private-pay and Medicare demand. These designs tend to feature smaller buildings with low bed capacities, smaller nursing units, and buildings with separate, distinct specialty units for short-stay rehabilitation patients, memory care patients, and general longer-term patients.

Nursing facilities are expected to experience increased competition from assisted living and home health care services for lower-acuity patients. More states are turning to less expensive long-term care options. Just as nursing homes are taking on higher-acuity patients discharged earlier from hospitals, assisted living facilities with lower cost structures are intercepting the demand for lower-acuity intermediate care that would previously have been satisfied by nursing homes.

Although there is no national program through Medicaid or another federal assistance authority to pay for assisted living services, the Center for Medicare & Medicaid Services (CMS), under the U.S. Department of Health and Human Services, has been granting Medicaid waivers to an increasing number of states. The waivers permit states to receive federal matching funds for Medicaid-eligible persons who would qualify for nursing home care, but are able to live as well or better in a lower cost, licensed assisted living facility.

The market generally prefers assisted living to nursing facilities since assisted living facilities serve a higher-functioning clientele and are often housed in newer, more spacious buildings with a more residential appearance.

Summary

Like nearly all service businesses, the nursing home industry has evolved from highly fragmented and unregulated small enterprises into ownership groups that control many facilities on a regional or national scale. This phenomenon is a response to changing social, governmental, economic, and technological forces. Increased life expectancy, achieved through healthier lifestyles, improved diagnostics, and evolving surgical and medication treatments, have lengthened the fragile final stages of life and created a greater demand for skilled nursing care. Social changes, including smaller family size, more working spouses, and the creation of the Medicaid and Medicare programs have also led to increased demand for institutionalized nursing care. These changes have been met with evolving governmental benefit, payment, and regulatory programs and greater reliance on cost-efficient health care providers in improved physical and operational environments.

Nursing facilities are continually offering increased levels of nursing care and rehabilitation therapy to patients because hospitals and their payors (Medicare and private insurers) want them discharged more quickly from hospitals. On the other side, nursing facilities are experiencing declining demand from lower-acuity patients, who increasingly prefer more attractive assisted living facilities and home healthcare alternatives. Over the past several decades, nursing facilities have become more dependent on government and private healthcare insurance payments.

The aging baby boom generation will place unprecedented strain on the U.S. economy as this segment of the population liquidates real estate and financial holdings to cover living costs during their retirement years. This change and the higher percentage of the U.S. population dependent on poorly funded Social Security and Medicare programs will present continuing problems for the industry in the future. Presumably, these risks are accounted for by the market.

Chapter 4

Assets of the Going Concern, Interest Appraised, and Ownership Structure

Most appraisal assignments relate to the sale or financing of nursing facilities. Typically, a combination of the fee simple interest in the real estate, tangible personal property or furniture, fixtures, and equipment, and intangible assets are included in the purchase price or as security for the mortgage or loan agreement. However, there are many instances in which the appraiser will be requested to estimate only the value of a specific interest in the real estate or intangible personal property assets. For instance, property tax assessments should exclude the value of the intangible assets. FHA-insured mortgages obtained through HUD are underwritten on the value of the tangible assets (real estate and major movable equipment), but this agency also requires the appraiser to estimate the value of the total assets of the business. The valuation of nursing facilities with a leased fee or leasehold interest may or may not include the tangible or intangible personal property.

A nursing facility's assets include:

- Real estate–fee simple, leased fee, or leasehold
- Tangible personal property–furniture, fixtures, and equipment
- Intangible personal property–including assembled work forces, licenses, certifications, approvals such as certificates of need (CON), patient records, goodwill, and management

Note that most appraisal engagements and sales transactions exclude current assets (working capital, cash, accounts receivable, etc.) from the purchase price consideration. Similarly, seller liabilities stay with the seller, and the buyer or successor in the business typically gains indemnity for the seller's liabilities. It is important to confirm what current assets and liabilities, if any, were included in the consideration.

Definitions of *going-concern* and *total assets of a business* follow:

Going-concern. A going concern is an established and operating business with an indefinite future life.[1]

Total assets of a business. The tangible property (real property and personal property, including inventory and furniture, fixtures and equipment) and intangible property (cash, work force, contracts, name, patents, copyrights, and other residual intangible assets, to include capitalized economic profit) of a business.[2]

Several terms are used to describe this value and will be used interchangeably in this book.

Business enterprise value is defined as:

Business enterprise value (BEV). A term applied to the concept of the value contribution of the total intangible assets of the continuing business enterprise such as marketing and management skill, an assembled work force, working capital, trade names, franchises, patents, trademarks, contracts, leases, and operating agreements.[3]

Real Estate Assets

Real estate interests may include fee simple, leased fee, and leasehold interests.

A fee simple interest is found when the ownership of the real estate and the operating rights for the facility are controlled by the same party or closely related parties, whereby agreements between related parties can or will collapse into a single entity for purposes of conveyance to a new party. *Fee simple estate* is defined as:

Absolute ownership unencumbered by any other interest or estate, subject only to the limitations imposed by the governmental powers of taxation, eminent domain, police power, and escheat.[4]

The leased fee interest is the interest held by the lessor or landlord. The interests of the landlord include the right to receive rent during the term of the lease plus the right to receive the leased assets back at the lease termination. Typically, nursing facilities are leased on an absolute net basis, whereby the tenant is responsible for expenses associated with the leased premises and the landlord has little or no responsibilities. The assets leased may include the real estate, tangible personal property, and intangible assets. Note that many nursing facility leases are vague or silent regarding successor rights to licenses, certifications, and other necessary intangible assets for the continuation of the

1. *The Appraisal of Real Estate*, 13th ed. (Chicago: Appraisal Institute, 2008), 29.
2. *The Dictionary of Real Estate Appraisal*, 4th ed. (Chicago: Appraisal Institute, 2002), 293
3. Ibid., 37-38.
4. Ibid., 113

business. In leases in which the tenant is required to cooperate with the landlord in transitioning the facility to the next operator, the landlord may be required to compensate the tenant for the tangible personal property. *Leased fee interest* is defined as:

> An ownership interest held by a landlord with the rights of use and occupancy conveyed by lease to others. The rights of the lessor (the leased fee owner) and the lessee are specified by contract terms contained within the lease.[5]

The leasehold interest provides the tenant with the rights to use the property to operate the facility, hopefully for a profit. The tenant may have the right to sublease the facility, changing this interest to a "sandwich" leasehold. The tenant, acting as the operator, will be the licensed entity and will possess the certifications, provider agreements, and other formal responsibilities in operating the nursing facility. Since most facilities are leased on an absolute net basis, the tenant is typically responsible for all maintenance and capital expenses during the lease term. The tenant will typically invest fairly substantial capital (working capital, replacement funds, and additions of building and equipment assets) in the enterprise over the lease term, so the lease should be long enough to fully recover the capital investment. Most leases include renewal or extension options, and some grant the tenant purchase options and first rights of refusal. *Leasehold interest* is defined as:

> The interest held by the lessee (the tenant or renter) through a lease transferring the rights of use and occupancy for a stated term under certain conditions.[6]

An expanded discussion of leased fee and leasehold interest valuation is included in Chapter 19, Valuation of Partial Interests.

Tangible Personal Property—Furniture, Fixtures, and Equipment

Personal property is defined as:

> Identifiable tangible objects that are considered by the general public as being "personal," e.g., furnishings, artwork, antiques, gems and jewelry, collectibles, machinery and equipment; all tangible property that is not classified as real estate... movable without damage to itself or the real estate.[7]

Nursing facilities require furniture and equipment in nearly every area of the building(s). Patients typically bring only

5. Ibid.
6. Ibid.
7. Ibid.

some of their personal items with them; beds and room furniture is typically provided by the facility. The operator may lease some equipment and fixtures such as vehicles, computer systems, dishwashers, and perishable décor items (plants and aquariums) that require frequent, specialized servicing. Outside providers, such as therapy companies and pharmacies, may provide their own exercise equipment and medicine carts. Further information on furniture, fixtures, and equipment is presented in Chapter 17.

Intangible Personal Property

Several definitions are fundamental to any discussion of intangible personal property.

> *Business enterprise* is defined by the Uniform Standards of Professional Appraisal Practice (USPAP) of The Appraisal Foundation as "an entity pursuing an economic activity."
>
> *Business assets* are "tangible and intangible resources other than personal property and real estate that are employed by a business enterprise in its operations."

The intangible assets of a nursing facility typically include:

- Licenses, certifications, and approvals (such as certificates of need) from government agencies and regulators
- Assembled workforces, including licensed, certified, and trained employees
- Patient records
- Goodwill
- Management
- Vendor contracts
- Trade names

Nursing facility operators enter into a series of agreements with government authorities. These agreements include a licensure agreement with the state agency responsible for licensure (typically within the state department of health) and provider agreements with the state agency that administers the Medicaid program (often contained within the state department of social services) and with Medicare. Other licensing and certifications are required at the facility level. Staff and consultants may need certifications issued at local, state, and federal levels. Local licensing and other regulations may be required for fire and safety, food services, and zoning compliance. Verification that the facility remains in compliance with various licenses, certifications, and other regulations is essential for the operator, investors, major creditors (mortgagee or landlord), and those underwriting and evaluating the assets of the business. The appraiser typically does not confirm or verify that all necessary licenses and certifications to operate the facility are current, but the appraisal report should include a stated assumption that those items are current and complete.

While licensed or certified staff and outside consultants (administrators, nurses, nurse aides, therapists, physician consultants, social workers, dieticians, etc.) are directly or indirectly employed by the operator of the facility, they also must adhere to the licensing laws and standards of their respective professional licensing agencies and professional organizations. Violations of laws and standards can result in disciplinary action against the facility and/or individuals, which will often have an adverse impact on the value of the assets of the going concern.

While it is beyond the scope of this book to examine the regulatory issues that are an essential part of nursing facilities, licensure will be addressed in Chapter 8, Site and Improvement Data and Analysis, and Chapter 13, Operating Expense Analysis.

Allocation of the Assets of the Business or Going Concern

USPAP does not specifically require that an allocation of assets be made, but it does require the appraiser to analyze the effect on value of non-real property items.[8] As required by Title XI of the Financial Institutions Reform, Recovery and Enforcement Act of 1989 (FIRREA), the market value of the real estate must be identified and valued separately. Methods for allocating the going-concern value of a nursing facility or any other real estate-intensive business continue to be debated. Under typical circumstances, the going-concern value for a highly profitable nursing facility will exceed the depreciated cost of the tangible assets, which suggests that there is intangible value. Chapter 18, Reconciliation of Value Indications and Allocation of the Going-Concern Value, will address value allocation issues.

In most cases, the whole is greater than the sum of its parts. The business could not operate if any one of its major assets were absent. If a facility loses its license because of inadequate care or a tenant terminates a lease taking the license (sometimes referred to as the *certificate of need*) and/or the patients and staff to a replacement facility, the value of the whole and the individual assets are suddenly and severely diminished. In fact, the value is often reduced to a small fraction of the physically depreciated cost if a new license for the building cannot be obtained.

---

8. *Uniform Standards of Professional Appraisal Practice, 2008-2009 Edition*, Appraisal Standards Board, The Appraisal Foundation, Standards Rule 1-4(g).

Ownership Structure Issues

The ownership of a nursing facility enterprise is often fragmented, with an operating entity in possession of the license(s), certifications, and business operations, while the ownership of the tangible assets (real estate and personal property) and the management are controlled by other related or unrelated parties.

In 2005, 66.0% of Medicare- and/or Medicaid-certified nursing facilities were owned by for-profit concerns; 27.9% were owned by private non-profits; and the other 6.1% were government-owned.[9]

In this legally complex and litigious business, the division of control and ownership can minimize some types of liability. The appraiser must properly identify the interest being appraised and identify the entity or entities that control that interest.

Figure 4.1 illustrates a basic ownership structure for a nursing facility. Note that ownership structures will vary considerably and are often restricted by state laws.

The typical structure for a multi-facility nursing home company will place each facility "owned" or leased from a third-party landlord into a separate real estate company and operating company. Each operating company will then contract for services with related or third-party management, therapy, pharmacy, and other service providers. The flow chart in Figure 4.2 illustrates a typical structure.

Figure 4.1 **Nursing Home Ownership Diagram**

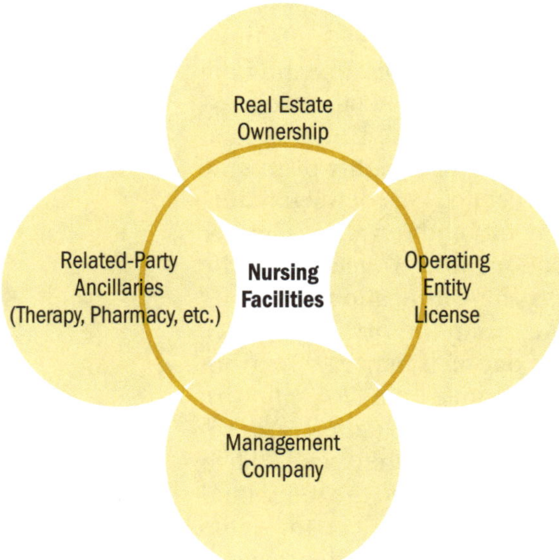

The operator is the licensed entity responsible for conducting all necessary and required activities of the nursing facility. These functions are managed at the facility level by a licensed administrator, who oversees the overall operations of the facility, and a licensed registered nurse, designated as the Director of Nursing (DON), who supervises the nursing staff. The licensed operator will be the entity certified for Medicaid and Medicare and will enter "provider agreements" with Medicare, Medicaid, private

9. Centers for Medicare & Medicaid Services, CMS, NHCompare database, available at http://www.medicare.gov/NHCompare.gov.

insurance companies, and other government agencies. Agreements are also reached with each patient directly. The staff is employed by the licensed operator although the operator may rely on third-party services to satisfy certain functions. Staffing issues will be examined in Chapter 13, Operating Expense Analysis.

Figure 4.2 **Typical Ownership Flow Chart for Multi-Property Skilled Nursing Facility Company**

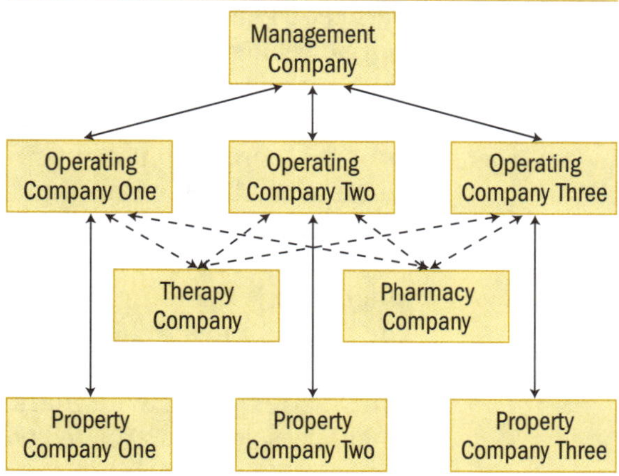

The operating entity may contract to lease the property from a related or unrelated owner. Likewise, it may contract with related or unrelated parties for management and ancillary (therapy and pharmacy) services. Note that leases and management and ancillary service agreements may or may not contain rates, escalator clauses, terms, or other conditions consistent with prevailing levels and terms in the market.

If the operating entity differs from the owner of the real estate, a lease probably exists. Related-party leases typically collapse into the operating entity when these interests are being conveyed to a third party through a sale and lease. Loans secured by property mortgages should somehow bind together the ownership interests in the tangible assets (real estate and furniture, fixtures, and equipment, or FF&E) and the operating rights that are associated with licenses, provider agreements, Medicare and Medicaid certification, certificates of need, and other valuable agreements. Also, landlords should have the ability to regain the operating rights at the termination of the lease. Foreclosure on the real estate interest is of limited value to the owner of the mortgage if the operator discontinues or transfers the business to a different location, rendering the existing building hollow and empty or without a license, staff, or patients.

The management of a nursing facility is often conducted off site through a management agreement with a related or third-party company. A discussion of management services and typical costs for management is presented in Chapter 13, Operating Expense Analysis.

Therapy services and prescription drugs are significant expenses for most skilled nursing facilities that provide for the dispensing of these services and products through licensed professionals. Since economics often prohibits full-time employment of these professionals at any given facility, operators typically contract with outside concerns to provide these services on an as-needed basis. The ownership of these providers may or may not be related to the operator. Many nursing home companies with many beds within a concentrated geographic area find it feasible to establish and operate therapy companies that not only provide therapy to patients in their facilities, but also to other nursing facilities on an inpatient basis or through outpatient programs at various venues. Some companies view their ancillary businesses as profit centers and will divert earnings from the facility's operating level by charging amounts that exceed the market rates. When analyzing the operations of a nursing facility, the appraiser should carefully compare third-party ancillary expenses with market levels. Excessive payments for ancillary services to related parties can misrepresent the financial condition of a facility; this practice can also reduce the debt service and rent coverage ratios required by operating covenants in mortgages and leases. Moreover, failure to adjust excessive charges from related parties will result in the underestimation of the market value of various property interests and rental value. Further discussion of ancillary expenses is presented later.

In a typical appraisal of the fee simple interest, the combined entities will be appraised as one. If the analyst is not careful, lenders, third-party landlords, and other creditors who have based their investment decisions on the "whole" will have an investment that is actually secured by something less than the whole and be exposed to elevated, and maybe unknown, risks.

Most sale transactions and financing structures will incorporate the assets of all the entities that control portions of the business enterprise into a single transaction. Considerable care should be taken by appraisers, analysts, and others who apply transaction prices to evaluate nursing facilities (and other going concerns) for investment decisions.

When examining related party, or even third-party, relationships, care should be exercised to determine if the party contracts are set at market levels. Some operators will shift profits from the facility level to real estate, management, or ancillary businesses. Accepting the operating statements without measuring the expenses reported against market levels may result in an inaccurate valuation.

For example, if a rent reset agreed to by an unrelated landlord and tenant requires the new rent to be based on a calculation using a market level of earnings, adjusting the tenant's related-party management fees and ancillary services contract to market levels is critical. A clever tenant may attempt to divert some of the earnings at the facility level to related parties to have a lower rent calculation.

In many instances, a landlord and tenant will dispute the ownership of the certificate of need or the right to the operating rights (license) at the termination of a lease or when exercising a purchase option. The value of a profitable facility without a license or certificate of need is often dramatically less than the value of that same facility with the license intact.

Landlords, lenders, and other creditors should carefully write their lease and loan agreements so that, in the event of lease termination or a creditor's action against the debtor, the operating entity will cooperate to facilitate a seamless transition that transfers the facility's license(s), certification(s), workforce, patient records, and other intangible assets to a succeeding operator.

Well-operated facilities with significant service revenue (income from therapies, the sale of medical supplies, etc.) can produce value that substantially exceeds the replacement costs of real and tangible personal property and the expense of obtaining licenses, approvals, a workforce, and management.

Valuing For-Profit and Non-Profit Nursing Facilities

As Tables 4.1, 4.2, and 4.3 show, 66.0% of all Medicare- and/or Medicaid-certified nursing facilities in the United States are controlled by for-profit concerns. For-profit entities control 68.0% of all certified beds and 67.1% of all occupied beds, based on

Table 4.1 **Percentage of Nursing Facilities Certified for Medicare and/or Medicaid in the U.S. by Type of Control in 2005**

Percentages of Total Certified Facilities				
Ownership Type	**Facilities**	**Licensed Beds**	**Occupied Beds**	**Occupancy**
For profit	66.0%	68.0%	67.1%	84.4%
Government	6.1%	6.7%	6.6%	84.7%
Non profit	27.9%	25.3%	26.3%	88.8%
Totals	100.0%	100.0%	100.0%	85.5%

Source: Centers for Medicare & Medicaid Services, CMS, NHCompare database, available at http://www.medicare.gov/NHCompare.gov.

Table 4.2 **Total Nursing Facilities Certified for Medicare and/or Medicaid in the U.S. by Type of Ownership Control in 2005**

Ownership Type	**No. of Facilities**	**Licensed Beds**	**Occupied Beds**
For profit	10,563	1,141,635	963,699
Government	971	112,257	95,096
Non profit	4,469	425,086	377,359
Totals	16,003	1,678,978	1,436,154

Source: Centers for Medicare & Medicaid Services.

survey data collected by the Centers for Medicare & Medicaid Services (CMS) in 2005.

Many studies suggest that non-profit nursing facilities experience fewer survey deficiencies and have higher nursing staff ratios and operating expenses. As Table 4.2 shows, government-controlled facilities have the highest percentage of Medicaid-only certified facilities. Non-profits have the greatest percentage of Medicare-only certified facilities. There is a net migration of patients from non-profit to for-profit nursing facilities.

Non-profit facilities tend to operate at higher expense levels, are less aggressive in their private-pay rate structures, and are often less profitable than otherwise similar for-profit facilities. Non-profit facilities have several operating advantages in that they are often exempt from local property tax, pay no income tax, and have access to lower-cost debt available through tax-exempt bond financing.

In appraising non-profit facilities, one of the first questions to resolve is how to treat the ownership. It may be necessary to appraise the facility under two assumptions. First, it can be appraised assuming it remains a non profit and will have certain tax and financing advantages, offset to some degree with higher operating expenses. Second, an assumption can be

Table 4.3 **Hospital-Based and Chained-Owned Nursing Facilities by Type of Control in the U.S. in 2005**

Ownership Type	No. of Facilities	Facilities Within Hospital	Total NFs by Control Type in Hospitals	Part of a Chain	Total NFs by Control Type That Are Part of a Chain
For profit	10,563	176	1.7%	6,468	61.2%
Government	971	343	35.3%	78	8.0%
Non profit	4,469	888	19.9%	1,825	40.8%
Totals	16,003	1,407	8.8%	8,371	52.3%

Source: Centers for Medicare & Medicaid Services.

Table 4.4 **Breakdown of Medicare- and Medicaid-Certified Facilities by Type of Ownership**

By Facility	For profit	Government	Non profit	Total
Medicaid-only	458	226	306	990
Medicare-only	293	57	507	857
Dual certification	9,812	688	3,656	14,156
Totals	10,563	971	4,469	16,003
Percentage of totals				
Medicaid-only	4.3%	23.3%	6.8%	6.2%
Medicare-only	2.8%	5.9%	11.3%	5.4%
Dual certification	92.9%	70.9%	81.8%	88.5%
Totals	100.0%	100.0%	100.0%	100.0%

Source: Centers for Medicare & Medicaid Services.

made that the facility is converted to for-profit ownership. In this case, the valuer will need to adjust the operating forecast to include taxes, higher interest rates, and lower operating costs, consistent with expense levels for comparable for-profit facilities in the same or similar market areas. Adjustments for occupancy characteristics and rates will also be needed. Converting from a non-profit to a for-profit facility, or vice versa, will impact a facility's Medicaid reimbursement in most states that apply facility-specific, cost-based reimbursement schemes. The valuation approach for a non profit ownership should be discussed and agreed on by the appraiser and the client when the appraiser is engaged.

Exposure and Marketing Time

News of an impending change in ownership often causes fear among nursing home staff and patients. For this reason, nursing facilities are often marketed quietly. Broadcasting the sale may cause some staff and patients to leave, thus impacting value. States must approve all changes of ownership (ChOWs) for licensed nursing facilities. The process varies by state, and in some states it can be quite lengthy. States must assure the public that the new ownership (licensed operator) is morally, ethically, and financially capable of meeting the obligations required. Because of the secrecy that surrounds the marketing of nursing care facilities, exposure and marketing time are difficult to measure objectively. In addition to actual sales data, interviews with operators who are active in the market or brokers who specialize in selling long-term care facilities can provide sufficient information to address these subjects in the appraisal report.

Summary

The appraisal of a nursing facility typically involves the valuation of the total assets of the business, including the real estate interest and the tangible and intangible personal property assets. Real estate interests may include fee simple, leased fee, and/or leasehold rights. Tangible personal property includes furniture, fixtures, and equipment. Intangible personal property usually includes assembled workforces, various local and state licenses, certifications, approvals, patient records, goodwill, and management know-how. These assets may be held by a single entity or the ownership may be fragmented between various related and unrelated parties.

The assets are generally divided for economic and legal reasons. In performing an appraisal or, for that matter, underwriting a financial transaction, it is important to identify, understand, and properly treat the assets being appraised. While the assets may be controlled by separate entities, the combining of these interests may be necessary for valuation purposes. Lenders often secure their loans by binding the assets of related parties to a single loan; real estate tax assessments are typically based on the fee simple interest, despite the presence of existing leased fee and leasehold interests. The reversion rights to personal property assets at the expiration of a lease are often disputed by the parties when the lease agreement is unclear as to the ownership rights. Current assets (working capital, cash, accounts receivable, etc.) and all liabilities are typically excluded from an appraisal assignment. For consistency purposes, the appraiser should verify the assets and liabilities that are included in the transactions that are used to develop comparable sale and lease data.

Chapter 5

Medicare Program and Reimbursement for Skilled Nursing Facilities

Medicare is a federal entitlement program that provides medical insurance coverage to most U.S. citizens age 65 or older. Coverage is extended to non-U.S. citizens who are permanent legal residents for at least five continuous years and are at least 65 years old (eligible, non-citizen residents). Coverage is also provided to U.S. citizens and eligible, non-citizen residents under 65 who are disabled and have been receiving either Social Security or Railroad Retirement Board disability benefits for at least 24 months. Also covered are those with amyotrophic lateral sclerosis (ALS), or Lou Gehrig's disease, and those who need continuing dialysis for kidney failure. The program has four benefit components (Parts A, B, C, and D). As of 2007, there were 44.0 million persons receiving Medicare coverage, of which 36.7 million qualified based on age and 7.3 million qualified through disabilities.[1]

Salient components of the four programs, as they pertain to skilled nursing coverage, are described as follows.

- Part A: This is the hospital coverage portion of the program, which also covers up to 100 days in a skilled nursing facility (SNF). For the first 20 days, Medicare covers the entire cost; for the remaining 80 days of potential coverage, a co-payment is required.
- Part B: This is optional medical insurance known as the Supplementary Medical Insurance (SMI) program. It pays a portion of doctors' bills and other outpatient expenses. Nursing facilities achieve limited Part B revenues through their patients not covered by Part A, mostly as reimbursement for covered therapy.

1. Centers for Medicare & Medicaid Services (CMS) Web site, Research, Statistics, Data & Systems.

- Part C: This part is known as the Medicare Advantage (managed care) alternative, whereby a person elects to substitute Medicare coverage for private health insurance coverage that mirrors or enriches the benefits that are offered by Medicare (Parts A and B).
- Part D: This is the recently added prescription drug benefit program, which is actually administered by private health insurance companies. Part D does not have a significant impact on nursing facilities.

The financial condition of the Medicare program is problematic since long-term program costs are not sustainable under current financing arrangements. Medicare has a board of trustees, which is required to issue annual reports on the financial status of the Medicare Trust Funds. These reports contain actuarial opinions concerning accounting information and cost projections prepared by the chief actuary of CMS. According to the 2008 report, Medicare's Hospital Insurance (HI) Trust Fund is expected to pay out more in hospital benefits and other expenditures than it receives in taxes and other dedicated revenues in 2008. The difference will be made up from general revenues, which pay for interest credits to the trust fund. The HI Trust Fund has been essentially lending its surplus collections to the U.S. Government for their general spending. At the current tax and spending levels, the growing annual deficits are projected to exhaust the fund's reserves in 2019.[2]

The underlying health care costs per Medicare enrollee are projected to rise faster than the wages per worker on which payroll taxes are based. As a result, Medicare's annual costs, which were 3.2% of GDP in 2007, are projected to reach 10.8% of GDP in 2082.[3]

A payroll tax increase from 2.9% to 6.44% or a 51% reduction in Medicare outlays immediately would be required for the Part A program to achieve actuarial balance over the next 75 years.[4] Any effort to solve the Medicare program will probably take a combination of stricter eligibility, reduced benefits, and higher taxes. Further delays in making adjustments to the program will only exacerbate the problem. By law, Medicare Parts B and D will remain adequately financed because the insurance rates will increase in step with expected cost increases.

Medicare and Medicaid are administrated through the Centers for Medicare & Medicaid Services (CMS), a component

---

2. *A Summary of the 2008 Annual Reports, Status of the Social Security and Medicare Programs*, prepared for the Social Security and Medicare Boards of Trustees
3. Ibid.
4. Ibid.

of the Department of Health and Human Services (HHS). The Social Security Administration is responsible for determining Medicare eligibility and processing premium payments for the Medicare program. CMS contracts with private companies, referred to as *Medicare intermediaries*, which are typically regional or national health care insurance companies. The intermediaries assist with processing claims and payments and provide call center services, clinician enrollment, and fraud investigation.

Further information on the various parts of Medicare coverage that pertain to skilled nursing care is provided in the remainder of this chapter.

Part A: Hospital Insurance

Medicare Part A is primarily financed by payroll taxes imposed by the Federal Insurance Contributions Act (FICA) and the Self-Employment Contributions Act. The taxes are paid into Medicare's Hospital Insurance (HI) Trust Fund. The tax is equal to 2.9% of wages, salaries, and other compensation for employment. For employees, 1.45% is withheld from their pay and an equal amount is matched by the employer. Self-employed individuals pay the entire 2.9%. Medicare does not tax other individual income from interest, dividends, distributions, or royalties. Prior to January 1, 1994, Medicare taxes were limited to a maximum amount of an individual's wages. Because of higher Medicare costs, the compensation limit was removed and Medicare taxes are now assessed against all wages, salaries, and other compensation in connection with employment.

The Part A premium is waived for patients if they or their spouses have 40 or more quarters of Medicare-covered employment. If the patient or spouse has paid into the HI Trust Fund for fewer than 40 quarters, the patient will be required to pay a premium to receive Medicare Part A benefits. As of October 1, 2007, the Part A premium is $233.00 per month for people who have 30-39 quarters of Medicare-covered employment and increases to $423.00 per month for people who have less than 30 quarters of Medicare-covered employment or are not otherwise eligible for hospital insurance.

Besides hospitalization coverage, Medicare Part A provides short-term coverage for those who require skilled nursing or rehabilitative care on a daily basis upon discharge from an acute care setting (a hospital) after a minimum hospital stay of three consecutive inpatient days. Unlike most Medicaid programs, Medicare pays the operator for restorative care, i.e., physical, speech, and occupational therapies, and for pharmacy and medical supply expenses, which collectively are referred to as *ancillary services*. Ancillary services are a significant profit center in most nursing homes. A single reimbursement method is applied nationally for this federal program administrated by CMS.

As previously noted, Medicare Part A provides up to 100 days in a skilled nursing facility. Medicare covers the patient's entire cost for the first 20 days of an eligible stay. For the remaining 80 days of potential coverage, the patient or the secondary insurer must make a co-payment. As of October 1, 2007, the co-payment was $128.00 per day. Many state Medicaid programs will pay the patient's co-payment if the patient also has Medicaid coverage. However, some states do not pick up the entire co-payment and the difference could result in uncollected revenues.

To receive skilled nursing care coverage under Medicare Part A, the beneficiary must:

- Have been receiving inpatient hospital care for at least three consecutive days
- Be admitted to the nursing facility within a specified time period (generally within 30 days) of that hospital discharge
- Need post-hospital extended care services for a condition that was treated during the qualifying hospital stay or for a condition that arose while he or she was in the SNF for treatment of a condition that was previously treated during the qualifying hospital stay
- Have a doctor certify that he or she requires skilled nursing and/or rehab on a daily basis that can only be provided on an inpatient basis
- Require skilled nursing or rehabilitation services, which means that services are ordered by a physician, require the skills of technical or professional personnel, and are furnished directly by, or under the supervision of, such personnel
- Require services that are reasonable and necessary for the diagnosis or treatment of his or her condition

If all of these requirements are met, the beneficiary would qualify for Part A. Once a beneficiary exhausts the 100 days of Part A coverage available in a benefit period or drops to a Medicare non-skilled level of care, the stay is no longer covered under Part A.

The nursing facility will bill Medicare no less than every 30 days or sooner if the patient is discharged before then, his or her benefits are exhausted, or the need for skilled care ceases.

Part B: Medical Insurance

Part B medical insurance is optional coverage that helps pay for some services and products not covered by Part A, generally on an outpatient basis. The premium is $96.40 per month and this amount can be paid by the individual, by his or her private supplemental health insurance company, or by the state Medicaid program. A new income-based premium scheme has been in effect since 2007, wherein Part B premiums are higher for beneficiaries with incomes exceeding $80,000 for individuals or $160,000 for married couples. Medicare Part B premiums are commonly deducted automatically from beneficiaries' monthly Social Security checks.

Part B coverage includes physician and nursing services, x-rays, lab and diagnostic tests, certain vaccinations, blood transfusions, renal dialysis, outpatient hospital procedures, limited ambulance transportation, immunosuppressive drugs for organ transplant recipients, chemotherapy, and other outpatient medical treatments administered in a doctor's office. Part B pays for some durable medical equipment (DME), including canes, walkers, wheelchairs, and mobility scooters. Part B coverage is subject to medical necessity.

Part B coverage is limited and nursing facilities generally receive most of their Part B revenues by providing therapies. In 2008 the maximum amounts were $1,810 annually for physical and speech therapy and $1,810 annually for occupational therapy. Because of these limitations, Part B Medicare revenues are typically substantially less than Part A revenues for most nursing facilities. Medicare reimburses 80% of its allowed charges and the beneficiaries pay the other 20% and any difference between the provider's charges and the charges Medicare allows. Medicare Part B has fixed fees on allowable or approved charges. The amount is often substantially less than the physicians' actual charges.

Part C: Medicare Advantage (Managed Care)

With the passage of the Balanced Budget Act of 1997, Medicare beneficiaries were given the option to receive their Medicare benefits through private health insurance plans instead of through the original Medicare plan (Parts A and B). These programs are known as *Medicare Advantage*, or Part C, plans and generally are referred to as private insurance or managed care within the operating statements of skilled nursing facilities. Medicare Advantage plans are required to offer benefits that either mirror those offered by the original Medicare plan (Parts A & B) or are richer than those that the beneficiary would receive through the original Medicare plan. Advantage plans can include Part D prescription drug benefits. According to the CMS, approximately six million individuals are enrolled in

Medicare Advantage programs; this equates to approximately 14.0% of all Medicare beneficiaries. The program is more popular in Western states and less popular in a scattering of less populated states.

Part D: Prescription Drug Plans

Medicare Part D went into effect on January 1, 2006. To receive this benefit, a person with Medicare must enroll in a stand-alone prescription drug plan (PDP) or Medicare Advantage plan with prescription drug coverage (MA-PD). These plans are approved and regulated by the Medicare program, but are actually designed and administered by private health insurance companies. Unlike the original Medicare plan (Parts A and B), Part D coverage is not standardized. In some states Medicaid will pay the beneficiaries' Part B premium for those with very low income and also pay for any drugs that are not covered by Part D.

In 2008 the Part D "base premium" was $27.93 per month. (Actual premium amounts charged to Part D beneficiaries depend on the specific plan in which they are enrolled and averaged $25 for standard coverage in 2008.) Part D also receives payments from states for the federal assumption of Medicaid responsibilities for prescription drug costs for individuals eligible for both Medicare and Medicaid. In 2008 state payments were estimated to cover 14% of Part D costs, but that percentage is projected to decline to 10% by 2014 as the state requirement decreases.

Medicare Part A Skilled Nursing Reimbursement

Medicare pays nursing facilities for Part A services using a prospective payment system (PPS). The Medicare Part A portion of PPS is a flat-rate, case-mix, prospective system with adjustments for differences in regional labor costs. PPS is based on a patient classification system known as RUGs III (resource utilization group), which classifies patients into 53 categories. Vital information used in RUGs III is taken from the Minimum Data Set (MDS 2.0). The reimbursements are based on wage-weighted staff time studies conducted during the 1990s. Rates are also adjusted for differences in regional labor costs based on labor indices applied to the labor portion of the rate. Medicare rates under PPS were developed from allowable costs using 1995 cost reports, when reimbursements were paid under a facility-specific, cost-based system. Medicare may eventually change PPS base rates to reflect a more recent reporting year, which would probably result in lower payments.

There are four components of PPS rates:

1. nursing
2. therapy
3. therapy, non-case mix
4. non-case mix

Table 5.1 presents the national rates for urban and rural facilities at 1.0 case mix indices for the nursing and therapy components.

Table 5.1 **Federal/PPS Unadjusted Rate Components—Effective October 1, 2009**

Proposed as of August 8, 2008, per *The Federal Register*, volume 73, number 154

		Urban	Rural
1.	Nursing @ 1.0 index	$151.74	$144.97
2.	Therapy @ 1.0 index	$114.30	$131.80
3.	Therapy, non-case mix	$15.05	$16.08
4.	Non-case mix	$77.44	$78.87

Note: These rates are adjusted annually, using the federal fiscal year beginning October 1st. Please consult *The Federal Register* at www.gpoaccess.gov/fr/

Each of the 53 RUGs only receives three of the four components. There are 23 RUGs that involve therapy or rehabilitation services, and rates for those RUGs include the sum of: (1) nursing, (2) therapy, and (4) non-case-mix. For the other RUGs, the rate is the sum of: (1) nursing, (3) therapy, non-case mix, and (4) non-case mix. The nursing case-mix indices range from 0.50 to 1.90, and the 23 therapy case-mix indices range from 0.43 to 2.25.

Tables 5.2 and 5.3 on the following pages profile the federal rate for each of the 53 RUGs for urban and rural areas effective October 1, 2008. The federal rates for rural facilities use the same case-mix indices, but apply the rural facility components shown above.

CMS has designed PPS so that the 53 RUG categories are independent rates. However, for practical purposes, Medicare Part A projections can be made in terms of an average RUG level for all Medicare patients. Since the urban and rural nursing and therapy components are different per diem amounts, it is impossible to precisely calculate a federal/PPS rate without applying both the nursing and therapy indices. Accordingly, the best way to resolve this issue in analyzing the distribution of patients within the 53 RUGs is to determine an average national case-mix index as well as the contribution ratio in the index of nursing and therapy services.

The federal rates must be adjusted for local wage index differences. CMS has developed a local wage index for each metropolitan statistical area (MSA) in the country. In addition, the

Table 5.2 **Medicare Prospective Payment Rates for Skilled Nursing Facilities, Associated Indexes and Labor Portions for *Urban* Counties, Effective October 1, 2008**

RUG-III Category	Nursing Index	Therapy Index	Nursing Component	Therapy Component	Non-Case Mix Therapy Component	Non-Case Mix Component	Total Rate	Labor Portion	Non-Labor Portion
RUX	1.90	2.25	$288.31	$257.18		$77.44	$622.93	$434.70	$188.23
RUL	1.40	2.25	212.44	257.18		77.44	547.06	381.75	165.31
RVX	1.54	1.41	233.68	161.16		77.44	472.28	329.57	142.71
RVL	1.33	1.41	201.81	161.16		77.44	440.41	307.33	133.08
RHX	1.42	0.94	215.47	107.44		77.44	400.35	279.38	120.97
RHL	1.37	0.94	207.88	107.44		77.44	392.76	274.08	118.68
RMX	1.93	0.77	292.86	88.01		77.44	458.31	319.82	138.49
RML	1.68	0.77	254.92	88.01		77.44	420.37	293.35	127.02
RLX	1.31	0.43	198.78	49.15		77.44	325.37	227.05	98.32
RUC	1.28	2.25	194.23	257.18		77.44	528.85	369.05	159.80
RUB	0.99	2.25	150.22	257.18		77.44	484.84	338.34	146.50
RUA	0.84	2.25	127.46	257.18		77.44	462.08	322.45	139.63
RVC	1.23	1.41	186.64	161.16		77.44	425.24	296.75	128.49
RVB	1.09	1.41	165.40	161.16		77.44	404.00	281.92	122.08
RVA	0.82	1.41	124.43	161.16		77.44	363.03	253.33	109.70
RHC	1.22	0.94	185.12	107.44		77.44	370.00	258.20	111.80
RHB	1.11	0.94	168.43	107.44		77.44	353.31	246.55	106.76
RHA	0.94	0.94	142.64	107.44		77.44	327.52	228.55	98.97
RMC	1.15	0.77	174.50	88.01		77.44	339.95	237.23	102.72
RMB	1.09	0.77	165.40	88.01		77.44	330.85	230.88	99.97
RMA	1.04	0.77	157.81	88.01		77.44	323.26	225.58	97.68
RLB	1.14	0.43	172.98	49.15		77.44	299.57	209.05	90.52
RLA	0.85	0.43	128.98	49.15		77.44	255.57	178.34	77.23
SE3	1.86		282.24		15.05	77.44	374.73	261.50	113.23
SE2	1.49		226.09		15.05	77.44	318.58	222.31	96.27
SE1	1.26		191.19		15.05	77.44	283.68	197.96	85.72
SSC	1.23		186.64		15.05	77.44	279.13	194.79	84.34
SSB	1.13		171.47		15.05	77.44	263.96	184.20	79.76
SSA	1.10		166.91		15.05	77.44	259.40	181.02	78.38
CC2	1.22		185.12		15.05	77.44	277.61	193.72	83.89
CC1	1.06		160.84		15.05	77.44	253.33	176.78	76.55
CB2	0.98		148.71		15.05	77.44	241.20	168.32	72.88
CB1	0.91		138.08		15.05	77.44	230.57	160.90	69.67
CA2	0.90		136.57		15.05	77.44	229.06	159.84	69.22
CA1	0.80		121.39		15.05	77.44	213.88	149.25	64.63
IB2	0.74		112.29		15.05	77.44	204.78	142.90	61.88
IB1	0.72		109.25		15.05	77.44	201.74	140.78	60.96
IA2	0.61		92.56		15.05	77.44	185.05	129.13	55.92
IA1	0.56		84.97		15.05	77.44	177.46	123.84	53.62
BB2	0.73		110.77		15.05	77.44	203.26	141.84	61.42
BB1	0.69		104.70		15.05	77.44	197.19	137.61	59.58
BA2	0.60		91.04		15.05	77.44	183.53	128.07	55.46
BA1	0.52		78.90		15.05	77.44	171.39	119.60	51.79
PE2	0.85		128.98		15.05	77.44	221.47	154.55	66.92
PE1	0.82		124.43		15.05	77.44	216.92	151.37	65.55
PD2	0.78		118.36		15.05	77.44	210.85	147.14	63.71
PD1	0.76		115.32		15.05	77.44	207.81	145.02	62.79
PC2	0.71		107.74		15.05	77.44	200.23	139.73	60.50
PC1	0.69		104.70		15.05	77.44	197.19	137.61	59.58
PB2	0.55		83.46		15.05	77.44	175.95	122.78	53.17
PB1	0.54		81.94		15.05	77.44	174.43	121.72	52.71
PA2	0.53		80.42		15.05	77.44	172.91	120.66	52.25
PA1	0.50		75.87		15.05	77.44	168.36	117.49	50.87

Table 5.3 **Medicare Prospective Payment Rates for Skilled Nursing Facilities, Associated Indexes and Labor Portions for *Rural* Counties, Effective October 1, 2008**

RUG-III Category	Nursing Index	Therapy Index	Nursing Component	Therapy Component	Non-Case Mix Therapy Component	Non-Case Mix Component	Total Rate	Labor Portion	Non-Labor Portion
RUX	1.90	2.25	$275.44	$296.55		$78.87	$650.86	$454.19	$196.67
RUL	1.40	2.25	202.96	296.55		78.87	578.38	403.61	174.77
RVX	1.54	1.41	223.25	185.84		78.87	487.96	340.51	147.45
RVL	1.33	1.41	192.81	185.84		78.87	457.52	319.27	138.25
RHX	1.42	0.94	205.86	123.89		78.87	408.62	285.15	123.47
RHL	1.37	0.94	198.61	123.89		78.87	401.37	280.09	121.28
RMX	1.93	0.77	279.79	101.49		78.87	460.15	321.11	139.04
RML	1.68	0.77	243.55	101.49		78.87	423.91	295.82	128.09
RLX	1.31	0.43	189.91	56.67		78.87	325.45	227.11	98.34
RUC	1.28	2.25	185.56	296.55		78.87	560.98	391.47	169.51
RUB	0.99	2.25	143.52	296.55		78.87	518.94	362.13	156.81
RUA	0.84	2.25	121.77	296.55		78.87	497.19	346.95	150.24
RVC	1.23	1.41	178.31	185.84		78.87	443.02	309.15	133.87
RVB	1.09	1.41	158.02	185.84		78.87	422.73	294.99	127.74
RVA	0.82	1.41	118.88	185.84		78.87	383.59	267.68	115.91
RHC	1.22	0.94	176.86	123.89		78.87	379.62	264.91	114.71
RHB	1.11	0.94	160.92	123.89		78.87	363.68	253.79	109.89
RHA	0.94	0.94	136.27	123.89		78.87	339.03	236.59	102.44
RMC	1.15	0.77	166.72	101.49		78.87	347.08	242.20	104.88
RMB	1.09	0.77	158.02	101.49		78.87	338.38	236.13	102.25
RMA	1.04	0.77	150.77	101.49		78.87	331.13	231.07	100.06
RLB	1.14	0.43	165.27	56.67		78.87	300.81	209.91	90.90
RLA	0.85	0.43	123.22	56.67		78.87	258.76	180.57	78.19
SE3	1.86		269.64		16.08	78.87	364.59	254.42	110.17
SE2	1.49		216.01		16.08	78.87	310.96	217.00	93.96
SE1	1.26		182.66		16.08	78.87	277.61	193.72	83.89
SSC	1.23		178.31		16.08	78.87	273.26	190.69	82.57
SSB	1.13		163.82		16.08	78.87	258.77	180.58	78.19
SSA	1.10		159.47		16.08	78.87	254.42	177.54	76.88
CC2	1.22		176.86		16.08	78.87	271.81	189.68	82.13
CC1	1.06		153.67		16.08	78.87	248.62	173.49	75.13
CB2	0.98		142.07		16.08	78.87	237.02	165.40	71.62
CB1	0.91		131.92		16.08	78.87	226.87	158.32	68.55
CA2	0.90		130.47		16.08	78.87	225.42	157.30	68.12
CA1	0.80		115.98		16.08	78.87	210.93	147.19	63.74
IB2	0.74		107.28		16.08	78.87	202.23	141.12	61.11
IB1	0.72		104.38		16.08	78.87	199.33	139.10	60.23
IA2	0.61		88.43		16.08	78.87	183.38	127.97	55.41
IA1	0.56		81.18		16.08	78.87	176.13	122.91	53.22
BB2	0.73		105.83		16.08	78.87	200.78	140.11	60.67
BB1	0.69		100.03		16.08	78.87	194.98	136.06	58.92
BA2	0.60		86.98		16.08	78.87	181.93	126.96	54.97
BA1	0.52		75.38		16.08	78.87	170.33	118.86	51.47
PE2	0.85		123.22		16.08	78.87	218.17	152.25	65.92
PE1	0.82		118.88		16.08	78.87	213.83	149.22	64.61
PD2	0.78		113.08		16.08	78.87	208.03	145.17	62.86
PD1	0.76		110.18		16.08	78.87	205.13	143.15	61.98
PC2	0.71		102.93		16.08	78.87	197.88	138.09	59.79
PC1	0.69		100.03		16.08	78.87	194.98	136.06	58.92
PB2	0.55		79.73		16.08	78.87	174.68	121.90	52.78
PB1	0.54		78.28		16.08	78.87	173.23	120.89	52.34
PA2	0.53		76.83		16.08	78.87	171.78	119.87	51.91
PA1	0.50		72.49		16.08	78.87	167.44	116.84	50.60

rural areas (areas outside MSAs) have separate state indexes, with a single index applied to all rural facilities in a given state. Wage index and other PPS rate information may be obtained through the Internet at:

http://www.cms.hhs.gov/SNFPPS/04_WageIndex.asp

As of October 1, 2008, the labor portion equaled 69.783% of the total federal rate, and this portion of the federal rate is adjusted to the wage index for the particular area. The labor portion of the Medicare rate has been declining for a number of years.

Medicare Part B Revenue

Medicare Part B revenue is received from Medicare through private-pay and Medicaid patients with Part B coverage. Part B coverage provides for limited amounts of physical, occupational, and speech therapy, other therapy services, examinations, pharmaceutical sales, personal care services, and special food and beverage sales. Part B reimbursements are based on a fee schedule. Therapy caps as of October 1, 2007, were $1,810 for combined physical and speech therapy and $1,810 for occupational therapy per year per patient.

About 75% of Supplemental Medical Insurance (SMI) Part B and Part D expenditures are paid from federal general fund revenues, with most of the remaining costs covered by monthly premiums charged to enrollees. Part B and Part D premium amounts are based on methods defined in law and increase as the estimated costs of those programs rise.

Contractual Allowances or Revenue Adjustments

Most financial statements will show revenue adjustments for Medicare, Medicaid, and managed care. These adjustments net out the difference between the facility's customary rate (rack rate) and the amount they actually receive from the payor. This accounting process is outdated and was established when the federal government required facilities to charge private-pay patients rates that equaled or exceeded the reimbursed amounts for similar services from Medicare and Medicaid. It is easier to work with net revenue amounts so, when contractual allowances appear in an operating statement, the appraiser or analyst can simply show the net revenue to avoid confusion. The operating statement might look like Table 5.4.

Table 5.4 Example of Operating Statement With Contractual Allowances

Medicare Part A revenue	Total	$/Per Diem
Medicare Part A routine	$1,578,453	$315.69
Less routine contractual	(178,593)	(35.72)
Part A physical therapy	287,542	57.51
Less physical therapy contractual	(35,875)	(7.18)
Part A speech therapy	65,875	13.18
Less speech therapy contractual	(25,478)	(5.10)
Part A occupational therapy	74,852	14.97
Less occupational therapy contractual	(35,879)	(7.18)
Part A prescription drugs	78,589	15.72
Less prescription drugs contractual	(47,835)	(9.57)
Part A medical supplies	25,789	5.16
Less medical supply contractual	(17,589)	(3.52)
Net Medicare Part A revenue	$1,769,851	$353.97

Medicare Part C (Medicare Advantage or Managed Care)

Managed care patients are typically patients covered by private insurance, and for most nursing facility patients that coverage is primarily through Medicare Advantage alternatives. However, there are patients who are too young for Medicare benefits or do not otherwise qualify for Medicare's long-term care benefits, but have private health insurance coverage for long-term care. Generally, nursing facility operating statements will lump Medicare Advantage, private managed care, and other types of private, long-term-care-insured patients (days and revenues) into a single classification, which is often referred to as *managed care or private insurance.*

Medicare contracts with private insurance organizations to provide a certain set of medical services to Medicare beneficiaries. These private insurers receive fixed, prepaid premiums from Medicare (CMS) for each enrolled Medicare beneficiary who has enrolled in the company's "Advantage" program. The private companies receive a flat, monthly payment, regardless of the patient's medical needs. The payments are adjusted annually and vary by region.

The qualified managed care program then contracts with health care providers (physicians, pharmacies, hospitals, nursing homes, home healthcare agencies, etc.) to provide enrollees with health care services that equal or exceed the services they would receive under Medicare. In skilled nursing facilities, managed care patients generally receive the same levels of service as Medicare patients, thus there is considerable expense attributable to therapy, pharmacy, and medical supplies associated with these patients. The popularity of managed care alternatives varies geographically, with the greatest "penetration" occurring in Western states, Florida, and some of the more populated Northeastern states, and the least penetration in rural and less populated states.

Managed care payments are typically set through negotiations between the private insurance company and the nursing facility. The rates are typically lower than Medicare payments for the same level of service, but the facility may incur less expense for managed care patients. As an example, Medicare requires the nursing facility to provide prescription medicines to Part A-covered patients at the facility's expense, whereas that same patient under managed care coverage might have these medicines covered through a separate drug plan. Historical and current actual, average per-diem rates represent a reasonable guideline for estimating managed care revenues. The appraiser should investigate the number of managed care contracts. Facilities that rely heavily on just one or a few contracts may be vulnerable to lapsing contracts or difficult rate negotiations. Some managed care companies will only approve a limited number of facilities in a given market–usually low bidders that produce the best patient outcomes–and exclude the other facilities. Other insurance companies will approve any facility willing to accept their rates and terms. Experience suggests that managed care revenue carries elevated business risk.

Table 5.5 shows the penetration of managed care in the Medicare-eligible population.

Medicare Part D

A patient who chooses Medicare Part D enrolls in a stand-alone prescription drug plan (PDP) or Medicare Advantage plan with prescription drug coverage (MA-PD) administered by a private health insurance company. Most nursing homes will not incur any revenue or operating expense associated with Part D.

Summary

Medicare is the federal program that provides medical insurance coverage for U.S. citizens aged 65 and older and some younger persons with disabilities. The program has four benefit components (Parts A, B, C, and D). Part A provides hospitalization coverage, along with limited skilled nursing benefits. Part B is an optional coverage that pays for certain physician, outpatient, and therapy expenses, including limited amounts of therapy that can be received at a nursing facility once Part A benefits expire. Part B coverage requires an individual to pay a

Table 5.5 **Medicare Managed Care Enrollees as a Percentage of Medicare-Eligible Beneficiaries, as of January 1, 2009**

Greater Than 25%	% Enrolled	Between 25% & 15%	% Enrolled	Less Than 15%	% Enrolled
Oregon	40.6%	Wisconsin	24.9%	Kentucky	14.3%
Pennsylvania	37.4%	New Mexico	23.4%	Oklahoma	13.8%
Arizona	36.8%	Michigan	23.1%	South Carolina	13.8%
Hawaii	36.4%	Washington	22.8%	Georgia	13.8%
Rhode Island	36.0%	West Virginia	22.5%	Indiana	13.3%
Minnesota	34.5%	Louisiana	21.2%	Virginia	12.8%
California	34.2%	Tennessee	21.2%	Arkansas	12.8%
Colorado	32.8%	Alabama	20.1%	Iowa	11.9%
Nevada	30.4%	Missouri	19.1%	New Jersey	11.6%
Utah	28.4%	Massachusetts	18.8%	Nebraska	10.9%
Florida	28.0%	Texas	17.4%	Washington D.C.	10.4%
New York	27.9%	North Carolina	16.7%	Kansas	9.7%
Ohio	25.9%	Montana	15.8%	Illinois	9.5%
Idaho	25.6%	Connecticut	15.0%	Mississippi	8.8%
				Maine	8.7%
				North Dakota	7.6%
				Maryland	7.2%
				South Dakota	6.7%
				Wyoming	5.5%
				New Hampshire	5.3%
				Delaware	4.5%
				Vermont	3.1%
				Alaska	0.7%

Source: Centers for Medicare & Medicaid Services, January 2009

monthly premium. Medicare Part C, or Medicare Advantage, is an alternative to traditional Medicare whereby a person elects to substitute Medicare coverage with private health insurance coverage that mirrors or enriches the benefits that are offered by Medicare (Parts A and B); this is often referred to as managed care. Part D is the recently created prescription drug plan, which offers Medicare recipients limited drug insurance coverage.

Medicare Part A is critical to the profitability of most nursing facilities. It pays short-term coverage for those who require skilled nursing or rehabilitative care after a qualified discharge from a hospital. The facility provides the Part A patients with routine services (room, board, and nursing care) and ancillary services, which include physical, speech, and occupational therapies, plus prescription drugs, medical supplies, and miscellaneous diagnostic and transportation services.

Medicare Part A uses a flat-rate, case-mix, prospective payment system (PPS) with adjustments for differences in regional labor costs. There are four components to PPS rates: nursing, therapy, therapy–non-case mix, and non-case mix. The nursing component is paid through one of 53 patient classifications, known as resource utilization groupings (RUGs). There is a therapy payment for 23 of the 53 RUGs and that amount varies by the intensity of the prescribed therapy. The other 30 RUGs receive a "therapy non-case mix" rate, which is the same for all 30 non-therapy RUGs. The non-case mix payment is the same for all 53 RUG categories. Again, all nursing facilities within a wage market receive the same rate for each specific DRG classification.

Part B reimbursements are based on a fee schedule and are subject to annual limits. Therapy caps as of 2008 were $1,810 on combined physical and speech therapy and $1,810 on occupational therapy per year, per patient.

Medicare Advantage (Part C), which allows patients to opt out of Medicare in favor of approved private managed care coverage, allows the insurance companies to negotiate payments directly with nursing facilities.

Chapter 6

Medicaid Program and Reimbursement for Skilled Nursing Facilities

Medicaid is a federal-state partnership administered at the state level, which provides health care benefits to low-income individuals and families who fit into various eligibility groups. Among the groups of people served by Medicaid are eligible low-income parents, children, seniors, and people with disabilities. While less than 10% of the Medicaid enrollees are elderly, expenditures for this group exceeds 25% of the total program spending. Medicaid is the largest source of revenue to the nursing home industry, and the amount, manner, and timeliness of the reimbursements profoundly impacts the operational and financial management of all certified facilities. Medicaid does not pay benefits to individuals directly, but instead sends benefit payments to health care providers. Typically, residents pay the facility directly from whatever income they have, usually just Social Security and maybe some other pension, and Medicaid will make up the difference.

This chapter focuses on the nursing home component of the Medicaid program. It presents an overview of key factors in state and federal financing, eligibility, and reimbursement principles. Key reimbursement issues that affect revenue, operating expenses, and earnings forecasts will be emphasized. Each state has different financing, eligibility, and reimbursement rules. Descriptions of each program would consume the pages of a very lengthy book and will not be presented here. However, many states apply similar financing, eligibility, and reimbursement principles and the information presented here will provide a fairly comprehensive overview and outline for any appraiser navigating through these issues in a particular state.

Financing the Medicaid Program

The federal government matches state Medicaid spending on an open-ended basis, using a calculation called the *federal medical assistance percentage (FMAP).* The FMAP, or federal match, is calculated annually for each state by applying a formula that compares the average per capita income levels for the state with the national average income level. FMAPs range from 50% in the wealthier states to almost 77% in the poorest state. On average, the federal government covers 57.2% of total Medicaid costs (see Table 6.1).

Table 6.1 **Federal Medical Assistance Percentages Effective October 1, 2008—September 30, 2009 (Fiscal Year 2009)**

State	Match	State	Match	State	Match
AL	67.98%	KY	70.13%	ND	63.15%
AK	50.53%	LA	71.31%	OH	62.14%
AZ	65.77%	ME	64.41%	OK	65.90%
AR	72.81%	MD	50.00%	OR	62.45%
CA	50.00%	MA	50.00%	PA	54.52%
CO	50.00%	MI	60.27%	RI	52.59%
CT	50.00%	MN	50.00%	SC	70.07%
DE	50.00%	MS	75.84%	SD	62.55%
DC	70.00%	MO	63.19%	TN	64.28%
FL	55.40%	MT	68.04%	TX	59.44%
GA	64.49%	NE	59.54%	UT	70.71%
HI	55.11%	NV	50.00%	VT	59.45%
ID	69.77%	NH	50.00%	VA	50.00%
IL	50.32%	NJ	50.00%	WA	50.94%
IN	64.26%	NM	70.88%	WV	73.73%
IA	62.62%	NY	50.00%	WI	59.38%
KS	60.08%	NC	64.60%	WY	50.00%

Source: *Federal Register*, November 28, 2007, vol. 7, no. 228.

The federal share of the states' Medicaid expenditures in 2006 was 21.5% of total state expenditures. Excluding federal matching funds, Medicaid spending consumed 16.8% of states' general fund expenditures.[1] Payments to hospitals and nursing facilities are the two largest expenses in the medical assistance portion of the Medicaid program, representing more than 40% of the total program cost. In 2005, states funded 42.8% of the Medicaid medical assistance program (see Table 6.2).

Medicaid is the second-largest program in the budgets of most states; education is the largest state expense. State revenues have generally not grown as rapidly as the costs of Medicaid programs and, unlike the federal government, most states prohibit deficit spending. As a result, states are under in-

1. National Association of State Budget Officers, *State Expenditure Report, 2006*

Table 6.2 Total (Federal and States Combined) Medical Assistance Program Expenses, 2005 (Dollar Figures in Billions)

Service Category	Total Expense	Percent of Total
Hospital, inpatient, and outpatient	$67.9	22.6%
Nursing facilities	**58.9**	**19.6%**
Mental health facility services	8.2	2.7%
Physicians' services	10.1	3.4%
Prescribed drugs	30.7	10.2%
Medicaid - managed care (MCO)	41.5	13.8%
Home and community	22.9	7.6%
Personal care services	9.4	3.1%
Medicare Part A & B premiums	7.8	2.6%
All other medical assistance programs	43.3	14.4%
Total Medicaid medical assistance	$300.7	100.0%
State's share		42.8%

Source: *2005 Medicaid Financial Management Report*, CMS Web site.

creasing pressure to reduce spending growth through Medicaid cost containment strategies, including increasing beneficiary co-payments, restricting eligibility, limiting benefits, and reducing payments to providers.[2]

Medicaid spending is projected to increase at an average annual rate of about 8% from fiscal 2008 through fiscal 2017, according to the most recent estimates by the Congressional Budget Office.[3]

States fund their share of Medicaid from general and specific taxes. Because few states are constitutionally allowed to borrow money, they are under great pressure to control costs and increase revenues. Provider taxes have grown popular in recent years as a technique for states to increase matching funds from the federal government for nursing facilities. *Provider taxes*, or *quality assurance fees*, are specific taxes charged to nursing home operators; these tax revenues then can be used to garner increased federal matching funds. The taxes and the augmented federal match are then redistributed to the nursing home operators in the form of increased reimbursements. In its simplest form, the provider gives the state $1 and the state receives $1 from the federal government (50:50 match). The state then returns $2 to the provider. The taxes are typically assessed as a bed tax (i.e., a flat tax per licensed bed), a tax per patient day, or a tax based on a percentage of non-Medicare revenue. Under all three systems, the taxes are applied uniformly across all Medicaid-certified facilities. An example of a provider tax calculation follows.

1. Assume a state charges all nursing homes an annual tax equal to $1,000 per licensed bed.

---

2. Kaiser Family Foundation / statehealthfacts.org
3. *The Basics*, National Health Policy Forum.

2. The state receives a 72% federal match [$1,000/(1.0 – 0.72) = $3,571].
3. Now assume that 75% of the statewide patient days are paid for by Medicaid. The net payment derived from the provider tax could be as much as $5,094 per bed for an all-Medicaid facility, calculated as follows:

Provider tax (paid by facility, state's share)	$1,000
Federal match (($1,000 divided by (100% – 72%), or $1,000 /.28)	$3,571
Total provider tax revenue	$4,571
Redistributed provider payment for 75% statewide ($4,571 divided by 75%)	$6,094
Less bed tax	(1,000)
Provider tax net gain (100% Medicaid)	$5,094

The states shown in Table 6.3 did not use some type of provider taxes for FMAP for nursing facilities in their 2008 state budgets.

In 1991, the U.S. Congress reigned in states' abuses of provider taxes. Prior to 1991, nursing facilities were "held harmless" or they were guaranteed to be made whole by the state after paying their provider tax. For example, if a facility paid $100,000 in "bed taxes" but only received $50,000 in reimbursement enhancements, the state would pay the provider the other $50,000 as a hold harmless payment. Facilities that have little or no Medicaid census do not benefit from this form of tax, but facilities with high Medicaid census have come to rely on the enhanced reimbursements allowed by provider taxes. Now, providers cannot be guaranteed that a portion of the tax amount will be returned after the federal matching funds are received. As of 2008, CMS limits the FMAP (federal match) from provider tax revenue to 5.5% of the total routine revenue from all nursing facilities in the state, excluding the Medicare revenue. CMS will not allow Medicare revenues to be subject to provider taxes, at least not directly.

Another technique used by a few states, and one that is being curtailed by federal law, is known as *intergovernmental transfer payments (IGTs)*. These schemes collect funds from state, county, and local government entities. For example, many states require their counties to transfer certain local tax revenues to help fund the state's Medicaid program. This practice is perfectly legal as long as the local funds do

Table 6.3 **List of States That Had No SNF Provider Tax During Their Respective 2008 Fiscal Years**

Alaska	Idaho	South Dakota
Arizona	Iowa	Texas
Colorado	Kansas	Virginia
Delaware	New Mexico	Washington
Florida	North Dakota	Wyoming
Hawaii	South Carolina	

not exceed 60% of the state share for purposes of receiving Medicaid matching funds.[4]

In summary, funding the Medicaid program will increasingly challenge fiscal policies as Medicaid spending growth is expected to increase at rates that exceed the combination of population growth and inflation, outstripping growth in GDP and tax revenues. Therefore, the prospects for any significant improvement in Medicaid reimbursement are grim.

Medicaid Eligibility

Medicaid eligibility varies by state, but generally requires that individuals meet an income test and deplete nearly all of their assets. During 2005 there were approximately 940,000 Medicaid recipients receiving nursing facility care at any point during the year.[5] To qualify for Medicaid benefits at a nursing home, a single person or surviving spouse who has a qualifying medical need must spend down all assets other than his or her home, personal furnishings, a burial plot, and $2,000 to $3,000 in cash. Medicaid applies a lien against the patient's residence for payment of the balance of care charges if the patient does not return home after a stay at a nursing home. Living spouses are granted some economic protection to limit catastrophic financial loss. Once a patient's income (social security and pensions) is less than the private-pay rate and the patient has depleted all assets, that person can be eligible for Medicaid. Some people attempt to preserve much of their wealth for their families by using trusts and other financial devices to shield assets, allowing the patient to qualify for Medicaid prematurely. As long-term care costs continue to increase more rapidly than inflation, there is a growing interest in creating *Medicaid trusts.* These strategies place additional burdens on federal and state budgets and challenges lawmakers to develop legislation to end abuses.

Medicaid Rate Setting

The Centers for Medicare & Medicaid Services (CMS), under the U.S. Department of Health and Human Services, has established general financial and operational guidelines for nursing home care which states must incorporate into their laws. States must apply and receive approval from CMS prior to adopting a reimbursement system or making changes to an existing system. According to a BDO Siedman study of Medicaid reimburse-

4. *The Basics*, National Health Policy Forum.

5. *The State Long-Term Health Care Sector 2005: Characteristics, Utilization and Government Funding*, published by the American Health Care Association.

ments conducted for the American Health Care Association, the average per-patient shortfall in Medicaid reimbursements in 2007 was $13.15 nationally, or $4.4 billion in total.[6]

In nearly every state, all facilities participating in Medicaid are required to submit annual or even biannual cost reports. One exception is Kentucky, which no longer requires Medicaid providers to submit cost reports. Cost reports present a standardized financial accounting of the operations of the facility and typically contain detailed census, revenue, operating expenses, and capital costs. These cost reports provide the appraiser with an unparalleled opportunity to obtain highly detailed census, revenue, operating expense, and capital cost data. The information is presented in a chart of accounts and signed by an officer of the nursing home, who certifies that it is entirely truthful under the laws of the state and federal fraud statutes. The Medicaid cost reports are available for the public to review under the Freedom of Information Act (FOIA). Any member of the public, including appraisers and other interested observers, may request and receive these reports through the state agency responsible for the financial management of the Medicaid program.

Cost reports can be very valuable in developing sale and lease comparable data, operating expenses, and construction cost comparisons. They can also be a gold mine for property and mortgage lenders as many states require operators to disclose their financing rates, terms, and lenders as well as lease terms and landlords. Some states will provide the cost reports for every facility in an electronic format at little expense to the party making the FOIA request; other states will only provide hard copies of reports from individual facilities. The request may take weeks or months to be filled, so careful, upfront planning is needed in order to benefit from this information.

Types of Medicaid Payment Systems

Most states employ a prospective payment system that pays operators predetermined Medicaid rates over a prescribed period. No final cost settlement is employed to reconcile differences between the actual final allowable costs and the actual reimbursement. A few states continue to use a retrospective payment system for some or all of the cost components. Retrospective payment systems make an interim payment to the provider over a rate period. The interim payment is an estimated rate that is typically based on the previous costs of the individual facility.

6. *A Report on Shortfalls in Medicaid Funding for Nursing Home Care*, BDO Seidman, LLP and Eljay, LLC for the American Health Care Association, September 2007.

After the actual costs of the provider are reviewed by the state or its intermediary, a final cost settlement is made to reconcile the difference between the interim payment and the actual allowable cost incurred during that same time period.

Payment systems have a variety of rate calculation methods but most are flat-rate systems or facility-specific systems.

Flat-Rate Reimbursement Systems

Flat-rate reimbursement systems are typically based on the prior expense history of the entire state or a geographic portion of the state where costs are perceived to be fairly typical. The specific allowable cost of a facility will not have a material impact on the reimbursement because regional or state averages are applied. Some states will adjust reimbursement rates according to the acuity level of the Medicaid patients at the facility. For example, Texas uses the TILE system, recognizing 14 different patient classes, and each TILE has a specific rate that all facilities in the state receive, regardless of the actual cost, location, or other variables. Some states incorporate flat-rate principles in reimbursing certain costs, such as administrative and capital costs, and reimburse other costs, such as nursing care, using facility-specific principles.

Facility-Specific Reimbursements

Facility-specific reimbursements are typically based on actual facility annual expenses as reported in state-standardized Medicaid cost reports. Typically, states will develop cost ceilings for various cost centers, categories, or groupings. Often, cost centers are divided into:

- Direct patient care (nursing, ancillary, and social services)
- Support services (administrative, management, activities, dietary, housekeeping, laundry, maintenance, and utilities)
- Capital (property tax and insurance, mortgage interest, depreciation, tangible asset rent, and return of equity)

Reimbursement ceilings are normally set at a specific amount above a mean or median (e.g., 115.0% of the mean or the 65th percentile of a defined group of facilities). To encourage cost control, many states allow providers to earn a small profit through a cost-savings incentive, whereby the state and operator share the difference between the cost ceiling and the actual allowable cost, if the cost is below the ceiling or some other target. Many states place limits on "ownership" costs–management fees, central office expense, administrator/owner compensation, etc.–since these are possible avenues for "expensing" their profits.

Many states are moving toward case-mix reimbursement for patient care costs, whereby the patient care component of the reimbursement can be adjusted according to the intensity of care (acuity) required. Intensity or acuity levels involve "grading" the patients' care needs, and this grading is generally referred to as *case mix.* Case mix allows the state to allocate resources more fairly to facilities that provide higher or lower levels of care than average. It is important to analyze trends in case-mix indexes for the subject and expense comparables as there is a correlation between the index, Medicaid revenues, and nursing expenses.

Types of Medicaid Payments

Capital Cost Reimbursements

Capital costs are of paramount importance in valuation and loan underwriting since this component of the reimbursement typically represents the single largest source of Medicaid revenue to compensate the owner/operator for depreciation, debt service, and/or rent. There are three basic forms of capital reimbursement: two that rely on actual historical capital costs and one that is a fair market rental system. Capital reimbursement will be discussed shortly.

A simplified facility-specific rate calculation follows.

Example of a Facility-Specific, Prospective Medicaid Rate Calculation

	Allowable Expense	Ceiling	Amount Paid
Patient care expense	$58.00	$60.00	$58.00
Support and general expense	54.00	51.00	51.00
Subtotal	$112.00	$111.00	$109.00
Inflation adjustment (4.0%)			4.36
Capital			10.00
Total reimbursement			$123.36

In this example, the allowable patient care expenses fall below the ceiling and thus the facility will receive the entire expense in the rate. The support and general expense of $54.00 exceeds the ceiling or limit and, as a result, the reimbursement will be limited to the ceiling amount of $51.00. The direct and indirect components are inflated to reflect cost increases from the prior year to the current year. States apply a variety of inflation trending factors that often relate to overall budget constraints. The capital reimbursement, which is not subject to inflationary adjustments, is added last.

Direct and Support Cost Reimbursements

Most facility-specific systems reimburse the direct and support components (i.e., operating expenses) based on their actual costs. This is known as *cost-based* or *dollar-for-dollar* reimbursement. If a facility spends $1.00 for nursing care, dietary, laundry, etc., it will be reimbursed $1.00. Simply put, costs drive revenue. The significance of this concept is that there is no opportunity for profit (beyond capital reimbursement or possibly shared cost-saving incentives) in a purely "cost-based" reimbursement system. Also, if costs exceed the cost ceilings, reimbursement may be less than costs. Ceilings are often set at a percentage of some average for peer groups of facilities of similar size in the region.

Minimum occupancy requirements also should be examined, especially if low occupancy performance is a persistent operational condition. Because of ceilings and minimum utilization requirements, a facility might spend $1.00 but receive a lower reimbursement. For instance, a 100-bed facility with an annual property tax expense of $50,000 and an actual occupancy rate of 85% incurs an expense that equals $1.61 per patient day (PPD). However, if the minimum utilization factor is 95%, the divisor increases from 31,025 to 34,675 patient days, reducing the reimbursement for taxes to $1.44 PPD. The calculation for minimum utilization is shown in the following example.

Minimum Utilization Calculation—Property Tax Component

Actual annual property tax	$50,000
Potential patient days (100 beds × 365 days)	36,500
Actual census @ 85% occupancy	31,025
Actual property taxes PPD ($50.000/31,025 PD)	$1.61
Minimum utilization calculations:	
Minimum allowed patient days @ 95% occupancy	34,675
Reimbursable property taxes ($50,000/34,675 PD)	$1.44

Many states have found it feasible to offer operators cost-saving incentives to keep costs down by sharing the difference between the ceiling and the actual allowable costs. An example of shared-cost savings is shown below.

Example of Medicaid Cost-Saving Incentive Calculation

Indirect care cost ceiling	$75.39
Actual allowable indirect cost	$71.18
Inflation factor to actual cost	× 1.03
Inflation-adjusted indirect cost	$73.32
Difference between ceiling and cost	$2.07
Cost savings share to provider	× 50.0%
Cost savings incentive	$1.04

For states employing a facility-specific reimbursement system, some or all of the rate components may be adjusted, or rebased, as frequently as once every six months (as in Iowa) or very infrequently. For example, New York rates are based on 1983 allowable expenses, inflated to present levels using industry-wide multipliers. For periods in which rates are not rebased, but cost reports were filed, inflation multipliers are relied on to bridge the gap.

Additional concern is advised when analyzing Medicaid reimbursements in situations where rates have not been rebased for extended periods because the actual allowable expense may be vastly different from the amount being received. Eventually, a rebasing could cause a dramatic change in earnings. In cases where rates have not been rebased for many years, such as in Illinois and New York, the actual allowable operating expenses are often $20 to $40 greater or less than the current reimbursement set through trend costs at the facility years ago. In both Illinois and New York, rates tend to exceed current allowable expenses in large cities, while reimbursements to facilities in downstate Illinois and upstate New York are typically well below actual costs.

While the operator realizes "profit" or "losses" in a current period, a rate rebasing could eliminate a substantial portion of the short-run profit or loss. Capitalizing this short-run profit or loss in perpetuity will result in a misleading value conclusion. In many situations, an operator can create an illusion of higher or lower value through a short-term mismatch of rate and expenses. Eventually, the Medicaid rate will be matched to the actual allowable expense, canceling any superficial earnings or losses. The following example illustrates the "profit illusion."

Assume that an operator is currently receiving a $123.36 Medicaid rate, which includes:

Patient care expense	$58.00
Support and general expenses	51.00
Subtotal	$109.00
Inflation adjustment (4.0%)	4.36
Capital	10.00
Total reimbursement	$123.36

Consider these other facts:

- The Medicaid rate is based on the state's review of the operating expenses filed with the provider's cost report from one year ago (one-year lag), adjusted for inflation, unallowable expenses, and ceilings.
- Assume that the facility operates below the ceiling and receives 100% of actual allowable expenses, but does not

receive any cost-saving incentives since none are provided for in the system.

- Now assume that a borrower presents a profit and loss statement for the past year (the year after the period used to set the current rate), showing improved earnings through better management and cost cutting.
- The nursing expenses have been reduced to $53.00 per patient day through staffing changes, and the support and general expense is reduced to $47.00 through staff cuts, reduced worker's compensation insurance premiums, and lower food costs through group purchasing.
- The expense reduction of $9.00 per patient day falls to the bottom line on the current operating profit and loss statement.
- The next Medicaid rate setting will occur in just a few months and will use the actual allowable expenses from the past year–$53.00 for direct care and $47.00 for support and general expenses.
- Based on the current-period expenses, the estimated new Medicaid rate will be $110 before inflation and $114.00 after inflation trending.

Patient care expense	$53.00
Support and general expenses	47.00
Subtotal	100.00
Inflation adjustment	4.00
Capital	10.00
Total	$114.00

The current and rebased Medicaid rates from this example are compared as follows.

	Current Rate	Rebased Rate
Patient care expense	$58.00	$53.00
Support and general expense	51.00	47.00
Subtotal	$109.00	$100.00
Inflation adjustment	4.36	4.00
Capital	10.00	10.00
Total	$123.36	$114.00

The principle above is illustrated in the three-year cash flow analysis in Table 6.4. The first-year expenses set the stage for the current-year rate. Because the current-year operating expenses were reduced, the facility shows a substantial increase in net operating income over the previous year. However, going forward one year, the Medicaid rate will be reset to the current expense levels.

Table 6.4 Imbalanced Revenue and Earnings Caused by Annually Rebased, Facility-Specific Medicaid Reimbursement

	Previous Year P&Ls			Current Year P&Ls			Following (Stabilized) Year P&Ls		
	Patient Days	$/PPD	Total	Patient Days	$/PPD	Total	Patient Days	$/PPD	Total
Private pay	10,000	$134.62	$1,346,154	10,000	$140.00	$1,400,000	10,000	$145.60	$1,456,000
Medicaid	30,000	117.49	3,524,571	30,000	123.36	3,700,800	30,000	114.00	3,420,000
Total revenue	40,000	$121.77	$4,870,725	40,000	$127.52	$5,100,800	40,000	$102.40	$4,876,000
Operating expenses									
Nursing		$58.00	$2,320,000		$53.00	$2,120,000		$55.12	$2,204,800
Indirect expenses		51.00	2,040,000		47.00	1,880,000		48.88	1,955,200
Reserves		0.48	19,200		0.50	20,000		0.52	20,800
Total operating expense		$109.48	$4,379,200		$100.50	$4,020,000		$104.52	$4,180,800
Net operating income			491,525			1,080,800			695,200
Capitalized value @ 13.5%			$3,640,928			$8,005,926			$5,149,630
Value per bed			$30,341			$66,716			$42,914
Cash flow available for debt service using a DCR of 1.5			$376,333			$376,333			$376,333
Loan amount at 75% loan to value						$6,004,444			
Annual debt service with a mortgage constant of 8.00%						$480,356			$480,356
DCR						2.25			1.45

Medicaid rate calculations	Current-Year Rate	Following-Year Rate
Nursing	$58.00	$53.00
Indirect care	51.00	47.00
Total operating expenses	$109.00	$100.00
Plus inflation @ 4%	4.36	4.00
Plus capital payment capital	$10.00	$10.00
Total Medicaid rate	$123.36	$114.00

Taking this example further, the table shows the prior, current, and "Medicaid-stabilized" rate developments, facility revenue, and operating expenses and valuations, assuming a single year's net operating income is capitalized. Obviously, the final year net operating income, using the Medicaid-stabilized rate, provides the best basis for valuation using direct capitalization.

Medicaid Capital Payments

Medicaid capital items include some combination of the following components:

- Building depreciation
- Mortgage interest
- Mortgage amortization
- Building rent
- Return on equity
- Equipment interest
- Equipment depreciation
- Equipment rent

Some states include property taxes and insurance in the capital rate but, in terms of net operating income or EBITDAR, the property taxes and insurance components of the Medicaid rate have corresponding expenses that are considered as operating expenses in most financial analyses. The contributions from the certificate of need and intangible assets are excluded from the capital reimbursement in most states regardless of their value or historical cost basis.

There are essentially three general forms of capital reimbursement: fair market rental, flat rate, and historical costs.

The fair market rental systems pay a "market" or "fair" rate of return on a predetermined value or cost of the real estate and/or personal property assets. The asset value is either determined from a cost approach appraisal or is a state-mandated value, such as a flat value per bed, adjusted for depreciation using building (asset) age. The rate of return applied to the recognized capital basis is the same rate for all properties. Some states will apply different return factors depending on the year the asset was established. The return factor covers interest, depreciation, rent, and/or a return on equity and it is typically not related to actual asset costs or financial obligations. Typically, changes in ownership or additional capital improvements will have little or no impact on the "rent" until a revaluation is performed or the effective asset age is adjusted.

The following example shows a typical capital payment calculation using the fair market rental system in a state that uses a flat, per-bed basis for real estate, minus depreciation.

Fair Market Rental Calculation

Replacement cost new			$49,383
Number of beds		×	120
Total replacement cost			$5,925,960
Less depreciation			
Average building age	25		
Depreciation (1.0% per year)	25.0%		
Total depreciation			$(1,481,490)
Allowable capital basis			$4,444,470
Market rental factor		×	9.0%
Fair market rental			$400,002
Total patient days			40,000
Capital reimbursement rate			$10.00

Historical capital cost reimbursement systems rely on the actual cost of the assets, actual interest cost, actual rental rates, and depreciation schedules. In July 1984, the federal government created a law that eliminated step-ups in the capital basis in the event of a change in ownership. New owners were mandated to receive the cost basis of the previous owner, despite possibly higher sale prices than the historic basis. This law was part of DEFRA, or the Deficit Reconciliation Act, and the industry generally refers to it as "capital limits subject to DEFRA." The law applied to Medicare for nursing facilities as well as Medicaid and Medicare capital reimbursement to hospitals. Medicare no longer reimburses nursing facilities and most hospitals on a facility-specific, historical-cost-based system. An example of the calculation of capital reimbursement under historical cost is shown below.

Example of Calculation of Medicaid Capital Reimbursement Using Historical Cost Basis

Calculation of allowable depreciation			
Asset	**Cost**	**Life**	**Allowed Depreciation**
Original building cost	$3,500,000	35	$100,000
Building addition	1,500,000	35	42,857
Roof replacement	100,000	15	6,667
Total allowable building capital basis	$5,100,000		$149,524
Calculation of allowable interest			
Allowable capital basis			
Total building capital basis	$5,100,000		
Land cost	100,000		
Total real estate basis	$5,200,000		
Allowable interest (interest only)	7.50%		390,000
Total allowable interest and depreciation			539,524
Total patient days			39,858
Total allowable per-diem reimbursement			$13.54

Staying with this example, assume there is a sale of this facility, and the allocated price for the real estate is $7,000,000 and the debt incurred to finance the purchase is $6,000,000. In this case, the new ownership will still receive depreciation payments based on $5,100,000 and interest reimbursement based on $5,200,000.

The majority of states continue to apply DEFRA principles to their capital reimbursement. Several states not only restrict the allowable capital basis to the historical (pre-1984) or even original costs, but require that once the asset has been depreciated and amortized out over the initial established period, then the interest and depreciation payments for that asset are discontinued or substantially limited. It is absolutely necessary to weigh the impact of this reduction in capital payments as assets reach the payment limits when valuing and underwriting facilities in states such as Connecticut and New York, where this type of capital reimbursement is practiced . Obviously, facilities with older physical plants are at greater risk for the exhaustion of capital payments under this system.

Returning to the previous example, Table 6.5 illustrates that once the interest and depreciation for initial construction is fully amortized after three years, the Medicaid capital reimbursement is reduced significantly. In this example, the Medicaid capital rate declines $9.28 per Medicaid patient day after three years; the reduction in reimbursement will be $278,489 per year if the facility has 30,000 Medicaid days. Since there are no off-setting expenses, this reimbursement loss falls to the bottom line and has a profound impact on operating and financial ratios.

The federal government relaxed the DEFRA rules in 1985, one year after they were established. The new law was referred to as COBRA, or the Consolidated Omnibus Budget and Reconciliation Act. COBRA gave states the option to increase the capital basis after a change in ownership by as much as 50.0% of the increase in a construction cost index between the time that the seller's allowable capital basis was established and the date of the change in ownership.

The example that follows illustrates a facility-specific capital payment calculation under the COBRA rules. The example rests on these assumptions:

- The facility was built in 1987 at a recognized cost of $20,000 per bed and is sold in December 2007 for $44,000 per bed.
- The state will allow the new owner's capital basis to increase to the lesser of the actual price, the current capital ceiling of $38,000, or the original basis plus 50% of the Dodge construction index (2.30).

Table 6.5 **Total Allowable Per Diem Reimbursement, Historical Basis, Without Resetting Interest or Depreciation After Change of Ownership**

	Original Building	Building Addition	Roof Replacement	Totals	Reimbursement Rate
Asset age	32	12	10		
Allowed depreciation life	35	35	15		
Years of depreciation remaining	3	23	5		
Allowable basis	$3,500,000	$1,500,000	$100,000		
Allowable annual depreciation, going forward					
Year 1	$100,000	$42,857	$6,667	$149,524	$3.75
Year 2	100,000	42,857	6,667	149,524	3.75
Year 3	100,000	42,857	6,667	149,524	3.75
Year 4	-	42,857	6,667	49,524	1.24
Year 5	-	42,857	6,667	49,524	1.24
Year 6	-	42,857	-	42,857	1.08
Allowable annual interest, going forward					
Allowable basis ($100,000 land included in original building)	$3,600,000	$1,500,000	$100,000	$5,200,000	
Year 1	270,000	112,500	7,500	390,000	$9.78
Year 2	270,000	112,500	7,500	390,000	9.78
Year 3	270,000	112,500	7,500	390,000	9.78
Year 4	-	112,500	7,500	120,000	3.01
Year 5	-	112,500	7,500	120,000	3.01
Year 6	-	112,500	-	112,500	2.82
Total capital reimbursement, interest & depreciation					
Year 1					$13.54
Year 2					$13.54
Year 3					$13.54
Year 4					$4.25
Year 5					$4.25
Year 6					$3.90

- The three bases are calculated per bed:

Actual cost as of December 2007	$44,000
Current ceiling	$38,000
Original cost, inflated 65%	
[((2.3 – 1.0) × .5) × $20,000] + $20,000	$33,000
New basis	$33,000

Under DEFRA or COBRA, states may opt to continue to pay depreciation and interest under the originally established depreciation and amortization schedules or re-establish schedules to the sale date. Some states will not pay, or will limit payments, for equity on equity. Thus, providers are motivated to finance all of the cost recognized by the Medicaid system.

A question that often concerns appraisers, assessors, underwriters, and lenders is whether to appraise the nursing facility reflecting the existing capital cost basis of the current owner, or to assume an ownership change that would reset the capital basis when the COBRA method is applied by the state. The buyer and seller could have significantly different capital rates. The appraiser needs to explain the COBRA rule to the client and discuss the approach to be taken in the valuation. Market value (and market rent) assumes that a change in ownership occurs; a change in ownership will typically result in a higher basis, resulting in a greater reimbursement to the buyer. However, for loan underwriting purposes, the cash flow forecast will probably be developed without the impact of COBRA if the appraisal is not performed to finance an ownership change. It could be that the client will desire two cash flow forecasts: one assuming a sale of the assets and re-establishment of the basis and capital cost and the other assuming no sale and a continuation of the current capital reimbursement.

The appraiser needs to be consistent when developing sale price indicators. *Do unto your sales as you do to the subject.* The appraiser must realize that the net operating income of a sale (and the subject) may be different for the buyer and the seller. It is inconsistent to apply a rebased Medicaid capital rate to the net operating income forecast of the subject while not rebasing Medicaid rates in the development of price indicators from the comparable sales–e.g., capitalization rates, discount rates, and income multipliers.

Many states re-establish the interest rate, amortization period, and recognized mortgage balance under DEFRA, COBRA, or fair market rental rules, causing the seller and buyer to have different capital rates. For example, in Wisconsin Medicaid does not pay a return on equity. If the owner refinances an amount that is greater than the existing debt, the increased interest expense will be disallowed because the additional borrowing is considered equity. However, a new owner could be paid a substantially greater amount by borrowing the entire allowable capital basis.

The calculations shown in Table 6.6 relate to the facility described above. As this example shows, the "seller's internal value" or "value in use" could be vastly different from the market value–i.e., value to a buyer. This is an important issue for lenders, appraisers, and owners. The appraiser should understand the circumstances of the capital rate calculation for the valuation and clearly state the assumptions used and the direction taken in the valuation. The same consideration should

Table 6.6 Medicaid Capital Payments Under Old and New Ownerships Using COBRA Guidelines

	Seller	Buyer
Allowable basis, per bed	$20,000	$40,000
Amount financed	$15,000	$30,000
Interest rate	9.00%	9.00%
Annual debt service	$1,350	$2,700
Plus depreciation	500	1,000
Total capital payment	$1,850	$3,700
Number of patient days per bed	347	347
Medicaid capital rate	$5.33	$10.66
Difference		$5.33
Medicaid mix		75%
Net average daily rate difference		$4.00
Annualized capital payment difference		$1,388
Capitalized value difference @ 12.5%		$11,104

be given to the comparable sale data used in extracting direct overall capitalization rates and revenue multipliers.

Several states impose Medicaid depreciation recapture charges. Depreciation recapture is assessed to a seller when the sale price exceeds the Medicaid depreciated cost basis. A Medicaid depreciation recapture example follows.

Example of Medicaid Capital Depreciation Recapture Calculation

	Improvements	FF&E
Total allowed cost basis (all years)	$2,000,000	$300,000
Depreciation claimed (all years)	$1,500,000	$250,000
New ownership's cost basis	$4,000,000	$500,000
Total patient days claimed over entire ownership period	500,000	500,000
Total Medicaid patient days over the ownership	400,000	400,000
Percentage paid by Medicaid	80%	80%
Depreciation recapture liability to seller	$1,200,000	$200,000

While the existence of depreciation recapture impacts the net amount received by a seller, there is no direct evidence that demonstrates that this rule has any effect on value. However, evidence does suggest that owners are less willing to sell and more likely to lease the property to a new operator to avoid the depreciation recapture payment. Note that there have been cases in which the lender forecloses on the property, turns around and sells the property for more than the depreciated basis, and becomes liable for the depreciation recapture.

Summary

Medicaid is the nation's health program for eligible individuals and families with low incomes and resources. The program is a federal-state partnership, administered at the state level. States fund their share of the program through various tax revenues. Unlike Medicare, the federal government uses general funds for their share. States pay roughly 40% of the total Medicaid cost, while the remainder comes from the federal level. For nursing facilities, Medicaid is the payor of last resort and pays the portion of the nursing home bill that the patient is unable to cover with Social Security and pension income. To qualify for Medicaid benefits in a nursing facility, a person must have medical need, have spent down nearly all of his or her personal assets, and have less income than the nursing home charges.

Each state administers its Medicaid program in the manner it sees fit. However, the state must conform to certain federal guidelines and the state programs must be approved by the Centers for Medicare & Medicaid Services (CMS), the administrative agency for the federal government. Each state's reimbursements to nursing facilities, hospitals, doctors, and other medical providers are different.

Most states employ a prospective payment system that pays operators predetermined Medicaid rates over a prescribed period with no final cost settlement. A few states use a retrospective payment system for some or all of the cost components. This system calls for interim payments (rates) to the provider, typically based on the previous costs of the individual facility, and a final cost settlement at a later date based on reconciliation with the actual, allowable cost of the facility.

There are two general payment systems: facility-specific and flat-rate. Flat-rate reimbursement is typically based on the prior expense history of a class of facilities (determined by size, location, or other grouping). The specific, allowable cost of a facility will not have a material impact on the reimbursement, as group averages are applied. Some states will adjust reimbursement rates according to the acuity level of the Medicaid patients at the facility; this is generally referred to as case-mix indexing. Some states incorporate flat-rate principles to certain cost centers, such as administrative and capital costs, and reimburse other costs, such as nursing care, using cost-based, facility-specific principles.

Facility-specific reimbursements are typically based on actual, allowable expenses for a facility. The reimbursement rate is typically calculated by using the actual, allowable expense of the facility or a ceiling amount, whichever is less. Usually, the total reimbursement rate is the sum of rates for various cost centers, with rate limits applied to each center. The major cost centers are direct patient care (nursing, ancillary, and social services), support services (administrative, management, activities, dietary, housekeeping, laundry, maintenance, and utilities), and capital (property tax and insurance, mortgage interest, depreciation, tangible asset rent, and return of equity). Rates can be rebased as frequently as every six months or very infrequently. In states where there is frequent rate rebasing, it is crucial to balance the forecasted operating expenses with the reimbursement to avoid misrepresenting long-run, or stabilized, earnings. Any analysis of a Medicaid reimbursement system will require considerable study. The material in this chapter provides a general framework for learning a specific system.

Chapter 7

Regional and Neighborhood Influences

The values of nursing facilities are influenced by the same physical, social, economic, and political forces that affect all real estate. The forces that affect real estate in general warrant consideration, but not at the expense of diluting or avoiding meaningful analysis of the factors that influence nursing facilities specifically. Location and environment affect a nursing facility's ability to compete for patients and staff. In addition to general knowledge of a region and neighborhood, the appraiser needs quantifiable demographic and labor data, obtained through public and private sources, to measure objectively, describe, and analyze regional and neighborhood forces.

Special consideration should be given to the following socioeconomic data:

- Current and future population of elderly
- Average income levels
- Housing characteristics, including percentage of homeownership, average housing value, and age of housing stock
- The size of current and future skilled and unskilled labor pools, employment rates, and wage levels
- Proximity to hospitals, public transportation, and institutional facilities

Population drives demand and demographic forecasts are reliable predictors of the demand for future long-term care. There are rule-of-thumb relationships between the number of nursing home beds in a market and the number of elderly. In the calculation of certificates of need, many states base the number of beds needed primarily on ratios of beds to elderly persons. Excellent demographic data, breaking down current and estimated future population by age cohorts, is available in hard copy or electronic form from several reliable sources.

There is a close correlation between wealth levels in a market area and patients' dependency on Medicaid. Wealth levels can be inferred from median household and/or per capita income, poverty ratios, home values, the percentage of owner-occupied dwelling units, and educational attainment. There is also a correlation between levels of wealth and Medicaid mix, with facilities situated in market areas with lower household income, property values, and educational attainment levels experiencing a higher percentage of Medicaid patients. This phenomenon is observed on state, regional, and local levels. As an example, Figure 7.1 shows a regression analysis of quality mix percentages for all skilled nursing facilities in St. Louis County, Missouri, compared to the median home value in the zip code for each facility.

Wages, salaries, and employee benefits are the largest expenses in operating a long-term care facility. Ideally, facilities should be located near sources of relatively low-cost labor since most jobs in long-term care are low paying. Facility operators in urban areas must be concerned with public transportation, onsite parking, employee safety, and other factors that make it possible to attract and keep desirable employees. Insufficient staffing (quality and/or quantity) can limit the effective bed capacity, jeopardize the license of the facility, or curtail deployment of more profitable, higher-acuity care. Many operators contend that it is easier to get patients than staff.

The U.S. Department of Labor, Bureau of Labor Statistics (http://www.bls.gov) provides substantial information re-

Figure 7.1 **Median Home Value in Zip Code Areas of SNFs Compared to Quality Mix Percentage—All of St. Louis County, Missouri**

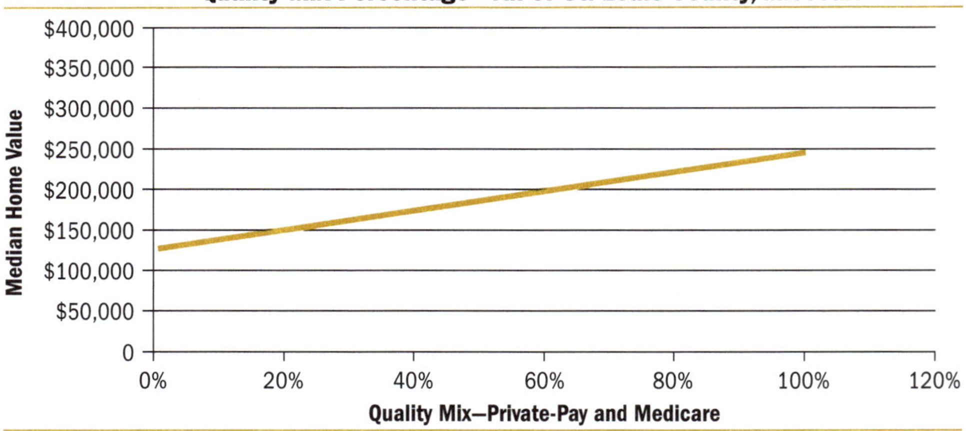

Sources: Tellatin, Short, Hansen & Clark, Inc., Claritas, Inc., and the Missouri nursing facility Medicaid cost reports.

garding national, state, regional, and county employment and unemployment as well as detailed wage and benefits statistics by occupation.

Hospitals play an important role in patient admission for nursing facilities. Hospitals are well-known landmarks with good access and capturing some of this exposure is generally positive for skilled nursing facilities.The trend toward a higher-acuity census in nursing homes is drawing these two providers closer geographically and financially. Until the early 1990s, nursing home development was usually found in residential settings. But with the rapid development of assisted living facilities, which target low-acuity, private-pay residents, and the expansion of Medicare benefits for rehabilitation stays, nursing home development has shifted towards a hospital-like design and locations associated with medical centers have become more desirable.

Locations that encourage relationships with hospitals for referrals, resource sharing, and medical community amenities are increasingly desirable for nursing facilities. Physicians have some influence in directing patients to nursing facilities and, therefore, will tend to favor patient referrals to facilities that are closer to physicians' workplaces and homes, all else being equal. Because employees at nursing facilities often rely on public transportation in urban and suburban areas, and hospitals are well served by public transportation, proximity to hospitals and transportation alternatives can be an advantage in recruiting and retaining employees.

Chapter 8

Site and Improvement Data and Analysis

Site Data and Analysis

The size of a nursing facility site will vary depending on its location in an urban, suburban, or rural area and on land costs. Besides the building, the site dimensions should include space for employee and visitor parking, deliveries, strolling areas for patients and guests, water drainage, landscaping features, and other environmental amenities. The terrain should be fairly level to accommodate the frail and often non-ambulatory clientele. In suburban and rural areas where public transportation is rarely a consideration, there should be adequate onsite parking available for two working shifts and guests (typically 0.4 to 0.6 spaces per bed). Urban sites may need to include a parking garage; zoning codes often will specify minimum parking requirements. Like residential property, a nursing home should be located away from areas with high levels of air and noise pollution.

The site should be identified with a legal description and property survey that satisfies the client. These documents should define the property boundaries, dimensions, land area, easements, and other site restrictions. The appraiser should read the legal description and review the site survey prior to and/or during the inspection to avoid errors or confusion later. Assessor's plat maps, aerial photographs, and site drawings on architectural plans may be accurate, but they occasionally are incorrect for various reasons.

Land ownership can be determined by reviewing public records. As discussed in Chapter 4, most nursing facilities have a multi-level ownership structure in which the fee simple interest in the real estate differs from the ownership of the business operations. A clear description of the ownership structure should be obtained from the management of the facility. Local real estate records should identify the real estate ownership, while state licensing agencies and Medicaid cost reports can be searched for license ownership.

The Uniform Standards of Professional Appraisal Practice (USPAP) require appraisers to investigate and consider any sale of the property within the past three years. They also require the appraiser to consider and analyze any current listing, sales contract, or sale option.

The zoning and other legal use restrictions and entitlements of the site should be considered in site analysis. Depending on the community, a nursing facility use may be allowed under a residential, institutional, or commercial zoning classification. Zoning is most critical to the analysis of a proposed facility and confirmation that the use will be permitted should be sought from the planning and/or zoning office of the governing jurisdiction. A facility on a nonconforming-use site may encounter special problems if the improvements are destroyed and rebuilding is not allowed. This could be catastrophic if certificate of need rules prohibit replacement facilities. Floodplain, wetlands, historic, conservation, and other restrictions on property rights should be investigated and considered relative to the site and the overall value of the property.

Utility service is especially important for nursing facilities as they are 24-hour, seven-days-a week businesses. Since most nursing facilities are required to have an emergency backup electrical generator, the availability of natural gas may be important. Many facilities opt for diesel fuel, so delivery access is important, as is the type of onsite storage. These days, most diesel fuel is stored in aboveground tanks that are incorporated into the housing structure of the generator. If an underground tank is present, the cost of removal should be considered in the valuation. Most buyers and lenders and many states require the removal of underground storage tanks.

The impact of excess and surplus land areas on value should be considered for the subject and comparable sales. Surplus land may be defined as additional land that can be used for expansion of the existing improvements, but cannot be developed separately or split off and sold. Surplus land does not have an independent or separate highest and best use and may or may not have additional value. The appraiser must ask:

- Is it economically feasible to expand the facility through additional bed capacity or additional common area?
- Can the building be expanded, replacing semi-private and ward patient rooms with private and/or semi-private rooms and adding revenue-producing functional space such as a larger therapy area with an outpatient component?

- Can an adult day care center or a specialty unit serving memory care, assisted living, sub-acute care, or other programs be added?

Certificate of need restrictions, Medicaid reimbursement, and competitive supply will govern the prospects of realizing additional value for surplus land. Note that if the surplus land has value, discounting that future value to present value needs to be considered since the opportunity to undertake the expansion may be years away.

Excess land is land that is not needed to support the use of the existing or probable future improvements.[1] Separating out the excess land should have minimal impact on the economic value of the nursing facility. Note that the sale of excess land may reduce the Medicaid capital basis and reimbursement and reduce property taxes.

If a condemnation calls for the partial taking of land and the lost land does not impact the access, visibility, or functionality of the site, and the taking does not impact the facility's census level, payor mix, rate level, or operating expenses, an effective argument can be made that the taking caused little or no difference in the value before and after the taking.

Improvements Description and Analysis

Nursing facility designs have evolved with the expansion of economic wealth, improved medical care, the increasing number of frail patients, competitive pressures from alternatives, and government reimbursements and regulations. Many facilities fail to meet patients' and families' expectations for privacy, comfort, and basic quality-of-life. These older facilities are becoming obsolete in markets where newer or renovated nursing facilities that offer greater privacy, therapy, and other quality-of-life design features are being developed.

Over the past 30 years, the typical nursing facility patient has become more frail. Prior to the creation of assisted living and home healthcare alternatives to nursing facilities, many patients were ambulatory at admission. Today, many of these ambulatory patients are choosing other alternatives. That leaves a higher percentage of nursing facility patients who are more frail or dependent on wheelchairs, which require different building designs. Patient needs and the use of physical, occupational, and speech therapies have increased substantially over the years, and these services have become a major source of profits. Rehabilitation patients are often younger and their lengths of stay

1. James H. Boykin, MAI, *Land Valuation: Adjustment Procedures and Assignments* (Chicago: Appraisal Institute, 2001), 238.

are much shorter as most will eventually return home after successful rehabilitation. To compete for these "profitable" patients, facilities are being developed or renovated to include separate rehab units, isolated from the long-term care patient areas.

The evolution of nursing facilities can be seen in statistics on gross building area per bed. The designs of many nursing facilities developed in the first decade of the Medicaid program (the 1960s) were influenced by states, which restricted capital reimbursements. Even today, Georgia continues to limit interest and depreciation payments to 280 square feet per bed. Some facilities compete with fewer than 225 square feet per bed. Over time, nursing facility building areas have increased to meet growing requirements for increased functional space coming from the Americans with Disability Act (ADA) and competitive market conditions. New nursing facility designs typically call for building areas with substantially more than 500 square feet per bed.

General Building Design Requirements and Construction Features

Each state develops minimum building specifications for licensed facilities that address the following general areas:

- Minimum construction standards
- Room sizes and dimensions
- Minimum areas for various functions and departments of the facility
- Minimum mechanical features, including heating, air-conditioning, ventilation, lighting, emergency lighting, and piping and plumbing fixtures
- Minimum fire and life safety requirements
- Distance from patient rooms to nurses' stations
- Bathing and toilet facilities

Skilled nursing facilities have four major function components:

1. Patient rooms
2. Nursing and therapy units
3. Common areas shared by residents
4. Support areas

Most nursing facility floor plans are based on building blocks that resemble letters of the alphabet.[2] Typical alphabet shapes

2. *Building Type Basics for Senior Living*, Perkins Eastman Architect, Stephen A. Kliment, 2004, page 121.

include A, B, C, E, F, H, I, L, P, T, U, V, W, and X. These building blocks account for most of the four functional components. Patient room areas are typically situated in peripheral areas, while common and support areas are concentrated closer to the building core.

Patient Areas

Patient areas include patient bedrooms, bathrooms, central bathing areas, and patient wing corridors. Newer nursing facilities are being developed with larger room sizes and more private rooms and toilets. Figure 8.1 depicts a typical patient or nursing unit, including patient rooms, circulation areas or corridors, and nurses' station, with adequate function design. The illustration is not to scale.

Patient Rooms

Patient rooms are the building blocks of a nursing facility. Most codes require a minimum size of 100 square feet for a semi-private room (two-beds) and 80 square feet for a private room, excluding toilet and storage space. To be fully wheelchair accessible, a room cannot be much smaller than 12 ft. x 12 ft., or 144 square feet. Room furnishings include hospital-type beds, chairs, night tables, wardrobes, privacy curtains, and closets. Patient rooms must have windows to the outside and privacy curtains between beds. A nurse call button or pull cord must be next to each bed and toilet.

While most facilities are designed with a high concentration of semi-private (two-bed) rooms, codes in many states still permit up to four beds per room. Rooms with three or more beds are referred to as *wards*. Wards are undesirable in most markets and are difficult to sell to private-pay patients. In those cases, wards may be functionally obsolete. More and more nursing facilities are being developed with increasing percentages of private rooms, as the patient-pay and Medicare markets are coming to expect these arrangements. Assessing the competiveness of nursing facilities should include an examination of the amount of each facility's mix of private, semi-private, and ward rooms. A nursing home will typically provide all necessary furniture, but a patient may be allowed to bring personal furnishings, subject to safety and facility policies. Most patients keep few personal possessions in their rooms other than items of clothing, books, small personal items, and photographs. Patient storage space is very limited, comparable to the amount of space found in a typical hotel room. Facilities must provide rooms that can be used for the isolation of residents with communicable diseases.

The photographs on page 93 shows some features of typical patient rooms.

Figure 8.1 **Typical Patient Area**

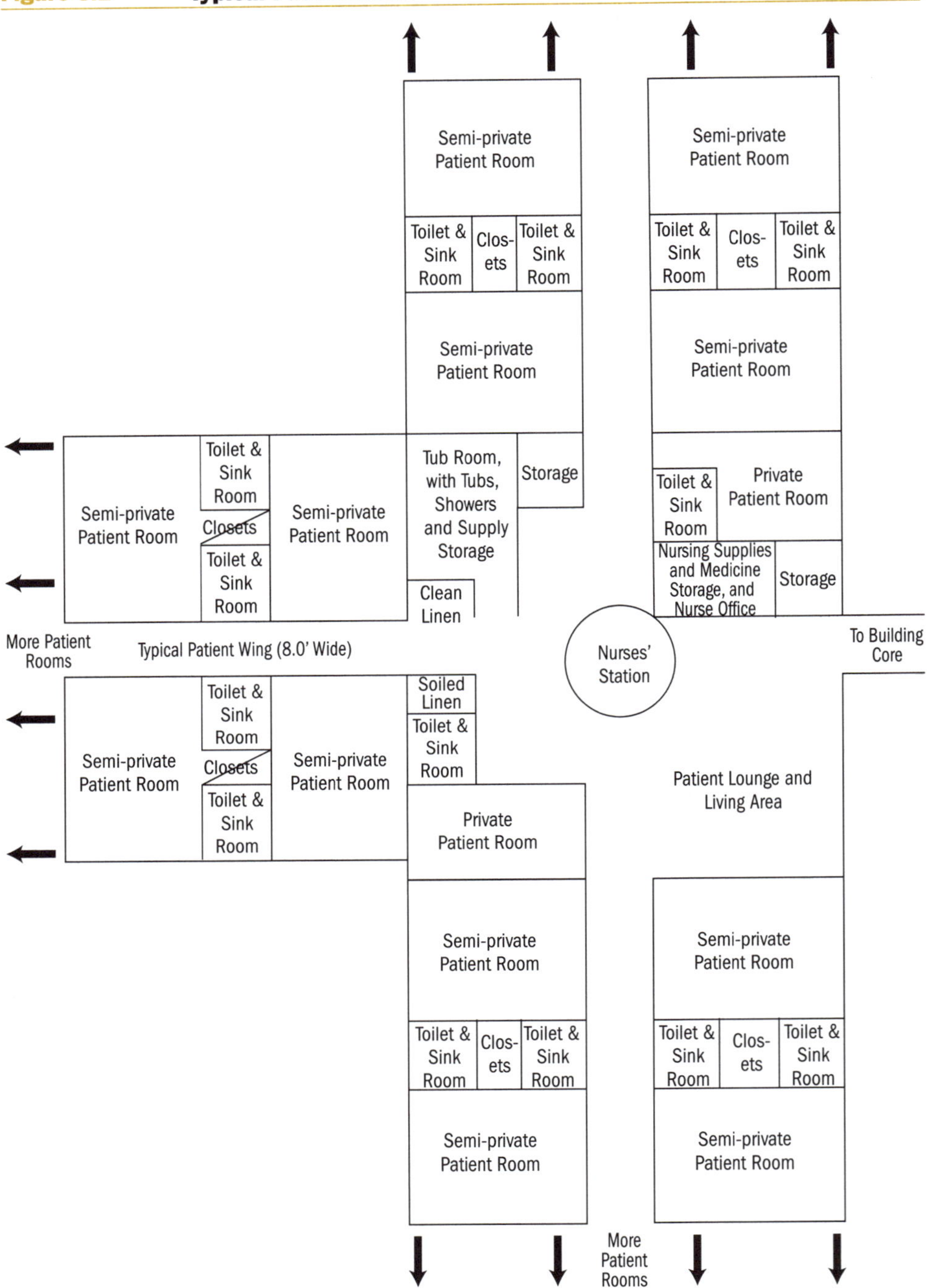

Source: Tellatin, Short, Hansen & Clark, Inc.

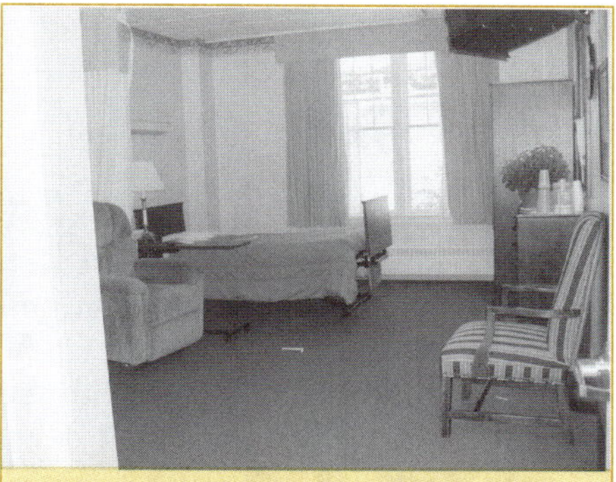

Private patient room in high-end facility with sitting area, carpeted floors, and attractive drapery

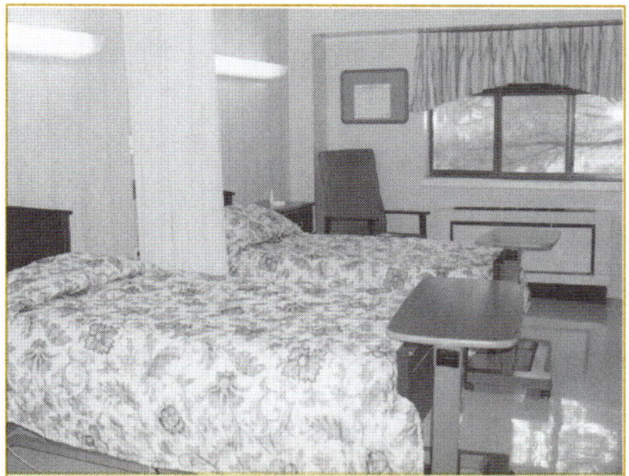

Typical semi-private patient room with side-by-side bed arrangement, vinyl tile floor finish, wall-mounted fluorescent lighting fixtures over the beds, minimal window treatment, vinyl wall coverings, little space for sitting and visitors, and privacy curtain between beds.

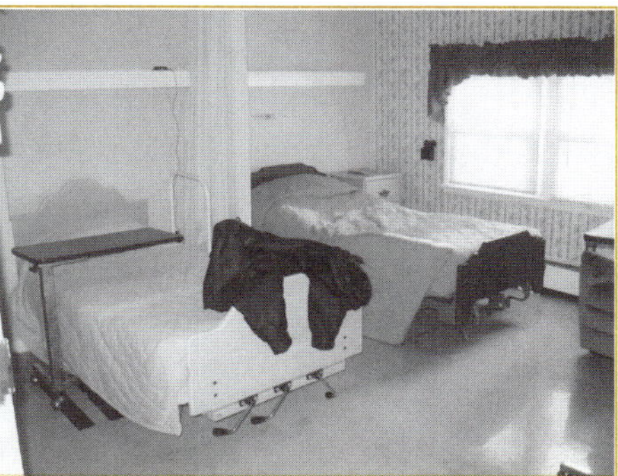

Typical semi-private patient room, with side-by-side bed arrangement, vinyl tile floor finish, wall-mounted fluorescent lighting fixtures, minimal window coverings, little space for sitting and visitors, and privacy curtain between beds. Note differences in beds.

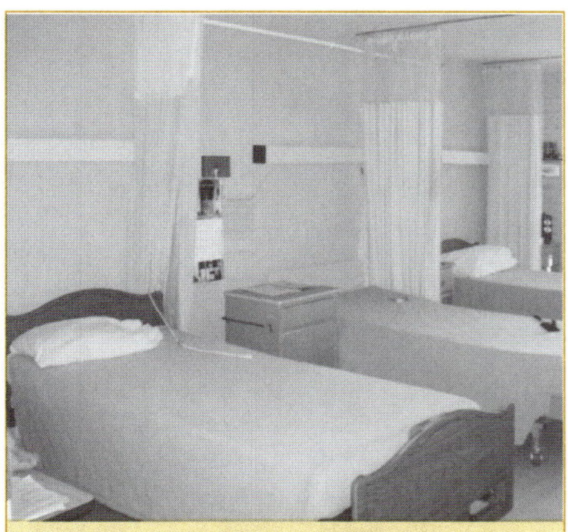

Typical three-bed patient room with side-by-side bed arrangement, vinyl tile floor finish, wall-mounted fluorescent lighting fixtures, minimal window coverings, little space for sitting and visitors, and privacy curtain between beds. Note differences in beds.

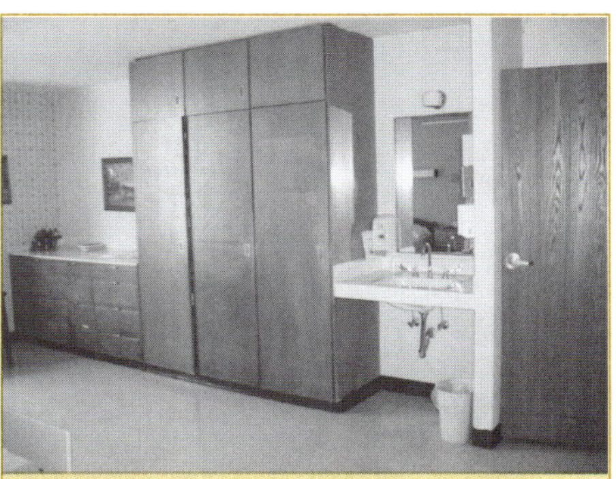

The same three-bed ward, showing the partition on the opposite wall with a wall wardrobe (center), matching lower chest of drawers, and an in-room sink (wheelchair accessible).

Patient Room Lavatories and Toilets (Wash Closets)

Lavatories are typically adjacent to patient rooms and often are shared by two rooms (semi-private). The market prefers private to semi-private or adjoining lavatories for obvious reasons. Some very old facilities may have patient rooms that have no adjoining toilets, requiring the patients to transfer through the corridor to use the lavatory or use a bed pan or portable toilet. This arrangement is considered functionally obsolete in most markets and may violate existing codes. Toilets should have wall-mounted grab bars and adequate room for wheelchair accessibility. Not all wash closets will be 100% handicapped accessible; however, a facility must have lavatories and toilets accessible to the handicapped in convenient locations. Older facilities will often have deficiencies in this area. Reviewing licensure surveys is helpful in assessing code compliance. Some lenders and FHA-insured mortgages will mandate that lavatories are upgraded to comply with current standards as part of the financing.

Private tubs and showers are typically not included in the patient rooms and are instead contained in central tub and shower areas, where the nursing staff has greater mobility in assisting with bathing. Individual room tubs are typically considered excessive functional obsolescence. Many patients are too frail to bath themselves and standard tubs and showers are too small to allow for staff assistance. Some higher-end facilities may include showers in the patient's bathrooms, but it is more a marketing feature than a functional feature. Newer construction designed to target shorter-term rehabilitation patients will include showers in patient rooms as these patients may be capable of self bathing. In some recently developed high-end facilities targeting only short-term rehabilitation patients, patient rooms are private and include a small "tea kitchen," a full bathroom, and more area for visitors. The degree of obsolescence found in a facility relates to the competitive market.

The photographs presented on the next page are representative of typical patient room lavatories and toilets.

Common Bathing Facilities

Nursing facility patients typically require staff assistance for bathing. Patient bathing is typically conducted in centralized tub and shower rooms located along patient room corridors. Tubs should be placed in a way that allows staff access to the patient at both sides and at the front of the tub. Special patient lifting equipment is often used to limit staff injuries and worker's compensation claims. Showers must be large enough for staff to

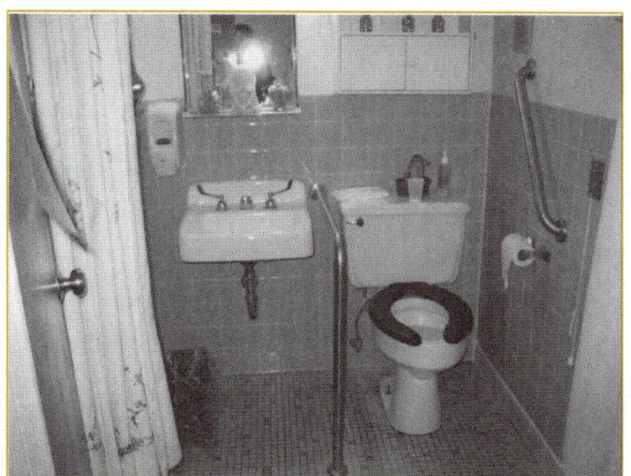

Typical toilet room located between two patient rooms contains a toilet (note grab bars) and a sink. The room is not handicapped accessible. Note ceramic tile floor and wall finishes. Many rooms have vinyl floor covers and drywall

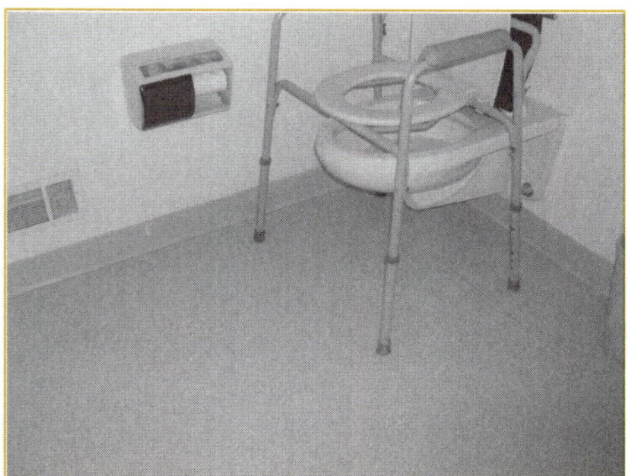

Typical toilet room serving a single patient room. This room is handicapped accessible, as evidenced by the larger floor area dimensions, and has vinyl floor covers and drywall wall finishes. The toilet is wall mounted to allow for easier housekeeping. In this case, the sink is situated in the patient room.

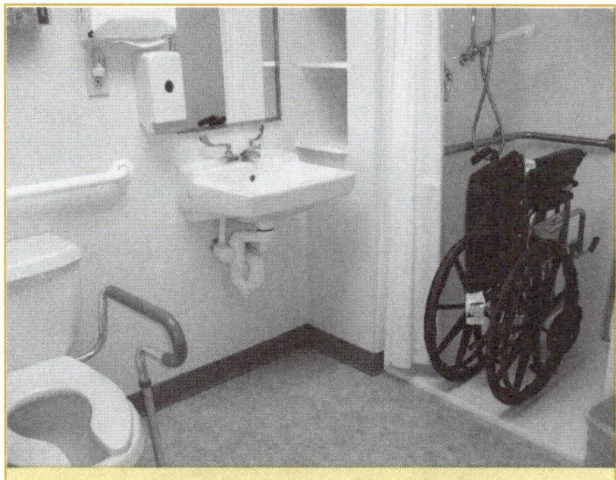

This patient room toilet also contains a sink and shower. This room is handicapped accessible and has vinyl floor covers and drywall wall finishes. The shower can be accessed from a wheelchair and has a flexible shower head. Note that showers in patient rooms are not often used for their designed intent because the patients are typically bathed in larger, common tub and shower rooms which provide staff more room to access the patient. Showers and tubs in patient rooms tend to become temporary storage areas.

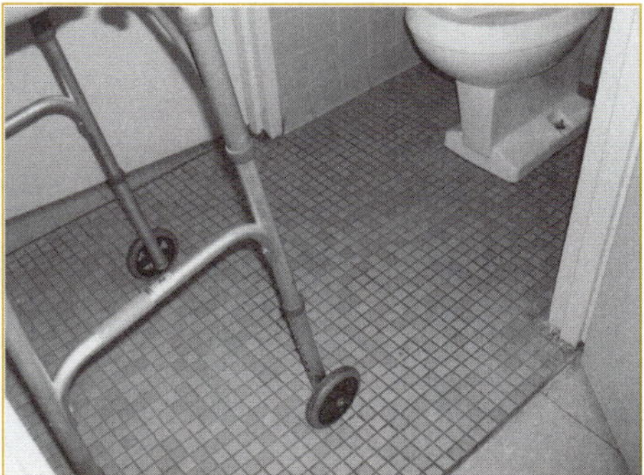

Typical toilet room located between two patient rooms. This room contains only a toilet and is not handicapped accessible. Note the ceramic tile floor and wall finishes, typical of 1960s construction. This toilet area is typical of older, lower-quality facilities that will be difficult to market to Medicare and private-pay markets.

bathe wheelchair patients. Centralized bathing facilities should have fixed partitions or fire-resistant curtains to provide a private compartment for each water closet, bathtub, and shower. Floor finishes typically include non-slip ceramic tile or sheet vinyl.

Corridors and Doors

Corridors are the backbone of patient areas and they receive heavy patient and staff traffic. Areas served from the corridors in the nursing units include patient rooms, clean and dirty utility rooms, clean and soiled laundry rooms, central bathing facilities, and nurses' stations. Other areas located in the nursing units may include day rooms, offices, activity areas, and dining areas. Representative photographs of patient wing corridors are shown on the next page.

Current standards require that corridors in patient areas have minimum widths of eight feet and be wider at elevators and other points of traffic concentration. Corridors in areas frequented by patients should have handrails along all walls. Doors to patient rooms and other areas that will remain open for long periods should open inward so as not to obstruct patient, staff, and equipment traffic. Many older nursing homes have narrow corridors, which may be nonconforming, but allowed under grandfather rules. Medicare and skilled certifications may be denied to patient rooms located off narrow corridors. Doors that patients pass through should be at least 44 inches wide, except for doors to bathing and toilet areas, which may be narrower. Doors between rooms and required corridors should be fire-rated, solid-core wood or metal doors.

Nursing and Therapy Units

Nurses' Stations

For obvious reasons, nurses' stations are the heart of a nursing facility. Each nursing unit should have a centrally located work station for the nursing staff with a work counter and storage space for patient charts. The station should be placed so that the nursing staff has unobstructed views down all patient corridors. Each state specifies the maximum distance between patient room doors and the nurses' station, usually 120 to 150 feet. A medicine preparation room and locked medicine room should be adjacent to each nurses' station. A private patient examination room is typically included in newer facility designs and located near the nurses' station. Each nursing unit must have a clean utility room and a dirty utility room that is directly accessible from a corridor of the nursing unit and is equipped with sinks. The nurses' station area should contain:

- Work counter
- Private office for the director of nursing
- Lavatory
- Medicine refrigerator
- Cabinets
- Locked medicine cabinet
- Provisions for proper temperature control

The maximum number of beds that a nursing unit may serve varies by state, but it is typically no more than 60 beds (restricted to a single floor). The optimum number of beds per nurses' sta-

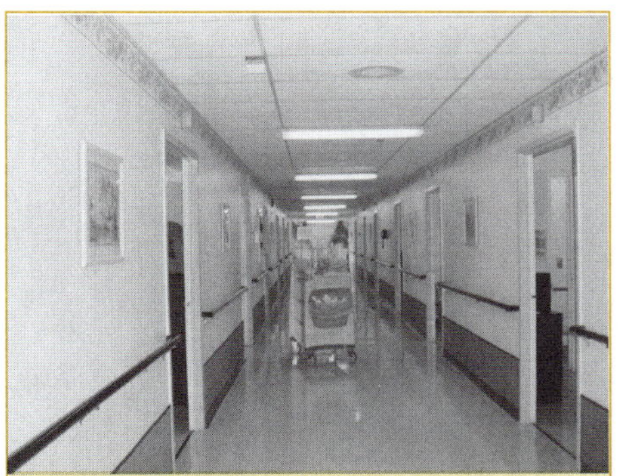

Typical corridor in a newer facility. Note the 8-ft. width (counting the 12-in. vinyl floor tiles and 2-ft. x 4-ft. ceiling tiles to measure). This corridor has an institutional look with a long, straight design, simple fluorescent lighting fixtures mounted below the suspended ceiling tiles, patient room doors flush with the corridor partitions, limited wall decoration, and simple handrails.

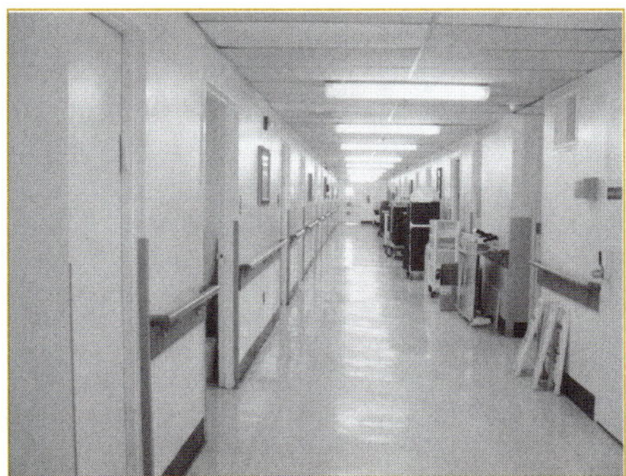

Typical corridor in an older building. Note 8-ft. width (counting the 12-in. vinyl floor tiles and 2-ft. x 4-ft. ceiling tiles to measure). This corridor also features an institutional look. The number of carts and other large objects in the corridor suggests that the facility lacks storage areas.

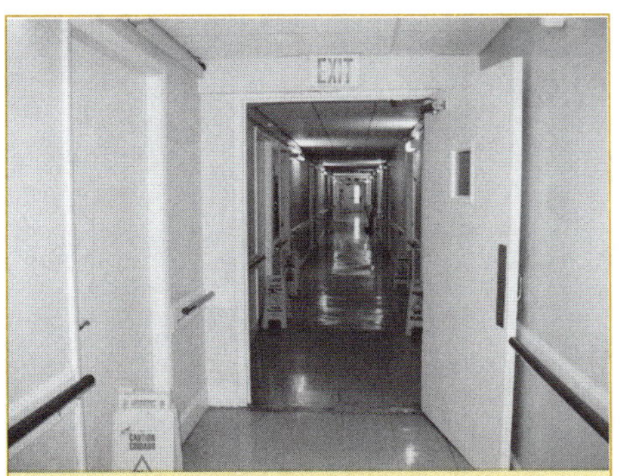

Corridor with 6-ft. width, which is substandard. Note the fire door below the exit sign and consider how difficult a rapid evacuation would be with such a narrow passage. Many states will no longer license beds in rooms accessed through narrow corridors.

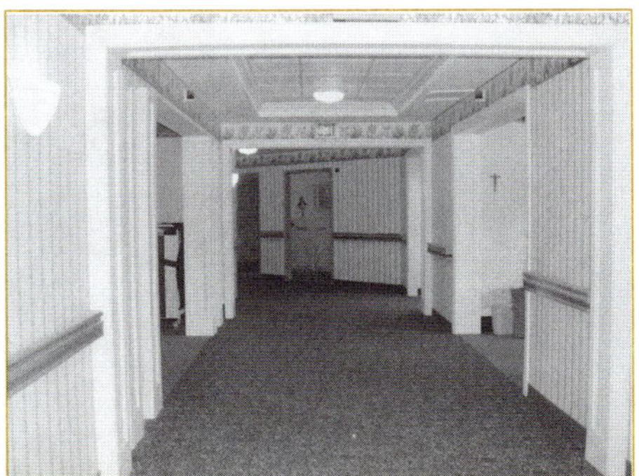

Corridor in a newer, high-end facility, with carpeted floor, vinyl wall coverings, incandescent wall- and ceiling-mounted lighting fixtures, and a mixed ceiling of finish drywall and recessed suspended tiles. Note the absence of equipment in the corridor.

tion may vary with minimum nursing-staff ratios imposed by the operator or state regulations. A day staffing-to-bed ratio of 1:7–i.e., one certified nurse assistant (CNA) for every seven occupied beds–may be the norm for a 7:00 am to 3:00 pm day shift. The evening shift may be reduced to a 1:10 or 1:11 ratio, and the night shift might be further reduced to 1:15. With these staffing ratios, a 60-bed unit with 90% occupancy could staff the day shift with eight CNAs, five or six CNAs in the evening, and three or four CNAs during the night. This staffing ratio will provide each patient with roughly 2.5 hours of CNA care daily; staffing is discussed further in Chapter 13, Operating Expense Analysis.

The following photographs depict a variety of older and newer nurses' stations.

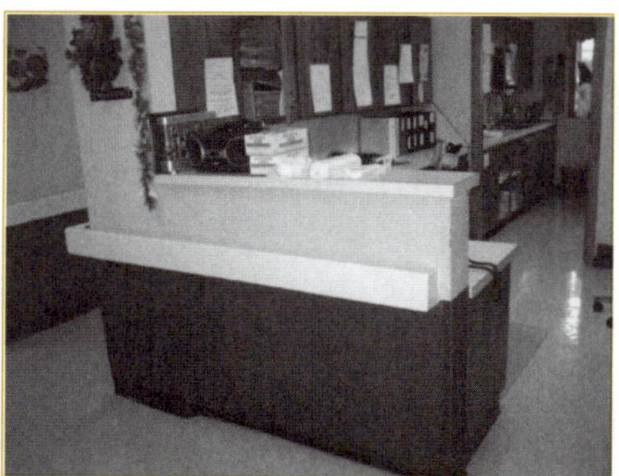

A nurses' station typical of an older facility with a high countertop. The door is open to a medicine room in the upper right corner of the photograph.

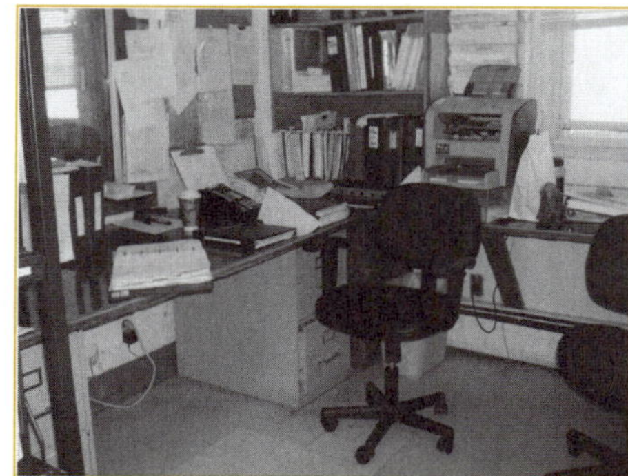

Nurses' station in an older (circa 1965) facility without significant renovation. This nurses' station lacks direct lines of sight down all patient room corridors.

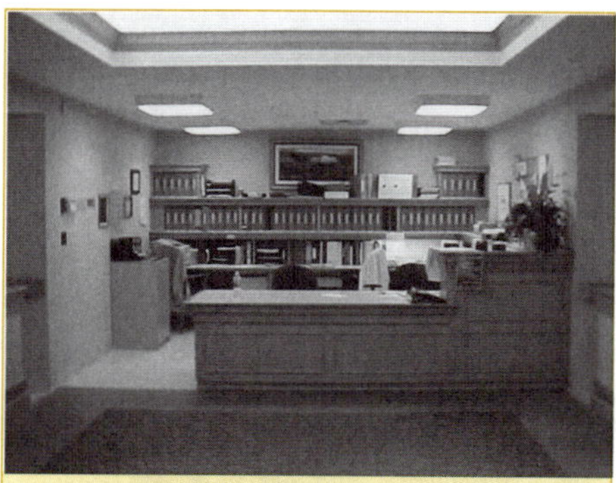

Nurses' station in a newer facility (circa 2005) with a lower countertop, visible to patients in wheelchairs, and an attractive patient records library.

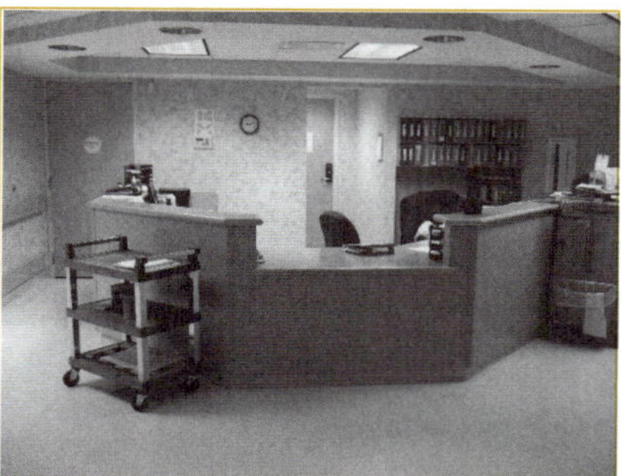

Nurses' station in newer facility (circa 2000) with medical storage and nursing office behind desk area, low countertop, and clean patient records storage area.

Therapy Areas

With the increase in Medicare coverage for nursing facility services beginning in 1989 and policies that favor discharging patients earlier from hospitals into lower-cost settings for recovery and rehabilitation, nursing facilities now require more space for physical and occupational therapy. Under current Medicare and managed care payment levels, rehab patients are highly profitable and competition for these patients can be very intense. Since most facilities compete aggressively for Medicare and managed care patients, who typically require therapy services, a large, well-equipped therapy area is very important.

An increasing number of facilities are being designed with separate entrances to designated parking areas for outpatient therapy patients. Facilities built before 1990 typically have limited, purpose-built therapy space, since Medicare benefits were once very limited for patients requiring skilled nursing and rehabilitation care. Some of these older facilities have added therapy areas by converting patient rooms or have expanded the building area to include a successful therapy unit. Therapy areas can be anywhere within the building and often are housed in lower levels or away from high-traffic areas. However, newer building designs tend to place therapy areas in prominent locations to promote a "rehabilitation" image. The therapy area should have a "gym-like" space with a privacy curtain for physical therapy. Ideally, it should also have a separate occupational therapy area (maybe in a separate room), which is a home-like setting that includes a domestic kitchen, bathroom, and furniture. Other separate areas for speech therapy and offices are also desirable. Many older facilities need to combine all the therapy functions into a single room due to lack of space, which often puts that facility at a competitive disadvantage in the market.

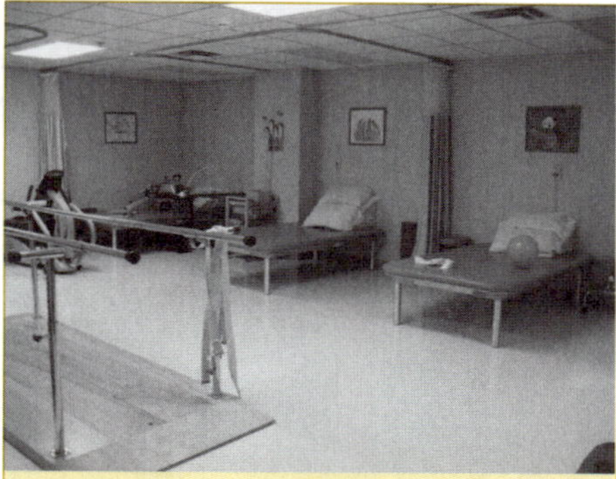

A typical, purpose-built physical therapy room, with adequate space and privacy curtains between the rehab tables.

Commons Areas Shared by Residents

Commons areas that are shared by all the patients typically include:

- Dining areas
- Day rooms
- Living rooms
- Recreational and activity rooms
- Personal care rooms (beauty shops–often contracted to an outside vendor)
- Smoking rooms
- Worship rooms

Dining experiences are important for patients and positive experiences are created with attractive settings, good service, and high-quality food. Older facilities tend to have a large central dining area or hall that may function as a multi-purpose room, offering one or two seatings and meals served on trays. Newer, upscale facilities tend to offer decentralized, smaller dining areas. Many facilities, especially newer ones, will incorporate a snack area, allowing patients limited or unlimited access to coffee, tea, small bakery items, and even ice cream. Such facilities often include private dining rooms for special occasions, parties, and family events. Dining areas often are featured in the center of a facility, merging various nursing units and creating a spacious atmosphere for visitors who do not travel beyond the common areas of the facility.

Day rooms are typically found in the middle or at the end of long patient wings and provide patients and visitors with informal sitting areas and tables for social activities. Living rooms typically are centralized, larger areas that may also be located near nurses' stations and should provide space for small group events, discussion groups, musical and other live entertainment, and TV and video watching. Small, newer facilities will have a theater room with newer video and audio equipment to provide a cinema-like experience; some facilities equip the entertainment area with a popcorn machine. Living rooms may include fireplaces, bookcases, and other home-like finishes.

Recreational activities, arts and crafts, libraries, and worship rooms are important areas for patients, their visitors, and staff. These areas tend to be centralized within a single-story facility or located on the main floor or a lower level of a multi-level building. Religion-sponsored facilities tend to place a worship area prominently within the facility. Such an area may become obsolete if the ownership changes and the religious component is de-emphasized. As new generations of patients enter nursing facilities, many facilities are adding or increasing access to computers in common areas, often locating this equipment in a library or day room. Recreational and activity areas are generally larger, open rooms where patients can assemble to share in programmed group activities, socialization, and therapies.

Nursing facilities almost always have a beauty shop to provide on-site personal grooming. These areas are typically a single room equipped with typical beauty and barber shop seating, counters, sinks, and cabinetry. These services are normally provided by outside, licensed professionals and patients must pay for them out of personal funds, as these services are not covered by Medicare, Medicaid, and private insurers. Depending on local and state laws concerning indoor smoking, facilities may provide a smoking area or room for patients and staff. Additional ventilation is important in these areas.

Representative photographs of common areas are shown on the next page.

Support Areas

Support areas include functional space for administrative, dietary, housekeeping, laundry, and plant operations. The administrative areas are often situated in the front portion of the building, near the main entrance, while the other support areas are found in the rear, at the side, or in the lower level, away from patient areas but accessible for shipping and deliveries.

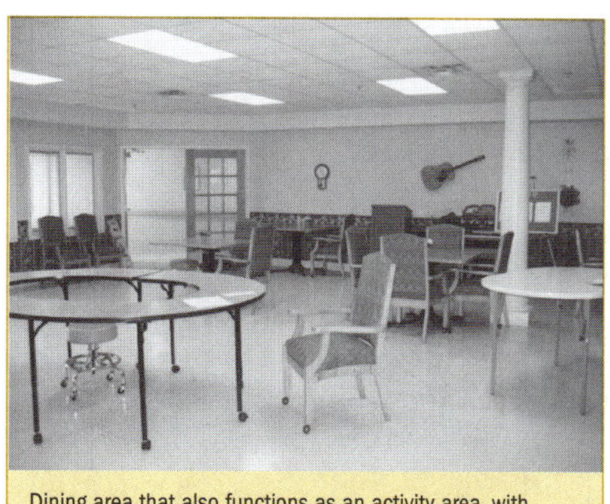
Dining area that also functions as an activity area, with simple features such as vinyl tile floors and suspended acoustical tile ceilings with recessed fluorescence lighting fixtures. Minimal and mixed furniture is provided.

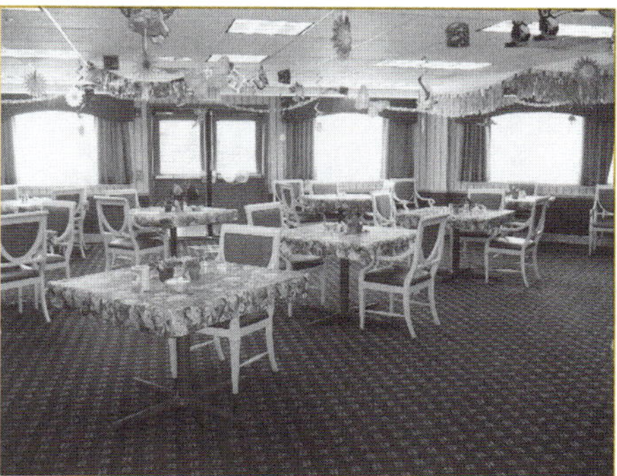
Dining room of a newer facility, featuring carpeted floors, matching furniture, and window treatments.

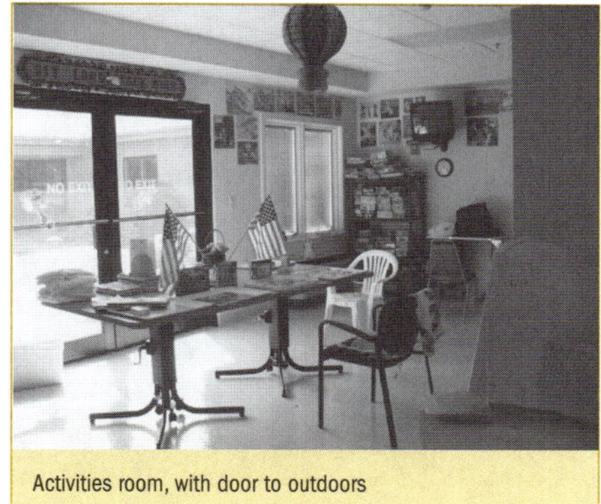
Activities room, with door to outdoors

Administrative Offices

Business offices, the administrator's office, and other office areas that house the accounting, marketing, social services, and administrative functions of the facility are typically clustered together in a suite-like arrangement. These areas are usually located near the main entrance of the facility to minimize traffic and activity in patient areas. Added traffic tends to confuse patients, is disruptive to the nursing staff, and increases the patients' risk of infection.

Construction in office areas is similar in quality and material to that of commercially leased general office space. Older nursing facilities tend to lack adequate administrative areas and often use a patient room or two for office space. This is not desirable since the rooms may be too large, include unnecessary closet and lavatory areas, and be located in patient areas away from other administrative areas.

Additional office-like space devoted to other departments can include in-service training rooms used to train nurse aides and conference rooms for staff meetings, family conferences, and other group functions

Main Lobby Area

The main entrance provides the first interior impression of the facility to the public, visitors, prospective patients, and their families. Located inside the front entry, this area will include a lobby, a waiting room, public toilet facilities, and public telephones. Newer facilities, designed to compete for private-pay patients, tend to enlarge these areas and include high-quality decorating. Construction is often similar to limited-service hotels. Older facilities were often built with little or no lobby and waiting room space. Some combined the lobby space with space used for other functions or with meeting areas where patients congregate near the front door. Newer designs attempt to minimize patient assembly near the front door as this makes a poor first impression on the general public and reduces the privacy of the patients.

Dietary Areas

The dietary area is a functional space that includes a large food preparation area, a dishwashing room, food storage areas, and a dietitian's office. For practical purposes, the dining area is adjacent to the kitchen. Kitchens typically are located on the side or at the rear of the facility to allow easy and quick food delivery.

The food preparation area is a large, institutional area with mostly stainless steel equipment, such as preparation tables, food rinsing sinks (with two or three compartments), washing sinks for pots and pans (typically three compartments), ovens, grills, ranges, exhaust hoods, toasters, mixers, blenders, convection ovens, microwave ovens, extensive refrigeration and freezer space (often walk-in units), serving tables, and other features. For sanitary reasons, dishwashing functions should be performed in a separate area of the kitchen or, better yet, in a separate room. Soiled dishes and utensils are processed from a receiving counter through a scraping area with a garbage disposal, pre-rinse sink, dish-racking counter, dishwasher, clean dish counter, and dish rack storage. The dietitian's office should be located in an area adjacent to the food preparation and storage areas.

Because of high demand for electricity and plumbing, kitchens, laundry rooms, and areas housing HVAC equipment are typically concentrated in a service wing to minimize costly distribution conduits.

Laundry Areas

Laundry functions are usually housed near housekeeping and maintenance areas. While this function may be near the dietary area, the space for these two functions should not overlap for hygiene reasons. Laundry facilities may be absent in some older facilities because outside vendors were once considered desirable. When facilities are dependent on outside contractors for this vital service, however, they have less control of the quality of the service. Older facilities in Texas and other states with warm climates used to encourage laundry functions to be housed in separate, onsite buildings. Laundry units in newer facilities must contain separate areas for soiled and clean laundry for sanitary purposes, with all laundry entering through the soiled room and laterally processed through the washers, dryers, and storage areas. Laundry equipment will typically include commercial-grade washers and dryers

Housekeeping and Maintenance Areas

Housekeeping and maintenance functions require the least permanent area in the building and are often housed in the least costly, most inconspicuous space–basements or unfinished space near mechanical rooms. Storage areas also are required for the warehousing of unused equipment, furniture, and personal items of patients. Most facilities have a great need for storage and lower-quality buildings, garages, or sheds are frequently used for additional storage. Employee break rooms are typically situated near the back-of-the-house functional space and near a rear entrance used by employees entering and leaving work, where the time clock is typically placed.

Mechanical Areas

Mechanical areas house heating and air-conditioning equipment (furnaces, boilers, chillers, and compressors), electrical distribution panels, indoor emergency generators, sprinkler valves, telephone equipment, hot water heaters, water softeners, and other equipment.

Figure 8.2 shows the layout of the core area of a typical nursing facility with adequate function design. The illustration is not to scale. Photos of support areas appear on page 105.

Exterior Features

The front elevation of the building will typically feature the main entrance and some surface parking. Other parking areas located along the sides or to the rear of the building are typically devoted to staff parking. The main entrance will often include a porte cochere. Newer facilities will typically include two sets of electric sliding entry doors to facilitate handicapped entry and energy efficiency. All patient rooms will contain at least one exterior window. Exterior evacuation doors are located at the terminus of each ground-level corridor. Unless the door is in an area with a secured perimeter, these exit doors are typically electronically locked to prevent patients from leaving the building, which is

Figure 8.2 **Typical Core Area**

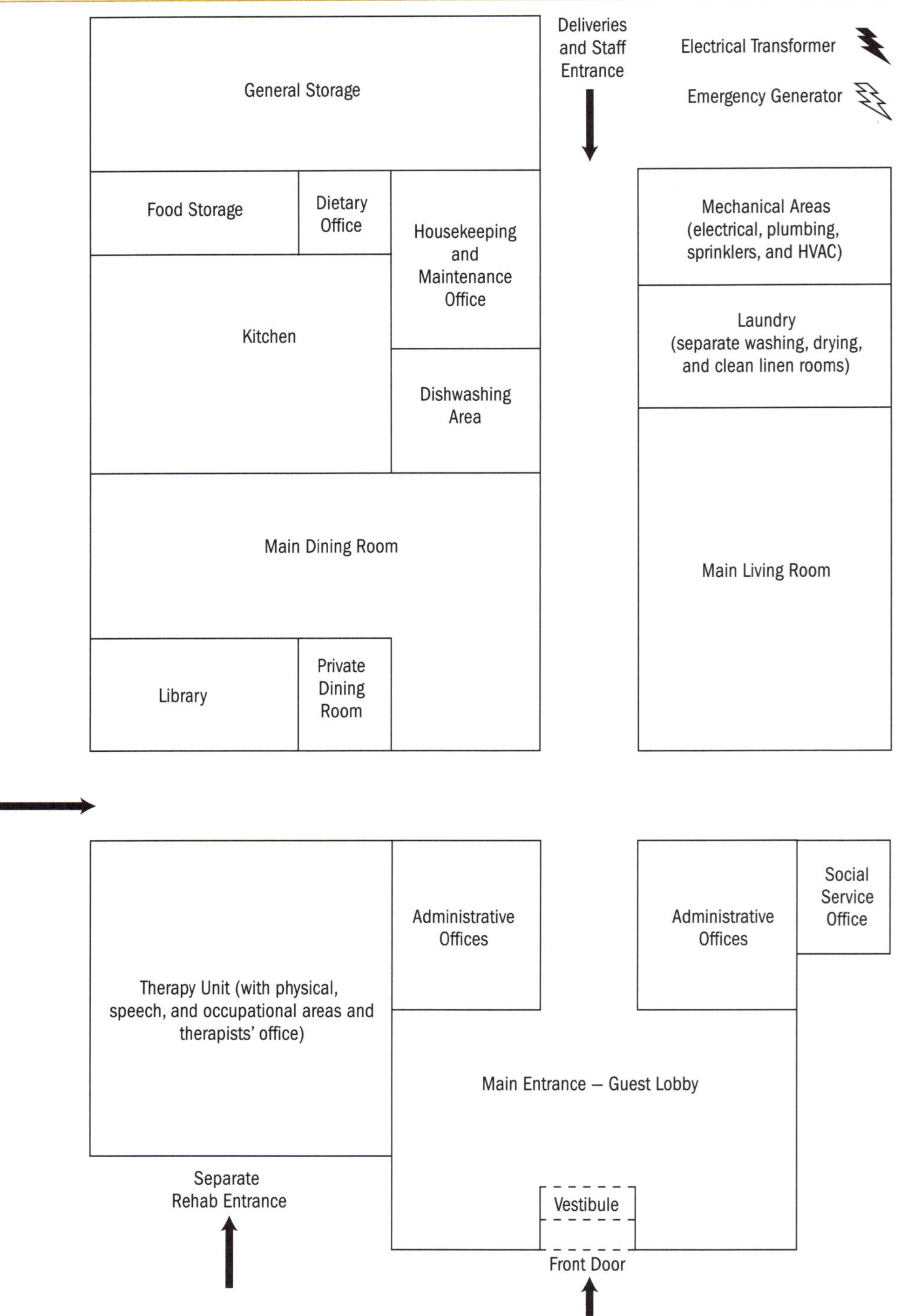

Source: Tellatin, Short, Hansen & Clark, Inc.

Drawing is not to scale

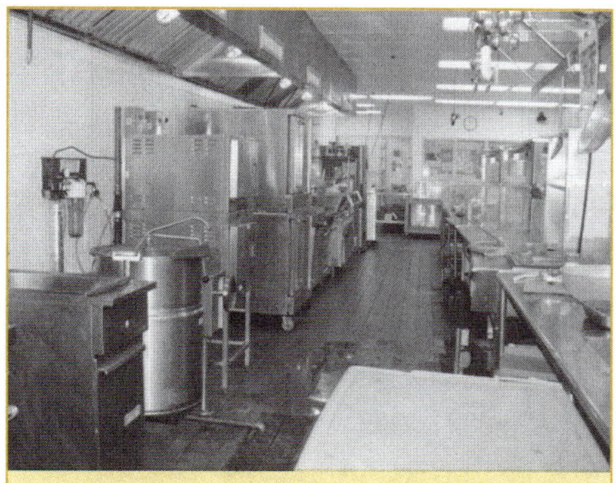
Typical kitchen features stainless steel equipment and quarry tile floor.

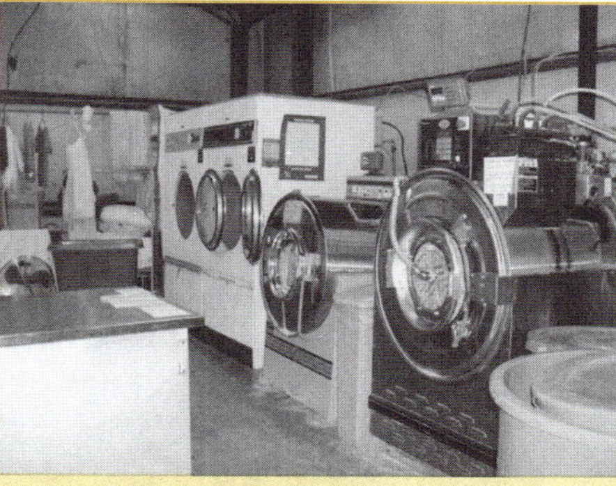
Laundry room with washers and dryers in the same room side by side. This arrangement is not acceptable in many states because of possible contamination from mixing clean and soiled linen.

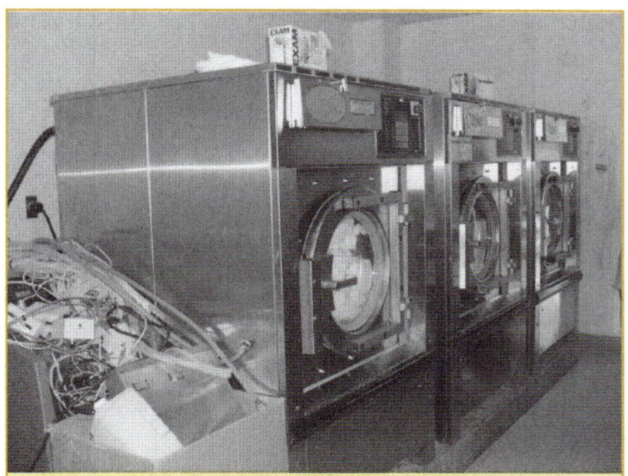
Laundry room with only washing units; dryers located in separate room. The washer room has negative air pressure, so air leaves the building through this room, drawing fumes outside the building.

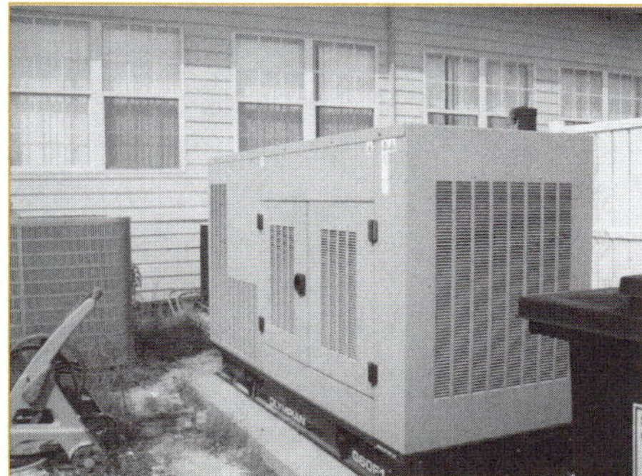
Emergency generators are usually located outdoors to reduce noise and air pollution indoors. In this case, the generators is situated just beyond the patient room windows.

referred to as *eloping*. Facilities that have memory care units or patients who wander often install surveillance cameras at exterior doors that are monitored and record activity. Landscaped courtyards, terraces, and patios are important outdoor features. Local climate, terrain, soil and other topographical factors will dictate landscaping features. Lawn furniture, gazebos, fountains, raised planting beds, and amenities for outdoor activities improve the quality of life for patients.

Most facilities will have a delivery door and a driveway at the rear of the building, adjacent to back-of-the-house functions (kitchen, mechanical, etc.). Emergency generators, trash dumpsters, electrical transformers, large air-conditioning equipment (cooling towers), lawn-maintenance equipment sheds, and other exterior components needed to support facility operations are typically located to the rear of the building, away from public view. Some facilities still rely on well water and their own sewage treatment systems. If this is the case, the appraiser should investigate the systems' compliance with current and known future regulations.

Special Construction Characteristics

Nursing facilities may require special building materials for the safety and well being of patients. Floors should be covered with finishes that can be cleaned and sanitized regularly. Carpeted floors should be confined to patient areas where incontinence occurs infrequently. Ventilation should draw clean air in through corridors and patient rooms and out through areas that can contain contaminated air such as soiled work areas, therapy rooms, tub and toilet rooms, janitor closets, and food preparation areas. Emergency lighting must be provided for exits, stairs, and patient corridors to facilitate emergency evacuations. Most facilities satisfy this requirement with an emergency generator capable of supplying power for other electrical needs as well. However, some states will accept battery lighting through a grandfather exemption. Elevators are required in facilities that have multiple levels that patients might have reason to enter. Elevators are not required for access to basements and penthouses that patients do not visit.

Life Safety Systems

Nursing facilities should be equipped with a sprinkler system, smoke detectors, heat detectors, fire extinguishers, pull stations, public address systems, and exit signs. Building inspection reports, local health and fire code inspection reports, and state licensure survey reports should be referenced to determine compliance. The facility's plant supervisor and/or administrator should have that information on file and the appraiser should request it early on.

Trends in New Design and Construction

To remain competitive, nursing facility designs are increasingly including larger room sizes, more function space, increased privacy, and a host of upgrades to interior finishes and mechanical systems. Some new design trends include:

- More private rooms or provisions for greater privacy in semi-private rooms
- Greater amounts of space for storing personal items in patient rooms
- Showers in patient room bathrooms
- Smaller, cluster-like patient wing units with separate, smaller dining, activity, and program areas
- Decentralized nursing staff–departing from the tradition of other-side-of-the counter nurses' stations

- Spa-like bath rooms
- Residential-type finishes vs. hospital-like appearance
- Specialty units for dementia, hospice, short-term rehab, and ventilator patients

Physical and Functional Assessment

Nursing facilities experience very high levels of wear and tear on interior finishes and mechanical systems because the buildings are open and doing business 24 hours a day. The area-to-occupancy ratio can easily be less than 200 square feet per occupant. This heavy use places intense demands on short-lived building components.

A critical review of the interior finishes (floor and wall coverings, lighting fixtures, doors, cabinetry, closets, and ceilings), and mechanical systems (heating and air conditioning equipment, fire alarms, communication systems, and life safety features such as sprinklers and emergency generators) should be conducted to determine current and future capital replacement costs as well as the facility's competitive position in the market.

The economic life of a nursing facility is generally considered to be 45 to 60 years. Facility life can be extended through substantial capital improvement programs should the competitive market, reimbursement levels, and regulatory conditions permit. Some states' certificate of need policies and/or Medicaid reimbursement systems encourage extending the life of existing facilities. If a state has a moratorium on licensing new beds, then nursing home operators and the market must make the most out of the regulated supply by stretching the remaining economic life of what might otherwise be an obsolete physical plant. Some Medicaid reimbursement systems discourage new construction by limiting capital reimbursements to a small fraction of the actual interest, depreciation, and return on equity for the development costs.

Functional obsolescence takes many forms in a nursing facility, and much of the obsolescence stems from its competitive, operational, and regulatory environment. Major items of function obsolescence include, but certainly are not limited to, the conditions described below.

- Patient rooms with three or four beds (wards) are more difficult to fill. Eventually the market catches up to this condition and vacancy rates will increase to a point where beds are removed from these rooms to create more competitive, semi-private rooms. Since the rooms were designed for three or four beds, wall-mounted bed lighting, nurse call stations, wardrobe space, cubicle curtain tracks, and floor area (square footage) are rendered excessive. Aside from curing the condition by moving some fixtures around, the downsizing of wards to semi-private rooms causes a form of functional obsolescence due to superadequacy.

- Patient rooms without toilets adjacent to the bedroom or toilets shared by two rooms could be a marketing disadvantage in markets where private toilets are the norm. This functional deficiency could prove to be incurable.
- Corridors less than 8-ft. wide are often found in lower-cost buildings erected in the 1960s or earlier. The regulatory standard has been eight feet for many decades and some states seek to delicense beds that are off narrow corridors. This condition is an incurable functional obsolescence caused by a deficiency.
- Small areas for physical and occupational therapy prove to be clinical and marketing disadvantages; this functional deficiency may be curable or incurable. Many nursing facilities have attempted to cure the deficiency by decommissioning several patient rooms or other functional space and renovating that area for therapy services. If the lost beds still remain on the license, the occupancy forecast should be adjusted accordingly.
- The absence of fire-protection sprinklers throughout the building is a functional deficiency that should be curable. Federal law now requires that all nursing homes become fully sprinklered by 2013 or they lose their Medicare and Medicaid certification. This item of obsolescence is curable and caused by a deficiency.
- The lack of common areas and program space for patient, staff, and visitors is a common problem

Effective Age and Remaining Economic Life

The concepts and estimates of effective age and remaining economic life are important to the valuation of nursing facilities as these estimates impact depreciation calculations in the cost approach, price adjustments in comparable sales analysis, and capitalization rate selection. Lenders will often consider loan amortization periods based on the facility's remaining economic life. The largest insurer of nursing facility mortgages is the Federal Housing Administration (FHA) which, through the Department of Housing and Urban Development (HUD), limits amortization periods for their fully amortization loan programs to 75% of the remaining economic life.

The definitions presented in this section are important to an understanding of effective age and remaining economic life.

Effective age is the age indicated by the condition and utility of a structure and is based on an appraiser's judgment and interpretation of market perceptions.[3]

The effective age may be different from the chronological age. A reduced effective age is achieved by replacing short-lived components and possibly some long-lived components. An increased effective age is caused by neglecting to replace fully deteriorated building components.

Economic life is the period over which improvements to real property contribute to the property value.[4]

Remaining economic life is the estimated period over which existing improvements are expected to continue to contribute economically to property value.[5]

According to *Marshall Valuation Service*, the economic life expectancy for a nursing facility (or "convalescent hospital") is as follows.

Typical Life Expectancy for Nursing Facilities

	Class A	Class B	Class C	Class D
Good to excellent	50	50	45	40
Low cost to average	45	45	40	35

Source: *Marshall Valuation Service*, Section 97, page 8

Marshall Valuation Service suggests that the typical life will likely be extended by good maintenance and the replacement of short-lived building components, which is true or can be assumed for most nursing facilities. *Marshal Valuation Service* does not provide figures for economic life, only typical life.

Extended economic life is the increased life expectancy due to seasoning and proven ability to exist.[6]

Nursing facilities erected between 1965 and 1970, in the first wave of development after the creation of the Medicaid program, will be approaching the end of their expected economic lives by 2010 to 2020, according to *Marshall Valuation Service* figures. With good functional features (semi-private rooms with at least adjoining lavatories, 8 ft.-wide corridors, and sufficient therapy areas) and regular replacement of short-lived building components, the economic life of the facility may be extended indefinitely. (A short-lived component is a building component with an excepted remaining economic life that is shorter than the remaining economic life of the structure as a whole.)

3. *The Appraisal of Real Estate*, 13th ed. (Chicago: Appraisal Institute, 2008), 412.
4. Ibid., 413.
5. Ibid., 415.
6. *Marchall Valuation Service*, Section 97, page 1.

Economic life can be shortened through external obsolescence.

> *External obsolescence* may be caused by economic or location factors. It may be temporary or permanent, but it is not usually considerable curable on the part of the owner, landlord or tenant.[7]

In addition to the typical external forces that affect most real estate, the remaining economic lives of nursing facilities are impacted by regulatory issues and Medicaid and Medicare reimbursements. Certificate of need restrictions may prohibit or severely limit the development of new facilities and impede competition, thereby extending the usefulness of the existing market supply. In addition, inadequate capital reimbursements from Medicaid may prevent economically feasible development of new facilities, thus providing a safer competitive environment for older, outdated buildings. State and federal finances may necessitate policies that extend the useful lives of nursing facilities to control cost increases.

On the other hand, state Medicaid waiver policies that favor shifting nursing facility patients into assisted living facilities can adversely impact the remaining economic life of marginally competitive facilities. Oregon and Wisconsin have experienced considerable nursing facility closures as a result of expanded assisted living programs.

Considering these and other issues, estimating the remaining economic life of a nursing facility can be problematic. A clear, objective assessment of the physical plant, its functional features, the facility's position in the competitive environment, and regulatory policy and reimbursement issues must be made to arrive at a well-reasoned remaining economic life estimate. Because many mortgages are tied to remaining economic life, this assessment is critical.

Summary

The site area requirements for a nursing facility are dependent on land costs. The relationship between land costs and building design differ in urban, suburban, and rural settings. The site for a nursing facility will need to accommodate the footprint of the building, satisfy employee and visitor parking needs, provide for deliveries and strolling areas for patients and guests, and address water drainage and other environmental issues.

Most of the nation's existing nursing home inventory consists of buildings designed specifically for that use. The inventory of facilities adapted from buildings originally erected for other

---

7. Ibid.

purposes, such as hospitals or large residences, is shrinking as dysfunctional designs and features and elevated age render them obsolete. Nursing facility buildings must comply with many state and federal standards, over and above local codes. Design, function, life safety features, construction materials, and mechanical systems have evolved along with continued growth in economic wealth and the higher acuity needs of the typical patient. The four functional areas of nursing facilities are: patient rooms, nursing and therapy areas, common areas shared by the patients, and support areas.

Patient rooms are typically designed for double occupancy and either have a private wash closet or share one with an adjoining room. The trend in new designs is to provide more private rooms with private toilets and showers. Depending on the competitive supply in a specific market, rooms with three or more beds (wards) or rooms that lack adjoining wash closets may be significantly obsolete. Newer facilities tend to incorporate greater percentages of private patient rooms in order to compete effectively for profitable Medicare and private-pay patients.

Nursing facilities are open and conducting business every hour of every day and, as a result, the building finishes and mechanical systems deteriorate more rapidly than they would if those items were exposed to typical residential or commercial use. Due to changes in market preferences, increasing patient acuity levels, and continued code upgrading, nursing facilities have obsolescence from many causes. In many states where there are certificate of need policies limiting the development of new facilities, the remaining economic life of older facilities may be extended; the older properties remain competitive as a result of the tight, controlled supply.

Chapter 9

Competitive Market Analysis–Supply and Demand

In market analysis, the current and future competitive supply of and demand for nursing facility beds is studied to forecast the most probable census levels, payor mix, and rates for the subject property:

- *Census levels (occupancy)* refers to the number of patients in the facility at a given time; census is measured in patient days over time and sometimes referred to as the *level of utilization.*
- *Payor mix* refers to the ratio of patients paying for their routine services privately or through Medicare, Medicaid, or other insurance.
- *Rates* refers to daily payments for routine services, which are reference points for the revenue forecast.

Estimated changes in supply and demand in the competitive market over a reasonable forecast period can be processed through a series of calculations to project future occupancy, mix, and rates for the subject.

Defining the Competitive Market

A competitive analysis begins by defining the competitive market area and primary and secondary competitive facilities. The competitive market area definition will vary with type of service (rehab, long-term care, or memory care), population density, distances, political and physical boundaries, and socioeconomic characteristics. The competitive market area is typically defined geographically. Patient origin data can be used to define the market area when such information is gathered and maintained by the management of the facility or through a state agency. At a minimum, the analyst should discuss patient origin with the management of the subject facility.

The market area may be different for Medicare and Medicaid patients. Generally, the market area of an urban or suburban facility should include the geographical area between the subject and the closest primary competitors in all directions. Often the market area will include only a portion of the city, county, or metropolitan area and may cross municipal and county boundaries. A rural facility's market area may include only other facilities in the same town (if any) plus the area halfway between the subject and the next closest facilities in every important direction. In rural areas, the entire county may constitute the primary market area if each surrounding county has only one or a few facilities. Market areas are often limited by state boundaries (because of Medicaid) and significant natural barriers.

Generally, area facilities can be identified as primary or secondary competition based on objective measurements such as occupancy and payor mix similarities, facility age, location qualities (based on demographic data), and health survey deficiencies, as well as subjective characteristics relating to the physical plant, location, and reputation.

Identifying primary and secondary competition within the defined geographic market area involves matching the major competitive qualities of the subject to the other facilities. Newer, high-end facilities with substantial Medicare and private-pay census may not compete with older facilities with substantial Medicaid census when there are other high-end facilities in the market. Similarly, a full-service Marriott hotel may not be competitive with a Super 8 motel even though they may be located within a few blocks of each other. Generally, occupancy levels and quality-mix figures provide a reasonable scale to grade and segregate primary and secondary competition. However, advice from the management of the subject and discussions with some of the competitors can also help the appraiser sort the market area supply between primary and secondary competition.

Sometimes competitive facilities are assigned a competitive weight factor. If a facility shares similar physical plant and location characteristics and most people in the market will consider both that facility and the subject, then a competitive weight factor of 100% may be appropriate for that competitor. On the other hand if a facility in the same general geographic market has significantly different physical plant qualities compared to the subject and the market would not seriously consider patronizing the other facility, it may be considered secondary competition and could be assigned a competitive weight factor of some amount significantly less than 100%. Competitive weighting involves varying degrees of subjectivity and both quantitative and qualitative analyses can be employed to refine the process. Based on interviews with various facilities in the market, the appraiser can learn to what degree the markets overlap.

Supply Analysis

Supply analysis should begin with identifying and inventorying the competitive supply. Supply is easily identified with online data from the Nursing Home Compare Web site maintained by Centers for Medicare & Medicaid Services, U.S. Department of Health and Human Services (CMS). This web site is: http://www.medicare.gov/NHCompare. The site provides fairly detailed health survey data, occupancy levels at the time of the last health survey, and nursing staff ratios. On the Nursing Home Compare site, the appraiser can search all Medicaid and/or Medicare-certified facilities in several geographically defined areas–within a specific city and radius. States also offer ways to easily identify competitive facilities through licensure inventory lists and/or Medicaid cost report databases.

In determining the competitive supply, the appraiser should consider the following criteria and discuss them in the appraisal report.

- Proximity of the competitors to the appraised property
- Commonality of primary market areas
- Physical quality (site and building)
- Reputation similarities
- Levels of care

The competitive supply should be surveyed to determine occupancy rates, payor mixes, rents and/or rates, physical and location qualities, services included in routine charge (or provided at an additional charge), and other physical or service differences that would impact rates or census performance.

Collecting relevant competitive facility data for a supply and demand analysis typically involves researching a combination of primary and secondary sources. Primary source data on competitive facilities can be gathered though face-to-face meetings, telephone interviews, and/or written surveys. Practical experience suggests that face-to-face interviews are extremely difficult to accomplish given the time demands placed on most facility administrators and social service personnel. The surveyor may wait a long time before conducting the interview. Telephone interviews are the most efficient technique, and even then the surveyor may need to be persistent. Written surveys often go unanswered and are not recommended. Distant interviews can be accompanied by personal observation–e.g., visiting each competitive facility to gain a feel for the location and physical plant characteristics.

It is wise to go into any interview armed with secondary data from Medicare's Nursing Home Compare Web site, including occupancy rates, care deficiencies, occupancy rate payor mix, case-mix, and possibly even the private-pay rate information contained within the Medicaid cost report from a recent reporting period. Greater cooperation is often obtained when the person being interviewed is informed that the surveyor has these reports and wants to "update" the information.

Medicaid cost reports form the bulk of secondary competitive market data. Cost reports are available to the public under the Freedom of Information Act (FOIA) through the state fiscal unit in the agency that administrates the Medicaid program. Each state is different, and the administration or management of the subject facility can help direct the appraiser to the proper contact(s) within the state. To supplement Medicare's Nursing Home Compare Web site and cost reports, other secondary data can be obtained from state occupancy surveys conducted by health planning agencies and local ombudsman. (An ombudsman is an official organization sponsored by the state and charged with representing the public's interests by investigating and addressing complaints.) These groups act as advocates for improvements in the long-term care system and assist people in selecting a nursing facility. Many people working in ombudsman organizations are volunteers. The web site for the National Long-term Care Ombudsman Resource Center is: http://www.ltcombudsman.org/static_pages/ombudsmen.cfm. Competitive facilities should be compared to the subject facility to determine their relative advantages and disadvantages. This sets the stage for projecting occupancy, mix, and rates for the subject. Actual occupancy levels, payor mix, and private-pay rates can provide a general guide for ranking the desirability of the subject relative to the competition, with superior facilities achieving higher private-pay rates and quality-mix ratios.

The following elements of comparison are significant:

- Location immediate surroundings, access, proximity to hospitals, average income and housing value levels, proximity to origin of demand (home, hospital, and relatives), and general reputation of the vicinity.
- Physical plant–overall appearance, age, maintenance, common area amenities, bed capacity, functional utility, and regulatory compliance issues.
- Ownership reputation of operator (sometimes measured by state surveys or interviews with hospital discharge planners), type of ownership (profit vs. non-profit), and affiliation with

hospital or religious institution. Actual results can be obtained from the most recent surveys of a facility (subject and comparable sales and rentals) or from the CMS Web site.

- Level(s) of care–acuity levels greatly affect rate and mix; higher-acuity facilities charge more since operating expenses are greater.

In interviewing the management of competitive facilities, experience suggests that some people, as a matter of choice or policy, will be unwilling to answer questions or may provide biased answers. Going into the interview with as much non-confidential information about the facility as possible will typically produce better results. The interviewer is more likely to receive accurate information after disclosing that he or she has the Medicaid cost report or other public information about the facility.

When the surveyor is denied the interview and the information, a second approach is to use a "mystery shopper." A mystery shopper will explain that he or she is interested in learning about the facility for a potential patient. Administrators often comment that their facilities are routinely mystery shopped. However, the mystery shopping approach often yields less than simply asking for the information. With either approach, it is suggested that the initial questions should cover the most critical items that cannot be gathered from public sources. Once those answers are obtained, less critical issues can be pursued. Facility staff has limited time, so being organized and setting priorities for the interview is recommended.

The following topics should be pursued in a competitive facility interview, in roughly this order:

Critical information not typically available from public sources:

- Private-pay rates (private, semi-private, and ward rooms, with and/or without lavatories)
- Additional charges for supplies and extra services
- Current occupancy rate or vacant beds
- Waiting list or difficulty "selling" any particular beds (private, semi-private, etc.)
- Current or past decertification or other regulatory action taken against the facility for sub-standard care

Reasonably important, albeit somewhat dated, information available from public sources (probably appropriate questions for mystery shopping):

- Current and/or recent historical payor mix
- Recent trends in total census and census by payor

- Hospital(s) providing the greatest numbers of Medicare and managed care admission referrals
- Building age(s), recent renovations, and likely future renovations
- Additional construction, bed additions or reductions
- Staffing difficulties and use of agency nurses
- Anticipated private-pay rate increases, how much and when; also, last increase date and amounts
- Confirm number of beds and type of ownership (for-profit, non-profit, religious-based, etc.)
- Patient acuity level preference (high, low)

Information that is good to know, but not critical:

- Any new facility developments, expansions, or closures in the competitive market
- Any changes in ownership (sales or leases) in the market or anywhere else
- Any scuttlebutt concerning the subject or other competitors in the market
- Identification of primary competitors for the subject
- Patient room mix (private, semi-private, wards) and occupancy levels for each room type
- Duration of facility management

Future Supply and Certificates of Need

Additions to the current supply can significantly affect the status quo or balance in a competitive market, causing permanent or temporary reduction in overall occupancy rates, quality mix (private and Medicare), and possibly private-pay rates. New facilities will often pluck key employees from the existing supply, causing professional staff wages to increase in tight employment markets. Because assisted living facilities are stepping into the traditional nursing home domain and siphoning off low-acuity private-pay patients, changes in assisted living supply and licensure policies that expand the level(s) of personal care allowed in assisted living should be addressed too.

Identifying new supply can be accomplished in a single step if the state has a certificate of need (CON) program for nursing facilities. In the absence of CON restrictions, identifying and estimating future competitive supply is more difficult, yet essential in performing a valuation. Usually the competitive market is aware of any proposed facilities. In interviewing managers at the subject facility and the competition, it is important to ask if they are aware of any proposed additions to the current competitive supply. Relying solely on information from the management of the subject is not advised; verification with third parties is more objective and thorough. Zoning or building departments are other sources of information concerning prospective supply.

New competitive supply is easily forecast where certificates of need (CON), or determinations of need policies are enforced. Certificate of need programs aim to restrain health care facility costs and allow for coordinated planning of new services and construction. Laws authorizing such programs are one mechanism by which state governments seek to reduce overall health and medical costs.

Many CON laws were put into effect across the nation as part of the federal Health Planning Resources Development Act of 1974 (PL 93-641, the Public Health Services Act, section XV). For decades state governments have played a visible role in guiding and regulating the development of nursing facilities. In the 1970s virtually every state established such certificate of need laws. In 1987 the federal incentive law was dropped, thus leaving to the states free to answer the question of how and what to regulate in this area. Despite numerous changes in the past 30 years, about 36 states retained some type of CON program, law, or agency as of January 2007 (see Figure 9.1).

The following Web site provides details and a direct link to each state's CON regulator: http://www.ncsl.org/programs/health/cert-need.htm. The CON agency is typically housed within a division of the state health department. The appraiser should be familiar with the state's CON rules as they apply to nursing homes and determine if (and how many) additional beds have been or will be approved for the primary and secondary competitive market of the facility being appraised. These additional beds should be included in the inventory for the periods in which the beds are expected to become available. If the future bed need of the market area has not been determined by the state for the analysis period selected, then the appraiser should make an effort to project future bed supply. In markets where demand growth is elevated, this estimate is crucial.

Keep in mind that when occupancy and rent levels in a market are high and demand is expected to increase, additional competition could follow. Occasionally competitive bed supply will decrease, allowing the subject facility to increase occupancy. A reduction in the supply of competitive beds could occur through voluntary or involuntary delicensing. Voluntary delicensing might occur if an operator simply decides to close all or part of the beds, usually for economic reasons. Sometimes these beds will be moved into a replacement facility outside the primary market served by the existing facility and/or the subject.

Figure 9.1 **Map of Certificate of Need States, 2006**

(Colored States Have Some Form of CON)

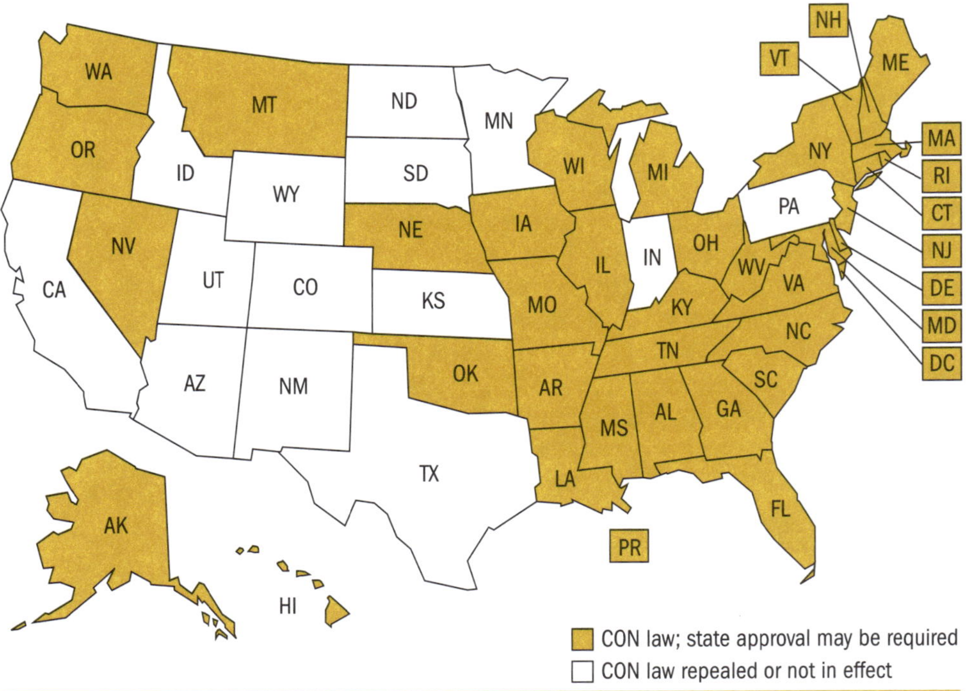

Compiled by NCSL, based on data from AHPA, June 2006

Bed transfer rules vary. Some states, such as Ohio and Missouri, have liberal rules that allow beds to be transferred within a county, while other CON states will require extensive CON review, with a low probability of approval. Involuntary delicensure generally occurs when a facility is in serious violation of health care regulations, and plans for correction have not been carried out. Licensure failure can occur swiftly and it may be permanent, leaving the ownership to seek an alternative for an empty facility.

Once the beds are removed from service (for whatever reason), states with CON bed need calculations can revisit their bed-need forecast for that planning area. Changes in competitive supply may occur in one segment of the market. For example, a facility may change Medicaid or Medicare certification to increase occupancy. Similarly, a hospital-based skilled nursing unit may be discontinued because that unit is no longer profitable under Medicare PPS, or a hospital may seek Medicare patients more aggressively to become profitable under Medicare PPS. Occasionally, freestanding, non-Medicaid facilities will certify for Medicaid to augment a deteriorating private-pay census level, placing the greatest pressure on less desirable facilities in the market.

Table 9.1 shows statewide average nursing facility occupancy rates, licensed beds per 1,000 population age 85 and older, occupied beds per 1,000 population age 85 and older, and average ADLs (activities of daily living) for each state. The data is grouped into states that require certificates of need for nursing facilities, states without any CON requirements or bed moratoriums, and states that have no CON regulations but impose moratoriums on additional nursing facility beds. The data shows that states without CON or moratoriums on new nursing facility beds have a lower occupancy rate (77.3%) than states with CON regulations in place (84.7%) and states without CON, but with bed moratoriums (89.1%). Similarly, non-CON states have a lower ratio of occupied nursing facility beds per 1,000 population age 85 and older than the other two groups.

Demand Analysis

Nursing facility demand is measured by occupied beds or patient days. The demand is best expressed in total patient days, but it is often measured by occupancy rate (total patient days divided by total potential patient days). Demand may be estimated as total bed demand (with all payor sources combined) or by each major payor source (Medicaid, Medicare, private-pay, and private insurance). This section presents techniques that analyze total demand, then segregate demand by payment type or payor mix (census mix).

Demand is influenced by macro and micro factors, with micro factors warranting the greatest attention. Micro demand analysis involves consideration of forces from within a local geographic area. Macro demand considers broader statewide and national forces. Macro demand may consider trends in total average daily census in Medicaid- and Medicare-certified skilled nursing facilities over a period of time, such as expressed in Figure 9.2, which was developed by the American Health Care Association (AHCA).[1]

This macro data shows that actual nursing facility bed demand declined slightly and steadily between 2000 and 2006. While the demand for nursing facility beds has declined, the use of assisted living has increased and the 75-plus population age cohort has also increased. This data implies that alternatives to skilled nursing facilities are increasing, and that this national trend should be considered in analyzing the local or micro market. The AHCA data shows a trend towards higher ADL (activities of daily living) dependency among nursing facility patients. From 2000 to

1. *Trends in Nursing Facility Characteristics*, American Health Care Association, Reimbursement and Research Department, December 2007.

Table 9.1 **Survey of Nursing Facility Certificate of Need Requirements, Occupancy Levels, Population-to-Bed Ratios, and Statewide Average ADLs**

State	Moratorium: Nursing Homes	Moratorium: CCRC Nursing Home Beds	Statewide Occupancy Rate 2006*	Beds Per 1,000 Population 85 Yrs. +†	Occupied Beds Per 1,000 Population 85 Yrs. +†	Average Number of ADLs per Resident, 1999‡
Continue to Regulate Under CON						
Alabama	no	no	87.5%	327.3	286.4	3.71
Alaska	no	no	88.3%	159.5	140.9	3.57
Arkansas	no	no	72.8%	434.9	316.6	3.62
Connecticut	yes	yes	90.9%	387.1	351.8	3.44
Delaware	no	no	81.1%	310.0	251.4	3.64
District of Columbia	no	–	92.4%	279.8	258.5	3.72
Florida	no	no	88.1%	166.8	146.9	3.75
Georgia	no	no	89.6%	338.1	303.0	3.66
Hawaii	no	no	92.8%	140.3	130.2	4.02
Illinois	no	no	75.0%	440.8	330.6	3.22
Iowa	no	no	77.8%	446.3	347.2	3.55
Kentucky	yes	no	89.3%	363.1	324.2	4.18
Louisiana	yes	yes	75.0%	540.2	405.2	3.34
Maine	no	no	90.4%	263.4	238.2	4.15
Maryland	no	no	87.1%	324.7	282.9	3.94
Massachusetts	yes	–	89.4%	360.7	322.5	3.75
Michigan	yes	yes	86.6%	261.1	226.1	3.7
Mississippi	yes	–	89.6%	361.6	324.0	3.57
Missouri	yes	yes	69.7%	461.9	322.0	3.54
Montana	no	–	73.7%	369.6	272.4	3.35
Nebraska	no	no	82.0%	405.6	332.6	3.45
Nevada	no	no	83.1%	187.9	156.2	3.52
New Hampshire	yes	no	90.1%	326.8	294.5	3.54
New Jersey	yes	no	87.6%	308.1	269.9	3.61
New York	no	no	92.8%	314.2	291.6	3.93
North Carolina	yes	no	87.6%	307.1	269.0	3.85
Ohio	yes	no	87.2%	420.2	366.4	3.76
Oklahoma	no	no	65.8%	450.7	296.6	3.43
Oregon	no	no	64.5%	171.7	110.8	3.85
Rhode Island	yes	yes	93.0%	350.5	326.0	3.4
South Carolina	no	no	90.3%	254.1	229.5	4.03
Tennessee	yes	yes	87.6%	366.3	320.9	3.89
Vermont	no	no	90.6%	284.5	257.7	3.94
Virginia	yes	no	89.2%	271.6	242.2	4.25
Washington	no	no	86.6%	201.8	174.8	3.86
West Virginia	yes	no	89.9%	292.2	262.7	4.13
Wisconsin	yes	yes	88.5%	335.1	296.5	3.48
Median for states with CON			84.7%	311.4	260.1	3.72
Eliminated CON Coverage: No Nursing Home Bed Moratorium						
Arizona	no	no	77.4%	146.4	113.3	3.67
California	no	no	84.8%	212.8	180.4	3.91
Idaho	no	no	75.0%	251.1	188.3	3.66
Indiana	no	no	69.8%	496.8	346.7	3.50
Kansas	no	no	76.4%	426.5	325.9	3.33
South Dakota	no	no	99.5%	334.1	332.4	3.44
Texas	no	no	72.2%	390.7	282.1	3.59
Wyoming	no	no	81.1%	355.9	288.6	3.31
Median for states with no CON & no bed moratorium			77.3%	292.6	226.1	3.55
Eliminated CON Coverage: Nursing Home Bed Moratorium						
Colorado	yes	–	83.0%	308.5	256.0	3.46
Minnesota	yes	–	91.4%	341.6	312.2	3.52
New Mexico	yes	no	86.7%	204.8	177.6	3.54
North Dakota	yes	no	91.8%	372.5	341.9	3.46
Pennsylvania	yes	–	91.1%	292.9	266.8	3.86
Utah	yes	no	70.9%	249.1	176.6	3.52
Median for states with no CON but bed moratorium			89.1%	298.6	266.0	3.56
U.S. (median)			83.5%	311.4	260.1	3.63

* National Center for Health Statistics, *Health United States, 2006, with Chartbook on Trends in the Health of Americans*, Hyattsville, MD: 2006

† National Center for Health Statistics and U.S. Census Bureau, *State Population Estimates, 2007*

‡ American Health Planning Association

Figure 9.2 **Trends in Certified Nursing Facilities, Beds and Patient Census—2000 through 2006**

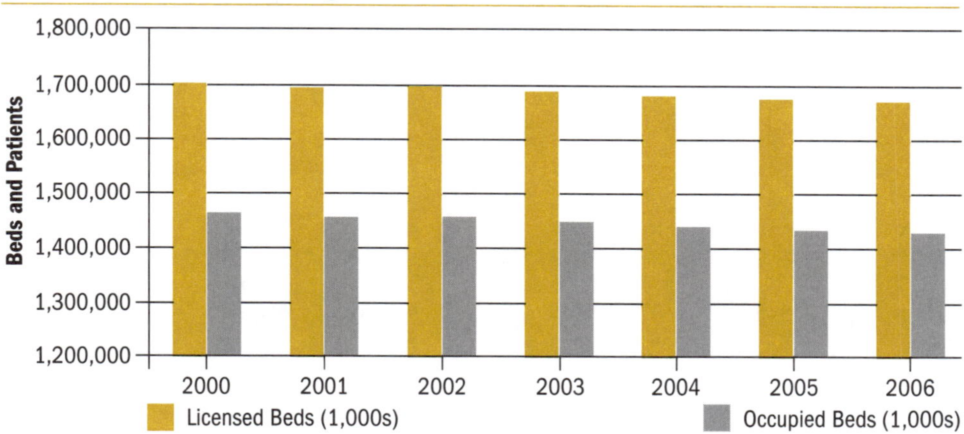

2007 the average number of ADLs increased steadily from 3.81 to 3.99.[2] One implication of this trend is that nursing facilities are receiving sicker patients and assisted living facilities are intercepting a greater amount of the lower-acuity demand.

Current demand is fairly easily determined by surveying occupancy characteristics in the competitive market. Generally, if a market has more than 10% vacancy, it is considered to be fully saturated, with all demand satisfied and little or no unaccommodated demand (displaced to other markets or unmet). Applying national or macro demand factors to a specific market will often result in an erroneous demand indication.

Demand can be estimated through a market saturation rate analysis. A saturation analysis is a comparative supply/demand analysis tool that is used to estimate demand, analyze supply/demand relationships, and calculate the *implied* occupancy rate. For a defined market area, the saturation rate measures actual demand (occupied beds) relative to qualified demand, which will be defined as total population over age 75. According to data from the American Health Care Association and Claritas, there were 79.3 nursing facility beds occupied for every 1,000 population aged 75 and over. However, this "saturation" ratio varies considerably from state to state. States with the highest ratio of occupied beds per 1,000 populations are concentrated in the Midwest while Sunbelt states tend to have lower ratios.

One way to measure demand using these statewide figures would be to apply the statewide "saturation" ratio total to the 75-plus population of the market area. Using a Greene County (Springfield), Missouri, example in which the market area

2. Ibid.

Table 9.2 **2006 Nursing Facility Occupied Bed Ratios Per 1,000 Age 75+**

State	Licensed Beds Per 1,000 75+ Population	Occupied Beds Per 1,000 75+ Population	State	Licensed Beds Per 1,000 75+ Population	Occupied Beds Per 1,000 75+ Population
Alabama	93.6	82.4	Montana	115.1	83.4
Alaska	39.2	33.8	Nebraska	131.1	109.0
Arizona	45.4	35.8	Nevada	46.2	39.0
Arkansas	134.1	97.1	New Hampshire	94.6	84.5
California	68.8	59.0	New Jersey	87.6	77.5
Colorado	89.3	74.5	New Mexico	62.4	54.1
Connecticut	115.9	107.1	New York	93.2	86.1
Delaware	87.7	75.9	North Carolina	86.3	76.4
District of Col.	85.0	79.2	North Dakota	125.1	114.8
Florida	53.5	47.5	Ohio	117.7	103.7
Georgia	99.6	88.9	Oklahoma	136.9	90.6
Hawaii	43.9	42.0	Oregon	52.2	33.6
Idaho	76.3	56.7	Pennsylvania	84.2	77.0
Illinois	133.0	105.4	Rhode Island	102.9	96.6
Indiana	148.1	119.5	South Carolina	73.9	68.8
Iowa	167.2	136.6	South Dakota	112.4	112.3
Kansas	137.5	117.2	Tennessee	107.7	95.4
Kentucky	104.8	95.9	Texas	115.1	85.6
Louisiana	145.8	108.5	Utah	75.8	53.8
Maine	73.4	66.8	Vermont	81.0	74.5
Maryland	91.1	80.0	Virginia	77.2	70.2
Massachusetts	109.9	99.7	Washington	62.1	53.8
Michigan	73.4	64.5	West Virginia	79.7	70.3
Minnesota	109.6	100.8	Wisconsin	101.1	88.7
Mississippi	108.8	97.5	Wyoming	102.7	83.8
Missouri	141.0	105.2	United States	93.1	79.3

Sources: American Health Care Association and Claritas

matches the county, a demand estimate for the county is estimated by multiplying the 75-plus population by the state ratio.

2007 Greene County 75-plus population	18,265*
Missouri "saturation" rate (percentage)	10.5%
Estimated nursing facility demand	1,918
Actual occupied beds, 4th quarter 2007	1,905†

* Claritas

† Missouri Certificate of Need Program, Department of Health and Senior Services, *Division of Regulation & Licensure (DRL) Quarterly Survey Report, Ending December 31, 2007.*

In this example, the implied demand, calculated by applying the statewide occupied bed ratio to the county population, closely matches the actual market demand. Because there is substantial bed vacancy in this market, suggesting that nearly all demand originating from within the area is satisfied, the implied saturation rate is 10.5% of the 75-plus population. The statewide bed-ratio data may be a fairly reliable demand indicator when existing demand from within a market is not overstated or understated by imbalances in adjacent markets. Adding to the bed supply may not be feasible in a market where the percentage of nursing facility beds relative to the elderly population substantially exceeds 10.5%.

Bed demand ratios can vary between rural and urban areas. Metropolitan markets may draw patients away from rural markets with facilities that specialize in certain diseases such as Alzheimer's. Metro markets may also have larger medical centers that offer more diverse services and patients' adult children may live in these larger communities where there are more employment opportunities.

The presence or lack of assisted living facilities can also skew demand figures. Still, applying statewide figures to measure a specific market demand may be more reliable than developing empirical saturation rates from one's own primary research of a smaller sample size.

It is often advisable to examine demand levels over the past few years to measure changes in market demand. Many states closely monitor nursing home occupancy data and make this information available to the public through state departments of health, often within the same division as the CON unit.

Nursing facility demand is largely driven by the elderly population, and current ratios of elderly population to occupied beds in a particular market should be calculated and compared to state or regional ratios. The typical ratio should then be applied to estimated future changes in population to determine the future bed need in the competitive market for the appraised facility. While elderly population growth and nursing home bed demand have been roughly parallel, this trend is diverging as increased use of home health care and assisted living nibble away at the edges of traditional nursing facility demand. The lowest-acuity nursing facility patients are finding their way into lower-cost, assisting living environments. Any demand assessment should examine a state's current and future use of Medicaid waivers, which may offer Medicaid patients assisted living and home health care alternatives. Private-pay patients requiring long-term care are increasingly being targeted by assisted living facilities where the costs are less, the environments are more attractive, and the patients' needs are met equally well.

Summary

The market analysis sets the stage for the development of occupancy, payor mix, absorption, and private-pay rate forecasts. Patients, their family and friends, and the medical community have the largest voice in selecting a facility. Generally, the competitive market area is limited to a geographic area that is within a short drive from the patient's home, family, friends, doctor(s), and hospital. The size of the area will depend on the density of the population and number of other facilities within or near the market area of the subject. Patient origin data may be available and is certainly helpful in delineating the market area and identifying the competition. The competitive supply may consist of all facilities located within the delineated market area of the subject, or the supply could reach beyond the market area. When the number of facilities in a market area is substantial, the competitve supply may be restricted to only those facilities that have qualities similar to the subject.

The appraiser should review certificate of need policies, bed need determination formula(s), and the inventory of existing and approved beds that are not yet built. This review should be able to identify all current supply and potential new supply for a few years in the future. Besides reviewing CON applications and approvals, reviewing building and zoning applications and interviewing the management of competitive facilities will identify developments in the pipeline.

The effects of any determinable change in competitive supply should be considered. Nursing facility demand is a function of population. In any given population, typically defined as a certain elderly age cohort, a certain percentage of the population will reside in a nursing facility. This percentage will vary by state and region and will be influenced by the amount and acuity levels for alternatives such as assisted living facilities and by Medicaid eligibility. Most markets with overall vacancy rates that exceed 5% to 8% should be considered nearly or fully saturated, and changes in demand will be closely tied to changes in the elderly population. In markets where there is little vacancy, some demand could be unmet.

Chapter 10

Projecting Occupancy

The projected occupancy of a facility should be based in the interplay of supply and demand and the relative competitive positions of the various facilities in the market. The historic and current census levels of the subject and the competition establish the basis for future demand estimates and projections. Changes in the demand should correlate to, but not necessarily parallel, the changes in the elderly population of the defined market. Developing an occupancy projection is a step-by-step process that includes estimating:

- Current supply
- Current demand
- Future demand
- Future supply
- Market share and penetration rates

In estimating occupancy and patient mix (private-pay, Medicare, etc.), the following definitions are used.

- *Fair market share* is the number of licensed beds in a facility divided by the total market bed supply.
- *Actual market share* is the number of occupied beds in a single facility divided by occupied beds in the market.
- *Market penetration rates* are calculated by dividing the occupancy rate of a facility by the occupancy rate of the identified competitive market.

To belabor the obvious, when competitive supply increases more rapidly than demand, occupancy levels in the market fall and the weakest competitors typically experience greater losses, through declining occupancy and quality mix levels and pressure on private-pay rates. Nursing facilities must also compete for labor, and there is anecdotal evidence that wage levels increase in markets where there are labor shortages and competition for staff increases with increased competitive supply.

Changes in competitive supply can occur not only from the entry of new facilities into the market, but from complete or partial closure of existing facilities and the repositioning of existing facilities that undergo substantial renovation or change in management. The demand will be redistributed within the market once the new beds are in operation. Total occupancy penetration rates for the existing competition will tend to decline during the absorption of the new facility. Upon stabilization, the new facilities will typically achieve superior occupancy, quality mix, and rate levels compared to the overall market.

Stabilized occupancy represents the occupancy level that a facility is expected to maintain relative to the occupancy levels in the market, considering the facility's physical plant and location. A facility with inferior physical plant and location attributes, relative to the market, is expected to sustain an occupancy rate below the market average. However, occupancy rates can be influenced by the bed capacity. For example, three identical facilities in a market may have different occupancy levels if the only difference is capacity. If two facilities contain 100 beds each and the third contains 90 beds, and all three facilities have 80 patients, the occupancy rate of the third facility is obviously higher.

Stabilized occupancy should exclude any temporary or abnormal relationship between supply and demand. The opening of a new facility in the market may cause the market occupancy to decline as the market sorts out a new balance. A temporary decertification or stop-placement order on a facility resulting from substandard care or serious survey violations that will be corrected soon may ripple through the market and displace demand over the short run. Normalizing these supply and demand conditions and other market abnormalities in the analysis will produce more creditable valuation results.

Case Study—Occupancy Rate and Total Census Forecast

The following case study presents a realistic situation in which there is demand growth and a new competitor enters the market. The subject property in this case is an existing, mid-market facility. This case study application shows the process of forecasting occupancy using market share and market penetration concepts. The case study will be continued later in the chapter to illustrate census mix forecasting principles The characteristics of the market are described as follows:

- The market is in the Midwest with a county population of 150,000, including 10,000 persons over the age of 75.

- Projected growth in population in the 75-plus age group is at 2.0% per year for the next five years—according to a demographic service projection.
- All nursing facilities and the two acute-care hospitals are located in the county seat, which has a population of 85,000.
- The state CON agency will approve additional beds when the county occupancy exceeds 94.0% of licensed beds and that new supply will not reduce countywide occupancy below 85%.
- Assisted living facilities and home health care are well established in the market and no further demand is expected to be shifted to these alternatives.

The significant distinguishing features of the competitors are summarized below.

- **Facility 1:** Newest facility in market with best plan; located in upper-middle income residential area and controlled by national chain
- **Facility 2:** Oldest facility in market, located in low-income, mixed-use area; cannot comply with physical requirements for Medicare and ownership changes frequently
- **Facility 3:** Newer, well-located "country club" facility operated continuously by local ownership; good reputation, but not aggressively seeking high-acuity patients
- **Facility 4:** Smaller, selective, faith-based facility located in established, middle-income residential area
- **Facility 5:** Regional facility has out-of-town, for-profit operator; aggressive in rates and average in quality; middle-aged physical plant is located on the edge of town in opposite direction from main growth
- **Facility 6:** Older, well-maintained building located near strong regional hospital which controls this facility; hospital favors discharging Medicare patients to this facility; the other local hospital does not favor one facility over another
- **Subject:** Older-than-average facility located in middle-income, stable area; for-profit ownership seeking high-acuity patients

In a balanced market, each competitor will capture its fair market share resulting in market penetrations of 100% for each facility. However, differences in locations, reputations, quality of care, physical plant, and management produce different penetration rates for occupancy and quality mix.

The following occupancy market share and penetration rates are calculated for the facilities within the competitive market.

Table 10.1 Characteristics of Facilities in the Competitive Market

Facility	Beds	Facility Effective Age (Years)	Physical Plant Quality Relative to Subject	Household Income in Facility Zip Code Area	Occupancy Rate, Past 12 Months	Private-Pay Mix, Past 12 Months	Medicare Mix, Past 12 Months
1	120	8	Superior	$65,000	97.5%	46.5%	22.5%
2	250	42	Inferior	$47,500	86.0%	5.0%	0.0%
3	90	12	Superior	$78,000	96.7%	82.9%	17.1%
4	60	32	Inferior	$60,000	96.7%	20.9%	10.0%
5	120	28	Inferior	$50,000	92.5%	18.0%	14.0%
6	240	23	Inferior	$55,000	97.1%	14.0%	22.5%
Subject	120	14	–	$60,000	95.0%	42.1%	13.2%
Total market	1,000				93.5%	26.7%	13.9%

Facility 2 has the lowest occupancy penetration rate and is considered inferior to the balance of the market because of its age and lower acuity level. Facilities 1 and 3 have the highest quality mixes and they are regarded as superior in age and location.

Using the total census market shares, market penetration rates, and occupancy rates for each of the existing competitors from the Table 10. 1, additional calculations can be made as shown in Table 10.2

Table 10.2 Occupancy Market Penetration of Competitive Market

Facility	Beds	Average Occupied Beds, Past 12 Months	Fair Market Share	Actual Market Share	Current Occupancy Rate	Market Penetration
1	120	117	12.0%	12.5%	97.5%	104.3%
2	250	215	25.0%	23.0%	86.0%	92.0%
3	90	87	9.0%	9.3%	96.7%	103.4%
4	60	58	6.0%	6.2%	96.7%	103.4%
5	120	111	12.0%	11.9%	92.5%	98.9%
6	240	233	24.0%	24.9%	97.1%	103.8%
Subject	120	114	12.0%	12.2%	95.0%	101.6%
Total market	1,000	935	100.0%	100.0%	93.5%	100.0%

Fair market share is calculated by dividing the licensed beds in a facility by the total beds in the market. The subject has 120 beds, divided by the 1,000 total beds in the market, which produces a fair market share of 12.0%. Actual market share is calculated by dividing the total census at a facility by the total census in the market. So, the actual market share for the subject is calculated by dividing its census of 114 by the total market census of 935 to arrive at 12.2% . Market penetration is calculated by dividing the occupancy rate of a single facility by the total market occupancy rate. The market penetration rate for the subject is 101.6%, calculated by dividing its 95.0% occupancy rate divided by the 93.5% occupancy rate of the total market.

The next step is projecting future demand, given the following facts:

- By using projections prepared by a demographic forecaster, the elderly population (age 75 plus) is estimated to increase 2.0% annually over the next five years.
- The total market census increased 1.9% between 2007 and 2008; the total average census for the prior year increased 2.1%.
- The estimated nursing facility market demand growth is forecast to equal the 2.0% annual rate of increase in the 75-plus population.
- A CON was recently granted for 100 additional beds in the market. A 100-bed facility is now under construction in a more affluent part of the primary market area, and the facility design will incorporate superior features relative to the existing supply—i.e., more private rooms, a separate rehab wing, all private toilets, and more common areas.
- The additional supply will reduce the county occupancy rate to 85.2% in the following year.

Using the market share and penetration rates that have been calculated, coupled with reasonable demand forecasts and adjustments in market preferences as a result of the new competition, the following market occupancy rates are projected for a four-year forecast period.

Table 10.3 Projecting Future Bed Demand Using Estimated 2.0% Annual Change in Elderly Population

Year	Historic and Current Average Census	Actual & Projected Annual Demand Growth	Projected Total Bed Demand	Total Bed Supply	Market Occupancy Rate
2006	898.7			1,000	89.9%
2007	917.6	2.10%		1,000	91.8%
Current (2008)	**935.0**	**1.90%**		**1,000**	**93.5%**
2009		2.00%	953.7	1,100	86.7%
2010		2.00%	972.8	1,100	88.4%
2011		2.00%	992.3	1,100	90.2%
2012		2.00%	1,012.1	1,100	92.0%

Table 10.4 shows that the subject has consistently achieved a slightly higher occupancy rate than the market average, as evidenced by its occupancy penetration rate, which exceeds 100% for the past three years. Since the subject has consistently out-performed the market and is rated superior to four of the six competitors, it is reasonable to expect that the subject will continue to achieve an occupancy penetration rate that is slightly greater than 100%. This reasoning yields the following occupancy forecast for the subject.

Table 10.4 Forecasting Subject Occupancy

Year	Market Average Census	Market Occupancy Rate	Subject Fair Market Share	Subject Actual Market Share	Subject Market Penetration Rate	Subject Occupancy Rate	Subject Average Daily Census
2006	898.7	89.9%	12.0%	12.4%	103.5%	93.0%	111.6
2007	917.6	91.8%	12.0%	12.4%	103.5%	95.0%	114.0
Now (2008)	**935.0**	**93.5%**	**12.0%**	**12.2%**	**101.6%**	**95.0%**	**114.0**
2009	953.7	86.7%	10.9%	11.2%	103.0%	89.3%	107.2
2010	972.8	88.4%	10.9%	11.2%	103.0%	91.1%	109.3
2011	992.3	90.2%	10.9%	11.2%	103.0%	92.9%	111.5
2012	1,012.1	92.0%	10.9%	11.2%	103.0%	94.8%	113.8

In this case study occupancy forecast, total patient days, the driver of revenue and operating expenses, is developed first. However, a valid alternative analysis is to eliminate the occupancy rate analysis and instead measure historical, current, and forecast total market bed demand and specific subject bed demand as indicated by average daily census or total annual patients days. These analyses will still express supply and demand relationships through fair market share and actual market share. The same conclusions should be reached if the data, analysis, and judgments are consistent. The same destination is reached regardless of the vehicle used.

Absorption: A Redistribution of Future Admissions

Absorption of a new facility depends on many factors, including:

- New beds as a percentage of total market supply–the absorption period extends as this percentage increases
- Average length of stay (turnover)
- Existence of pent-up demand
- Location
- Reputation of operator in community and/or established relationships
- Physical qualities

A simple and reasonably reliable method for estimating nursing bed absorption is through turnover analysis, which essentially redistributes the admissions and discharges in the market to include any new bed supply. The process begins by determining the number of nursing home admissions and discharges for the entire market for a given period, say, one quarter of a year. Admission and discharge figures are often available from a state department of health and many facilities will also track this data. Some high-level turnover data is shown in Table 10.5.

Table 10.5 **Nursing Facility Average Lengths of Stay, Discharge Rates, and Payment Sources at Admission**

Average length of stay (ALOS)–all nursing facilities:	272 days
Discharge rate per 100 beds	
All facilities	134.2 discharges/100 beds
Medicare-only facilities	339.2 discharges per 100 beds
Medicaid-only facilities	58.1 discharges per 100 beds
Percentage of discharges with ALOS of 90 days or less	68.0%
Expected source of payment at admission:	
Medicare	30.9%
Private-pay/insurance	25.1%
Medicaid	40.2%
Other	3.9%

Source: *The National Nursing Home Survey: 1999 Summary*, U.S. Department of Health and Human Services Centers for Disease Control and Prevention, National Center for Health Statistics, Library of Congress Catalog Card Number 88-600333.

Once the number of admissions and discharges are projected for the market, the appraiser can calculate the fair market share and estimate the penetration rate for the new facility. New facilities achieve higher admissions penetration rates during absorption periods because:

- New, relatively empty facilities have greater capacity.

- The physical plant is new and often more attractive than some or all of the competition.
- A new facility can actually draw patients out of other facilities with better physical and location features.
- A new facility can achieve higher ratios of Medicare patients and other rehab patients with substantially shorter average lengths of stay–thus, faster bed turnover.

As a new facility is absorbed, the admissions penetration rate tends to gravitate down to 100%, where it should remain for the long run, provided its average length of stay is similar to the market average. Discharges will continue to mount as the census increases and seasons. Initially the discharge rate lags behind the admissions rate, but it will eventually approximate the number of admissions after the occupancy level stabilizes. The nursing bed absorption calculation is shown in Table 10.6.

Table 10.6 Example of Absorption Calculation

Period	1st Q	2nd Q	3rd Q	4th Q
Total bed demand (1,200 bed supply with subject)	1,000	1,000	1,000	1,000
Estimated quarterly admissions rate for market (a)	300	300	300	300
New facility's admissions penetration rate (b)	200%	175%	150%	125%
New facility's fair share (c)	10%	10%	10%	10%
New facility's quarterly admissions (a × b × c)	60.0	52.5	45.0	37.5
Prior quarter-end census	0	52.5	82.7	97.3
Less discharges (30.0% of previous quarter census and 12.5% of current quarter admissions)	7.5	22.4	30.4	33.9
Net census at end of quarter	52.5	82.7	97.3	100.9
Occupancy rate of new facility at end of quarter (120 beds)	43.8%	68.9%	81.0%	84.1%

Based on these calculations, the new facility reaches a stabilized occupancy rate in the fourth or fifth quarter. This absorption calculation is a broad-brush technique that proves to be generally reliable. Absorption rates will be faster for Medicare, managed care, and rehabilitation patients as this group has a much faster turnover, or shorter length of stay, than long-term patients typically paying privately or receiving Medicaid. A more detailed absorption analysis can be performed with this model by running calculations for each payor source using the admissions and turnover rates for the respective payor sources.

Summary

Forecasting the occupancy level for a nursing facility will involve analyzing the existing and future competitive supply and demand in the market and measuring those forces against the relative physical characteristics, location, and reputation of the subject. This chapter explored the use of fair market share, actual market share, and market penetration rates. Fair market share involves dividing a facility's number of licensed beds by the total market bed supply. Actual market share is the average daily census of a facility divided by the average total occupied beds in the market. The market penetration rate is calculated by dividing the occupancy percentage of a facility by the occupancy rate of the competitive market.

In markets that have stable supply and demand conditions and where none of the competitors, or the subject, are expected to be repositioned in the market as a result of a major corrective action such as a building renovation or replacement of inept management, then the historic relationships of market share and penetration will probably continue. Where a change in supply is anticipated, either through an increase or decrease in competitive beds or a repositioning, the appraiser or analyst will need to exercise more judgment in applying penetration rates. In developing an absorption forecast for a new facility or an addition to an existing facility, census turnover and the redistribution of admissions are important considerations. New supply will compete for future admissions; patient transfers from other facilities are typically not expected to occur to any great extent unless there is a large quality gap. If patient transfers are anticipated, then an accelerated absorption process may occur.

Chapter 11

Payor or Census Mix Analysis

Estimating the most probable payor or census mix is essential in the valuation of a nursing facility. The four major sources of payment for skilled and intermediate nursing care are Medicare, Medicaid, private insurance (managed care), and private-pay or self-pay. Profitability levels vary among these groups, with Medicare generally being the most profitable and Medicaid the least profitable. Mix is typically represented by patient days, however, some reports use "revenue mix," in which the revenue from each payment source is compared to the total revenue. Payor mix is not only critical to the income capitalization approach, but it is also a significant element of comparison in the sales comparison approach and, indirectly, it can be a factor in estimating external obsolescence.

On a macro level, Medicare patients are becoming a larger component of the overall nursing facility census by patient days. Nevertheless, Medicaid and private-pay payor mixes and actual occupied beds declined between 2001 and 2007 (see Figure 11.1 and Table 11.1).[1]

Nursing home admissions often start out as Medicare or private-pay patients. In 1999, 30.9% of nursing facility admissions (at the time the patient entered the facility) were under Medicare, 25.1% were private-pay, 40.2% were under Medicaid, and 3.9% used other payment sources.[2] Eventually the Medicare benefits expire and/or the patient's personal funds are depleted and the patient must turn to Medicaid.

1. *Trends in Nursing Facility Characteristics*, American Health Care Association, Reimbursement and Research Department, December 2007.
2. *The National Nursing Home Survey: 1999 Summary*, U.S. Department of Health and Human Services Centers for Disease Control and Prevention, National Center for Health Statistics, Library of Congress Catalog Card Number 88-600333.

Figure 11.1 **Trends in Nursing Facility Payor or Census Mix From 2001 to 2007**

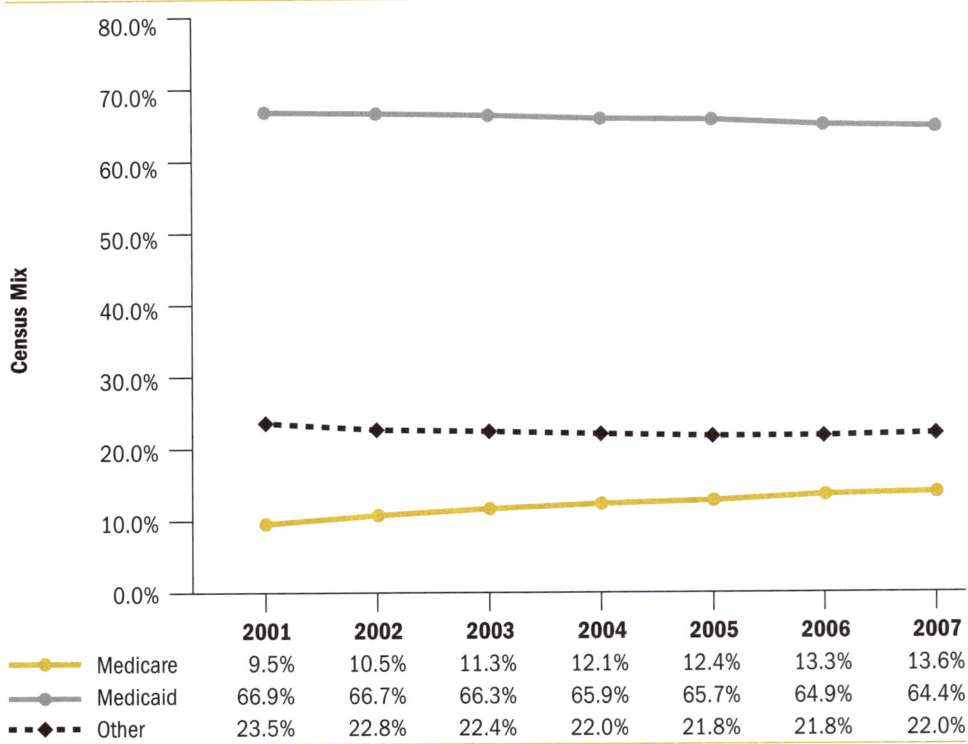

	2001	2002	2003	2004	2005	2006	2007
Medicare	9.5%	10.5%	11.3%	12.1%	12.4%	13.3%	13.6%
Medicaid	66.9%	66.7%	66.3%	65.9%	65.7%	64.9%	64.4%
Other	23.5%	22.8%	22.4%	22.0%	21.8%	21.8%	22.0%

Table 11.1 **Trends in Nursing Facility Census by Payor Between 2001 and 2007**

	Medicare	Medicaid	Other Payor	Total
2001	139,452	977,678	343,752	1,460,882
2002	152,279	971,398	331,894	1,455,571
2003	164,244	961,774	324,301	1,450,319
2004	174,696	949,586	317,105	1,441,388
2005	178,824	945,623	314,201	1,438,647
2006	190,283	927,110	312,229	1,429,622
2007	193,150	914,620	312,448	1,420,217

Source: *Trends in Nursing Facility Characteristics*, December 2007.

A brief review of issues in the Medicaid and Medicare programs that are relevant to census mix is presented below.

Medicare Part A is generally very profitable for a nursing facility. Chapter 5 covers the salient features of the Medicare program that relate to eligibility, coverage, and payments for skilled nursing. Briefly, Medicare will cover 100% of the cost of the first 20 days in a skilled nursing facility and co-pays for up to another 80 days. Over 30% of admissions into nursing facilities come from patients with Medicare coverage. Medicare provides short-term coverage for those who require skilled nursing or rehabilitative care on a daily basis upon discharge from an acute care setting (hospital) after a minimum stay of three days. Unlike most Medicaid programs, Medicare pays the operator for restorative care, i.e. physical, speech, and occupational therapies, and for pharmacy and medical supply expenses, which collectively are referred to as *ancillary services.* Ancillary services are a significant profit center in most nursing homes. A single reimbursement method is applied nationally to this federal program administrated by the CMS. Medicare Part B (medical insurance), C (Medicare alternatives) and D (drug benefits) are not components of the Medicare census. Medicare contracts with regional insurance companies (Medicare intermediaries), which process more than one billion fee-for-service claims per year.

Medicaid is the payor of last resort and it is the payor for the largest group of patients. Issues of reimbursements, eligibility, and program financing are presented in the Chapter 6. As a quick review, Medicaid is a federal-state partnership, administered at the state level, which pays for certain health care, including intermediate and skilled nursing care, for persons with need but without adequate financial resources to pay for these services themselves or through insurance. Since states finance part of the cost, they have a substantial role in determining regulations, eligibility, and reimbursement policies. Nursing facilities receive reimbursement checks from the state, typically in arrears and on a monthly basis, using pre-set, daily reimbursement rates that are often less than the actual costs to provide care.[3]

Nursing facilities also have private-pay patients plus some private insurance (managed care) hospice and VA patients. Private-pay rates are typically unregulated. In many states, private-pay rates must equal or exceed the Medicaid rates for the same level of service at the facility. Until private-pay patients exhaust their assets, they will not receive any direct medical assistance from Medicaid. Long-term care insurance policies are gaining favor with the elderly, but still represent a small percentage of the market. Conventional insurance, including managed care, is directing younger clients from hospital settings into skilled nursing facilities to complete their rehabilitation in these lower-cost environments. Some nursing facilities will identify hospice patients as a separate category. Generally, hospice patients receive Medicaid or are private-pay. Medicaid will pay the standard Medicaid rate for a hospice patient, and the patient may receive hospice services and supplies through an outside hospice organization.

---

3. *A Report on Shortfalls in Medicaid Funding for Nursing Home Care*, BDO Seidman, LLP and Eljay, LLC, for the American Health Care Association, September 2007.

Managed care and private insurance represent a growing component of the "other" payor category. Medicare Advantage is an alternative to regular Medicare whereby a person opts out of Medicare in favor of qualified alternative coverage from private companies. These companies negotiate directly with skilled nursing facilities to provide their enrollees with the same or "better" services than they would receive with Medicare benefits. Patients with commercial long-term care insurance and other forms of private insurance coverage are often included within the managed care and private insurance category. Generally, these patients represent a small fraction of the total census.

Managed care patients using Medicare Advantage generally receive the same levels of service as Medicare patients. Thus there is considerable expense for therapy, pharmacy, and medical supplies associated with these patients. The popularity of managed care alternatives varies geographically, with fewer participants in rural and less populated areas.

The Veterans Administration (VA) provides retired and disabled military service people with certain long-term care benefits. While there are some attractive, newer, freestanding VA nursing facilities, many VA patients chose private nursing facilities. Most nursing facilities do not accept VA patients citing inadequate reimbursements, and those that do typically have only a few patients at any given time. For census and revenue forecasting purposes, VA patients have an affinity to Medicaid.

Estimating Payor Mix

Nursing facility developers focus on locations and designs that will yield the highest percentages of private-pay, Medicare, and managed care patients (quality mix) in a specific market. The factors that influence payor mix are primarily economic and physical forces. All else being equal, facilities located in market areas that have high income levels and high residential property values typically achieve higher private-pay mixes. Physical plant characteristics, including age and condition, patient room mix (private, semi-private, and wards; private vs. semi-private lavatories), rehab space, and common area amenities for patients, visitors and staff are of paramount importance. Good advertising and public relations can promote a quality mix. Facilities controlled by hospitals can direct profitable discharges into their own facilities. Nursing facility administrators, directors of nursing, and social workers can improve the quality mix through community involvement in social and professional organizations oriented toward the elderly and the medical community.

Under stable market conditions, the current and recent payor mix relationships provide a sound indication of probable payor mix in the future. Significant and subtle shifts in census mix can result from changes in the competitive market. Changes in management or ownership that correct physical or operational weaknesses in existing facilities will often ripple across the competitive landscape. Conversely, the replacement of management or ownership that has achieved extraordinarily high census levels, often at the expense of financial success, may result in a redistribution of quality-mix patients to other facilities in the market. This often occurs when a non-profit facility that has underpriced its services and/or provided additional services changes to for-profit ownership. Generally newly opened facilities will reduce the private-pay and Medicare percentages of the existing nursing facilities in the market.

The payor mix projections can be analyzed in a manner similar to the analysis of occupancy rates, i.e., through an examination of supply, demand, penetration rates, market shares, etc. Since Medicaid is the payor of last resort, and the Veterans Administration and other payment sources are generally insignificant, payor mix analysis focuses on private-pay and Medicare. In most cases, the remainder of the census is Medicaid.

Private-Pay Mix Forecasting

Estimation of the private-pay mix of a facility begins by comparing the current and historical (i.e., two to three years) private-pay figures of the subject and the primary competitors in the market. Market share and penetration rates for the subject and competitors should remain fairly consistent as long as supply and demand remain stable and no facility undergoes major changes in physical quality or reputation, which can significantly alter its competitive ranking.

Future supply and demand should be factored into the payor mix analysis in much the same way as they are in the occupancy analysis, giving consideration to:

- Changes in demand
- Changes in bed supply, both in number and quality
- Development of assisted living facilities, which can attract low-acuity demand, especially private-pay residents
- Market share and penetration rates
- Rate levels and comparative value
- Attrition rate–general decline in private-pay census in the market
- Other factors

Changes in competitive supply not only stem from the development of new facilities, but from existing facilities being repositioned with substantial renovation and/or management changes. Moreover, existing facilities in the market can add beds or completely or partially eliminate beds. The market redistributes payor mix with changes in the quantity and quality of supply. Medicare and private-pay census and penetration rates for the existing competition have a tendency to decline after the arrival of new competition.

Case Study

The case study presented in the occupancy forecast in Chapter 10 is continued here to illustrate payor or census mix forecasting using market share and market penetration concepts. As indicated previously, this case study represents a realistic situation in a typical market where there is demand growth and a new competitor has entered the market. The subject is an existing, mid-market facility.

The subject facility is a 120-bed facility which currently and historically has captured 40 out of the 250 private-pay patients in a 1,000-bed market. The subject has a 16.0% private-pay market share (40/250). The location, physical plant, and management of the subject are above average, which is confirmed by its relative census characteristics. Assume the following:

- 250 of the 950 occupied beds in the market are private-pay.
- Total bed supply is currently 1,000 (95% occupancy).
- A CON was recently granted for 100 additional beds within the market, and that facility is now under construction in a more affluent area of the primary market area. The new facility will incorporate features superior to the existing supply, with more private rooms, a separate rehab wing, all private toilets, and more common areas.
- Demand is expected to increase steadily each year by 2.0% (total census and private-pay census).
- The new facility is expected to achieve a private-pay census of 45 patients at stabilization or a private-pay mix of approximately 50%.
- The 120-bed subject facility is expected to maintain its current private-pay market share (16.0%) among the existing supply.
- Based on these assumptions and the calculations in Table 11.2, the average private-pay census at the subject will decline from 40% to 33.6%, and the private-pay mix will decline from 42.1% to 38.0% in one year.

This subject facility's decline in private-pay mix, coupled with the declining occupancy rate, will have a significant adverse impact on cash flow. The impact resulting just from the lost private-pay census is shown as in Table 11.3.

In this case study, the subject facility will lose 2,482 total patient days, which will include a loss of 2,336 private-pay days. The other lost days may include a loss of Medicare and managed care days and an increase in Medicaid days as the market matriculates through market changes. If the average private-pay rate of the subject is not affected by competitive or inflationary pressures, the facility will experience a $430,490 decline in private-pay revenues between these two years. Assuming a marginal operating

Table 11.2 Forecasting Market and Subject Private-Pay Census

		Current (2008)	1 Yr. From Now
Current bed supply	a	1,000	1,100
Bed demand growth–2.0% annually			
Current total occupied beds in market	b	935	953.7
Market occupancy rate (b / a)	c	93.5%	86.7%
Subject occupied beds	d	114	107.2
Market private-pay occupied beds	e	250	255
New facility private-pay census at stabilization	f	0	45
Private-pay census allocated to balance of supply (e – f)	g	250	210
Subject private-pay census, currently	h	40	
Subject private-pay market share, next year @ current year's market share (h / g)	i	16.0%	
Forecasted private-pay market share for subject, excluding demand captured by new facility (= i)	j		16.0%
Subject private-pay census (g × i or j)	k	40	33.6
Subject private-pay mix (j / d)	l	35.1%	31.3%

Table 11.3 Impact on Revenues and Earnings Resulting from Change in Private-Pay Mix Caused by Additional Competition

		Current (2008)	1 Yr. From Now
Subject occupied beds	d	114	107.2
Total annual patient days	m	41,610	39,128
Total lost patient days	n		2,482
Subject private-pay census	k	40	33.6
Annual private-pay patient days (k × 365 days)	o	14,600	12,264
Lost private-pay days	p		2,336
Average private-pay rate	q		$184.28
Private-pay revenue loss (p × q)	r		$430,490
Reduction in operating expenses as a result of lower private-pay census ($175.00 × p)	s		$(373,760)
Private-pay marginal NOI loss (r – s)	t		$56,730
Marginal income capitalization rate	u		12.5%
Capitalized value difference (t / u)			$453,836
Other patient days lost (Medicare and Medicaid) (n – p)			146

expense of $175.00 per patient day, the lost private-pay census will result in a $56,730 decrease in net operating income or EBITDAR (earnings before interest, taxes, depreciation, amortization, and rent). The earnings loss is actually greater since the vacancy rate will increase and the facility's Medicare and/or Medicaid census may decline too.

If an appropriate overall capitalization rate for this marginal income is 12.5%, then the loss in value would be $453,836, before considering the impact of the lost Medicare census. The question of actual value loss would depend on whether the market had already priced the new competitor into the market. Issues relating to the forecasting of Medicare census are addressed later.

Private-Pay Attrition

In addition to potential private-pay losses from new competition, natural private-pay attrition is occurring in nearly every market. From a macro or industry-wide perspective, private-pay census mix has been declining steadily since the 1970s. "Other payor" patient census and mix, which are mostly private-pay, declined each year between 2001 and 2006 (see Table 11.4).

Table 11.4 **Trends in Private-Pay and Other Census between 2001 and 2007**

Year	Average Daily Census—Private-Pay and Other	Private & Other Census Mix
2001	343,752	23.5%
2002	331,894	22.8%
2003	324,301	22.4%
2004	317,105	22.0%
2005	314,201	21.8%
2006	312,229	21.8%
2007	312,448	22.0%

Source: *Trends in Nursing Facility Characteristics*, American Health Care Association, Reimbursement and Research Department, December 2007.

Private-pay attrition is attributable to several social and economic factors. Despite laws for combating asset-sheltering schemes, such techniques continue to erode the private-pay census. The cost of skilled nursing has out-paced general inflation as well as increases in Social Security and pension incomes for the elderly, causing a legitimate acceleration in the process of spending down assets. Moreover, assisted living and home health care alternatives continue to penetrate deeper into traditional nursing facility markets. Over the long run, these alternatives are expected to apply greater competitive pressures on nursing facilities, as they are generally preferred by residents, families, and "progressive" government policymakers. As more states roll out Medicaid waiver programs designed to move lower-acuity patients from nursing facilities into assisted living and other residential alternatives, the percentage of private-pay may increase, but at the expense of total census. It is important to consider these trends in the local competitive market in making census-mix forecasts.

Medicare and Managed Care (Private Insurance) Mix Forecasting

The same considerations and processing used in forecasting the private-pay census are appropriate in forecasting the Medicare and managed care mix for a nursing facility. Since Medicare and managed care are often more profitable than private-pay, new nursing facilities are being designed with a focus on maximizing Medicare and managed care patients with more private rooms, high-end therapy areas, etc. Although they make up a small percentage of the total census, Medicare and managed care are generally very profitable and volatile. Thus considerable care should be taken in estimating these components of the census. Unlike the private-pay mix, Medicare census is gradually increasing nationwide (see Tables 11.5 and 11.6).

Table 11.5 Trends in Medicare Census between 2001 and 2007: Includes Freestanding and Hospital-Based Skilled Nursing Units

Year	Average Daily Medicare Census	Medicare Census Mix
2001	139,452	9.5%
2002	152,279	10.5%
2003	164,244	11.3%
2004	174,696	12.1%
2005	178,824	12.4%
2006	190,283	13.3%
2007	193,150	13.6%

Source: *Trends in Nursing Facility Characteristics*, December 2007.

Table 11.6 Ratio of 65+ Population to Annual Medicare Patient Days

State	Average Medicare Census in SNF Beds—2005*	65+ Population—2005†	Annual Patient Days Paid by Medicare Per Person Age 65+	State	Average Medicare Census in SNF Beds—2005*	65+ Population—2005†	Annual Patient Days Paid by Medicare Per Person Age 65+
Alabama	3,056	608,154	1.8339	Montana	547	128,918	1.5482
Alaska	60	44,153	0.4958	Nebraska	1,113	236,305	1.7189
Arizona	1,463	747,704	0.7142	Nevada	489	271,172	0.6584
Arkansas	1,681	388,721	1.5782	New Hampshire	827	161,340	1.8716
California	11,902	3,894,444	1.1155	New Jersey	6,985	1,155,796	2.2059
Colorado	1,639	459,696	1.3014	New Mexico	665	233,490	1.0395
Connecticut	3,998	483,420	3.0184	New York	13,623	2,545,571	1.9534
Delaware	629	111,330	2.0622	North Carolina	5,567	1,055,819	1.9245
District of Columbia	259	68,395	1.3821	North Dakota	435	94,496	1.6813
Florida	13,448	3,025,779	1.6222	Ohio	10,170	1,544,733	2.4031
Georgia	3,610	869,355	1.5155	Oklahoma	2,135	474,106	1.6436
Hawaii	347	174,581	0.7255	Oregon	1,110	468,566	0.8645
Idaho	750	162,083	1.6886	Pennsylvania	9,103	1,936,102	1.7161
Illinois	9,540	1,540,572	2.2603	Rhode Island	850	153,869	2.0167
Indiana	5,594	781,093	2.6139	South Carolina	2,385	533,230	1.6324
Iowa	1,641	440,303	1.3603	South Dakota	448	110,653	1.4777
Kansas	1,462	358,716	1.4877	Tennessee	4,801	754,891	2.3211
Kentucky	3,089	529,375	2.1298	Texas	10,883	2,270,469	1.7495
Louisiana	2,446	536,772	1.6633	Utah	927	209,060	1.6184
Maine	1,008	194,376	1.8933	Vermont	398	82,887	1.7521
Maryland	3,596	651,873	2.0136	Virginia	4,120	870,215	1.7282
Massachusetts	5,953	870,833	2.4951	Washington	2,708	716,440	1.3798
Michigan	6,468	1,266,564	1.8641	West Virginia	1,266	283,888	1.6273
Minnesota	3,504	626,008	2.0428	Wisconsin	4,015	727,678	2.0141
Mississippi	1,678	358,105	1.7099	Wyoming	344	62,153	2.0209
Missouri	4,043	781,591	1.8882	**United States**	**178,824**	**37,055,843**	**1.7614**

Sources:

* *The State Long-Term Health Care Sector 2005: Characteristics, Utilization and Government Funding*, The American Health Care Association

† Claritas

Medicare demand is driven by hospital discharges. In 2006 there were 13.24 million Medicare discharges from all hospital types in the United States and 2.54 million Medicare admissions into skilled nursing facilities, showing that 19.2% of all Medicare discharges will be followed by a nursing facility stay that averages 26.4 days.[4]

Case Study

Continuing with the case study, the census mix forecast presented here relates to a typical nursing facility in a competitive market. The subject achieves a 16.7% Medicare market share (25/150). The location, physical plant, and management of the subject are above average, which is confirmed by its census characteristics.

Assume the following:

- 130 of the 950 occupied beds in the market are covered by Medicare.
- Total bed supply is currently 1,000 (95% occupancy).
- A CON was recently granted for 100 additional beds within the market. That facility is now under construction in a more affluent area of the primary market area and the facility design will incorporate superior features such as more private rooms, a separate rehab wing, all private toilets, and more common areas.
- Total demand and Medicare demand are expected to increase steadily each year by 2.0%.
- The new facility is expected to achieve a superior Medicare census because of its "state-of-the-art" rehab unit. The expected stabilized Medicare census for the new facility is 30.
- The 120-bed subject facility is expected to maintain its current Medicare market share among the existing supply.
- Based on these assumptions and the calculations in Table 11.7, the average Medicare census at the subject will decline from 15 to 11.8, and the Medicare mix will decline from 13.2 percent to 11.0 percent in one year.

This decline, coupled with the declining occupancy rate, will have a significant negative impact on cash flow. The impact from the lost Medicare census alone is shown in Table 11.8.

The case study shows that the subject will lose 1,168 Medicare patient days annually as the market adjusts to include the new facility that contains a "state-of-the-art" rehab unit. Assuming a marginal Medicare operating expense of $300.00 per patient day, the lost Medicare census will cause a corresponding $116,800 decrease in net operating income, or EBITDAR.

Putting all the pieces of this case study together provides a comprehensive view of the mechanical workings of a typical market when competition increases. Table 11.9 shows that the subject will lose Medicare and private-pay census along with a decline

4. Medicare Data Extract System, Centers for Medicare & Medicaid Services. http://www.cms.hhs.gov/Medicare

Table 11.7 **Forecasting Market and Subject Medicare Census**

		Current (2008)	1 Yr. From Now
Current bed supply	a	1,000	1,100
Bed demand growth–2.0% annually			
Current occupied beds	b	950	969
Market occupancy rate (b / a)	c	95.0%	88.1%
Subject occupied beds	d	114.0	107.2
Market Medicare occupied beds	e	130	132.6
New facility Medicare census at stabilization	f	0	30
Medicare census allocated to balance of supply (e – f)	g	130	102.6
Subject Medicare census, currently	h	15	
Subject Medicare market share, next year @ current year's market share (h / g)	i	11.5%	
Forecasted Medicare market share for subject, excluding demand captured by new facility (= i)	j		11.5%
Subject Medicare census (g × i or j)	k	15.0	11.8
Subject Medicare mix (j / d)	l	13.2%	11.0%

Table 11.8 **Impact on Revenues and Earnings Resulting from Change in Medicare Mix Caused by Additional Competition**

		Current (2008)	1 Yr. From Now
Subject occupied beds	d	114	107.2
Total annual patient days	m	41,610	39,128
Total lost patient days	n		2,482
Subject Medicare census	k	15	11.8
Annual Medicare patient days (k × 365 days)	o	5,475	4,307
Lost Medicare days	p		1,168
Average Medicare rate	q		$400.00
Medicare revenue loss (p × q)	r		$467,200
Reduction in operating expenses as a result of lower Medicare census ($300.00 × p)	s		$(350,400)
Medicare marginal NOI loss (r – s)	t		$116,800
Marginal income capitalization rate	u		12.5%
Capitalized value difference (t / u)			$934,400
Other patient days lost (private-pay and Medicaid) (n – p)			1,314

in total census. At the same time, some of the emptied private-pay and Medicare beds are now filled with Medicaid patients. That Medicaid demand would have settled for inferior facilities under prior market conditions. This case study does not explore managed care and other payor mixes, but the principles involved are the same.

Occupancy and Census Mix

Table 11.9 Impact on Subject Facility Census, Revenues, and Earnings Resulting From Additional Competition

	Current Average Census	1 Yr. From Now	Current Average Daily Rate	Average Daily Rate Forecasted	Change
Payor					
Private-pay	40.0	33.6	$184.28	$184.28	
Medicare	15.0	11.8	338.82	338.82	
Medicaid	59.0	61.8	147.13	147.13	
Total	114.0	107.2	$185.39	$179.87	$(5.51)
Annual Figures	**Annual Patient Days**	**Annual Patient Days**	**Current Annual Revenue**	**Forecasted Annual Revenue**	**Change**
Private-pay	14,600	12,264	$2,690,560	$2,260,070	$(430,490)
Medicare	5,475	4,307	1,855,045	1,459,302	(395,743)
Medicaid	21,535	22,557	3,168,377	3,318,741	150,364
Total annual patient days	41,610	39,128	$7,713,981	$7,038,113	$(675,869)
Ancillary revenues			72,818	68,474	(4,344)
Total revenues			$7,786,799	$7,106,587	$(680,212)
Total Operating Expenses					
Private-pay and Medicaid			$4,980,374	$4,830,963	$(149,411)
Medicare			1,505,625	1,460,456	(45,169)
Total operating expenses, including management and replacement reserves			$6,485,999	$6,291,419	$(194,580)
Net operating income - EBITDAR			$1,300,800	$815,168	$(485,632)

Managed Care

The typical nursing facility census will have just a small percentage of managed care and other private insurance patients. The same processes used to estimate private-pay and/or Medicare census can be applied for this payor group. As mentioned in Chapter 5, some states have high percentages of residents selecting Medicare Advantage programs or managed care alternatives. Facilities in these states will probably require closer scrutiny than facilities in states with little managed care penetration, which usually have a considerable rural population.

Medicaid Mix Forecasting

Medicaid is the payor of last resort and the Medicaid mix is estimated as the number of patient days remaining after deducting Medicaid, private-pay, and other days from the total projected patient days. While this payor often represents the largest component of the census, an analysis of the Medicaid mix can be the default to the private-pay and Medicare mix forecasts.

As Table 11.10 shows, Medicaid is gradually representing fewer patients and a declining percentage of the overall payor mix in nursing facilities.

The number of Medicare patients has been increasing as the number of Medicaid patients declines. The declining Medicaid numbers are evidence that Medicaid waivers are effective in diverting qualified patients from nursing facilities to assisted living and home health care alternatives.

Table 11.10 Trends in Medicaid Census between 2001 and 2007, Includes Freestanding and Hospital-Based Skilled Nursing Units

Year	Average Daily Medicaid Census	Medicaid Census Mix
2001	977,678	66.9%
2002	971,398	66.7%
2003	961,774	66.3%
2004	949,586	65.9%
2005	945,623	65.7%
2006	927,110	64.9%
2007	914,620	64.4%

Source: Medicare Data Extract System.

Other Payor Mix Issues

Nursing facilities that specialized in care for the developmentally disabled and mentally retarded (DD/MR) are often 100% Medicaid, and many of these facilities lack Medicare certification. For this facility type, there is little or no need to conduct a payor mix analysis. These facilities are typically licensed as intermediate care facilities (ICF-DD /MR) and their populations do not mix well with the typical skilled nursing facility patients. Developing supply, demand, and occupancy forecasts for this specialty, or for any other specialty facility or unit, should be limited to analysis of similar specialty facilities. Market areas for ICF-DD/MR facilities can span an entire metropolitan area or even an entire state.

In 1990 the Americans with Disabilities Act became law, and one of the significant outcomes of that law is known as the Olmstead Decision. This legislation mandates states to transfer suitable ICF-DD/MR patients from large institutional or nursing home settings into community group homes. An investigation into state plans to close their remaining large ICF-DD/MR facilities is critical to any analysis of an ICF-DD/MR facility. ICF-DD/MR facilities are typically housed in older buildings that have limited appeal for conversion into skilled nursing facilities, even if it is legally or physically possible. Thus, the remaining economic life of such a facility may be short and difficult to estimate, and sale data is scarce.

Facilities that specialize in Alzheimer's and memory care typically cater to long-term patients and Medicare and managed care typically represent a small proportion of the census of this patient type. These patients generate longer average lengths of stay and consequently have greater dependency on Medicaid. A competitive market analysis of facilities for this specialty group should only include other freestanding and specialty memory care units. Many general nursing facilities will mix these patients into their regular population, and many memory care facilities using assisted living platforms retain the residents beyond the point when they should be transferred to a nursing facility. Therefore, it may prove difficult to obtain an accurate census of the Alzheimer's and memory care market. The same principles applied to develop occupancy and payor mix forecasts for skilled nursing facilities are applicable to these special facilities.

Summary

Census or payor mix profoundly impacts revenues, earnings, and value and its impact can be measured in all three valuation approaches. There are four major sources of payment: Medicaid, Medicare, private insurance (managed care) and private-pay. Profitability levels vary between these groups, with Medicare generally being the most profitable and Medicaid the least profitable. Mix is usually measured by patient days, however, some reporting uses "revenue mix," in which the revenue from each payment source is compared to the total revenue. The techniques applied to estimate occupancy and total patient days are equally applicable to forecasting census and days for private-pay, Medicare, managed care, and Medicaid, using market share and penetration rates. Nationally, the average Medicare mix in nursing facilities is slightly less than 15%, Medicaid represents slightly less than 65%, and private-pay, managed care, and some miscellaneous payment sources represent the remainder. New competition often has the greatest impact on the Medicare, managed care and private-pay mixes of the existing supply. Omitting the impact of new competition may result in a crucial valuation error.

Chapter 12

Revenue Forecasting

Revenue is forecast by combining the occupancy and payor mix forecasts with daily routine rates and ancillary and miscellaneous charges derived from private-pay, Medicaid, Medicare, and other payors.

The valuation and treatment of revenue for other types of long-term care offered by independent or assisted living, rehabilitation, and long-term acute care hospitals, are not covered in this book. The combination of any of these other components of long-term care in a skilled nursing facility can significantly complicate the valuation. Many of the revenue issues affecting other long-term care uses also affect nursing facilities. Of course, Medicaid and Medicare reimbursements differ. If these other components are included in the subject facility, the revenues they produce should be developed through separate analyses of their respective competitive markets and reimbursement systems. Developing a separate set of operating expenses for these other components might be necessary too because Medicaid reimbursements may be tied to facility-specific, allowable costs. Moreover, application of the income capitalization and sale comparison approaches may require the appraiser to weigh the earnings from the various components to assess valuation indicators.

Routine rates are payments for room and board, nursing and personal care, social services, and activities. Routine revenues do not typically include payments for therapy services, physician services, prescription medicines, or hospitalization charges for residents at the nursing facility. Routine services are typically billed on a per-diem basis. Usually, private-pay and Medicaid rates cover routine costs, while ancillaries are provided at an additional charge.

Ancillary revenue includes income derived from therapies, certain medical supplies, certain medications, and charges for other services. The vast majority of ancillary revenue is reimbursed through Medicare Parts A and B and from managed care and other private insurance. Medicare Part A incorporates routine and ancillary reimbursement into a single rate; however, many nursing facility's financial statements will separate Medicare routine and ancillary revenues. For revenue forecasting, Medicare Part A typically includes routine and ancillary income.

Miscellaneous income is derived from non-care sources and typically includes changes for personal laundry, vending machine income, salon services, guest and employee meal sales, and charges for medical supplies not covered by Medicare, managed care, or Medicaid. Other revenue can also be realized from rentals for space leased to related or third parties adult day care programs, or outpatient therapy.

Medicare and some managed care payments will incorporate both routine service and ancillary charges into a single reimbursement rate. Since routine revenue is the primary income source for nearly all nursing facilities, this topic will be treated first. Ancillary and miscellaneous revenue will be covered next.

Chapters 5 and 6 provide considerable guidance in determining Medicare Part A and Medicaid reimbursements. Chapters 9, 10, and 11 present procedures for developing occupancy and census mix forecasts. The remaining components of revenue to be discussed are routine revenues from private-pay and other payors; ancillary revenues, which are typically achieved through Medicare Part B; and out-of-pocket receipts from private-pay patients.

A number of the revenue calculations presented in this chapter will be demonstrated with the case study that is developed throughout the book.

Routine Revenue—Private-Pay

Most nursing facilities express routine private-pay charges on a per-diem basis. While Medicare and Medicaid pay in arrears, private-pay charges can be collected at the beginning of a billing period; billing cycles are usually monthly. Typically, nursing facilities charge the same rate to all private-pay patients receiving the same level of care in the same type of room. Rate increases are usually applied to all private-pay patients at the same time, not on anniversary dates. Rate or rental concessions are not offered to induce admissions. Facilities do occasionally have difficulty collecting all of the private-pay charges, especially when a patient is transitioning from Medicare to private-pay or Medicaid. Those unpaid charges are expensed as bad debt and, depending on the Medicaid reimbursement system, bad debt expenses may not be allowable in the Medicaid reimbursement rate calculation.

Private-pay rates are unregulated in most states and are only subject to competitive market forces. Minnesota and North Dakota restrict routine rates to amounts that are no greater than the Medicaid rate for the facility. Private-pay rates are allowed to be less than Medicaid rates. However, this has not always been the case. Federal rules have relaxed a long-standing requirement that prohibited private-pay rates from being lower than the Medicaid rate for the facility for the same level of care. This rule is applied differently by different states, with many requiring private-pay rates to equal or exceed Medicaid rates. There is very little evidence to suggest that Medicaid-funded residents receive consistently lower-quality care than private-pay patients within a given nursing home.[1]

To develop private-pay revenue forecasts, the appraiser first estimates private-pay patient days and an average private-pay rate. The estimate of private-pay patient days is part of the occupancy rate and private-pay mix forecasts. Comparing Medicaid and Medicare rates for routine services is typically unnecessary since these rates are determined by specific formulas and are not directly established by competitive market forces.

Overall, the cost of care within a skilled nursing facility has steadily increased while "non-skilled care" costs have remained relatively flat (see Figure 12.1). For example, in 2008 the average annual rate for a private nursing home room was $76,460, compared with a 2004 average annual rate of $65,185. This increase represents 4.07% compound annual growth over that period and means that Americans can expect to pay over $10,000 more per year than five years ago.[2] As the previous data shows, the average difference between the private and semi-private SNF room rate in 2008 was $20.58 per day.

Private-pay rate forecasts are developed by analyzing past and current rates for the subject and comparing them with rates at comparable facilities in the market. It is important to learn what services and supplies are included in the basic rate as these can vary substantially within markets. Most nursing facility operating statements will not separate private and semi-private room revenues and that information may not be available. Understanding the historical private-pay mix between private and semi-private rooms becomes increasingly important when

---

1. National Bureau of Economic Research, white paper no. 12361, July 1, 2006, "Nursing Home Quality as a Public Good," David C. Grabowski, Jonathan Gruber, and Joseph J. Angelelli.
2. Genworth Financial, *2008 Cost of Care Survey*, April 2008, Home Care Providers, Adult Day Health Care Facilities, Assisted Living Facilities and Nursing Homes.

Figure 12.1 **Five-Year National Trend in Average Annual Private-Pay Skilled Nursing and Assisted Living Costs**

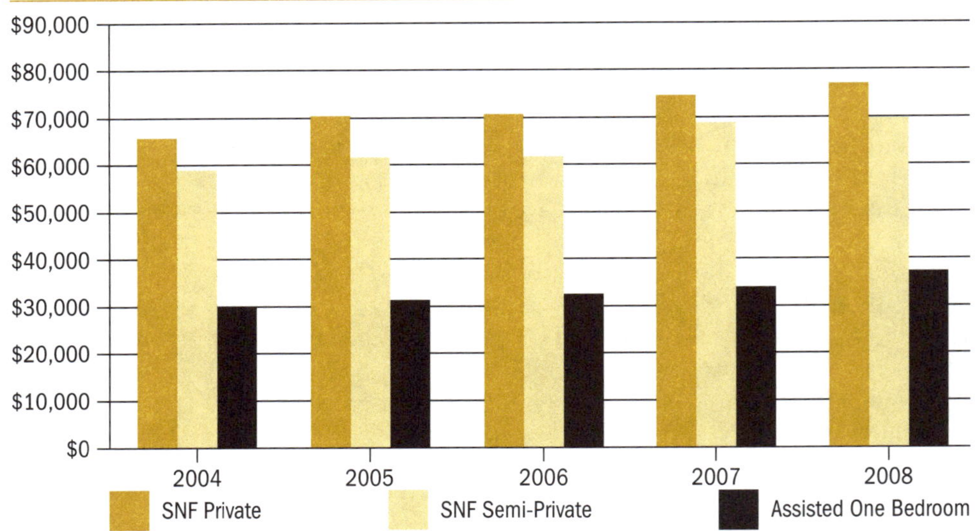

Source: Genworth Financial, *2008 Cost of Care,* April 2008, Home Care Providers, Adult Day Health Care Facilities, Assisted Living Facilities, and Nursing Homes.

there is a high ratio of private rooms and/or the gap between the private and semi-private rates is substantial. In the absence of actual historical information, the room mix can be obtained by questioning the administrator or the bookkeeper. It is rare to find any significant private-pay census within ward rooms, unless a facility has few private and semi-private rooms. In that case, the facility usually has a low private-pay census mix.

Most facilities will charge a fixed rate to all patients for a specific room type, regardless of the acuity of care. Some facilities will scale charges according to acuity, but this system requires additional charting and billing and often proves counterproductive. Some facilities will place patients with heavier or lighter care needs in a unit or wing of the building that is staffed for a different level of care, and rates may vary for beds in those units. Again, obtaining historical census and revenue information for the various private-pay acuity levels may be nearly impossible.

Trending historical private-pay rates for inflation is one technique that may be useful in forecasting revenue. This method is most reliable when the forces of supply and demand are in balance, causing no undue pressure on rates, and the future room mix and acuity levels are expected to be consistent with the past. Rate indications from historical trending are less reliable when there is an anticipated change in room or acuity mix, or the facility is undergoing a renovation that results in market repositioning. Also, a change in the competitive market can place pressure on rates. These issues should be weighed when considering the use of historical trending in the development of the private-pay revenue forecast.

Comparing the current private-pay rates of the subject to the rates of competitive facilities is a familiar process for appraisers–i.e., a rent comparison. However, the elements of comparison differ. Elements of comparison pertinent to private-pay rates include

- Physical plant considerations, which are real-estate driven
- Location considerations, which are also real-estate driven
- Quality of care, which relates more closely to intangible components of value

Most, if not all, of the information needed to conduct a comprehensive comparison of market-determined rates can be obtained with a reasonable amount of research and review of public documents.

Physical Plant Comparison

Physical plant conditions can be assessed by touring the competitive properties, reviewing property assessment records, interviewing management, or even reviewing building plans filed at the state's health department. The following physical plant factors should be considered in analyzing private-pay rates and other rates that may be set by competitive market forces (e.g., private insurance):

- Overall age, condition, cleanliness, and quality of the facility. For obvious reasons, newer facilities with higher-quality finishes and fresher appearances should command higher rates than older, lower-quality facilities with exhausted appearances, everything else being equal.
- Site and landscaping. The facility's exterior often makes a lasting first impression, and a favorable or unfavorable appearance relative to the competition that can show up in rates as well as occupancy and census mix levels.
- Common area amenities for patients and the design, layout, size, and attractiveness of dining, living, congregating, therapy, and other public areas. Rate premiums can be achieved when facilities provide greater common space areas for patients and their visitors. Facilities designed to include smaller living, dining, and lounge areas spread out into "neighborhoods" that create a less institutional atmosphere are viewed more favorably than facilities with large rooms centered around the building core. Designs with small din-

ing or event rooms for private gatherings, libraries, theater rooms, craft rooms, snack parlors, and other specific-purpose areas, where patients and visitors can gather for personal and recreational activities, can not only elevate census and quality mix, but also command higher rates.

- Patient rooms–sizes, privacy, toilet and bathing facilities (private or shared), furniture, storage, and decorating. Patient room size affects rates for many of the same reasons room size affects hotel room rates and apartment unit rents. For many patients, personal possessions are reduced to fit the space in a patient room. Since most patients will occupy a bed in a semi-private room, their privacy correlates to the distance between the beds. However, the market does not measure rates by dollars per square foot and most facilities do not mention room square footage in their marketing materials. Rate differences based on size are subjective.

Rooms with private toilets rather than shared, adjoining toilets command rate premiums. In fact, facilities with both arrangements often attach a premium for rooms with private toilets. Furnishings, interior finishes, storage, and exterior views may also affect rates.

Location Comparison

Location assessment requires knowledge of the area and of demographic data. The immediate surroundings, general reputation of the neighborhood, and proximity to the patients' familiar "stomping grounds" are important. Proximity to medical centers, cultural facilities, and access points are additional factors that can distinguish one facility from another enough to impact rate levels.

Nearby medical services may provide patients and their families with a sense of security and will certainly reduce transportation time. Facilities in locations that are more convenient for physicians and other medical professionals may be able to capitalize on this advantage and achieve higher rates. Accessibility can affect rates in other ways too. The surrounding environment–adjacent and nearby land uses, property value levels, etc.–plays into the desirability of nursing facilities just as the environment influences rent and occupancy levels for other types of real estate. A nursing facility situated in a neighborhood dominated by commercial or industrial uses may be less desirable than otherwise similar facilities located in areas with higher concentrations of residential, medical, public, and/or cultural land uses. While many of these factors are difficult to describe objectively, and difficult to translate into rate differences, household income levels and residential and commercial property values are objective measures that may correlate to rate variances among competitive facilities in a market.

Quality and Levels of Care (Intangible) Comparison

Quality of care differences can be identified by reviewing online health surveys, which show survey deficiencies and nursing staffing ratios. A review of Medicaid cost reports may also reveal staffing levels and costs. The Medicare and Medicaid cost reports will also show food and dietary costs, which may be indicators of patient satisfaction, although costs do not necessarily equate to value or quality. The following factors can be used to distinguish differences in quality of care and care levels.

- Level of care. Higher-acuity patients require more staffing and those greater costs are passed through.
- Nurse staffing ratios. Differences in staffing affect expenses and possibly quality of care. The differences in nursing expenses should be reflected in the rates.
- Health care survey results. Quality of care can be objectively measured by comparing the number and severity of health care deficiencies and the staffing ratios reported in annual healthcare surveys.
- General reputation of operator. Reputation is a subjective measure, but the occupancy rate, census mix, and even rate levels are often tell-tale signs of the reputation of the facility.
- Quality of food and type of food service.
- Quality of rehabilitation services. Rehab services may be affected by the physical capacities of the plant.

Quality of Care Assessment Using Government Survey Data

While state governments oversee the licensing of nursing homes, CMS, under the Department of Health and Human Services, monitors states and requires that Medicare- and Medicaid-certified facilities meet minimum requirements established by the U.S. Congress. CMS partners with each state to determine if the minimum quality and performance standards are being met through onsite inspections. These inspections are typically conducted by employees of the state's health department or department of human services. All Medicare- and Medicaid-certified nursing facilities are surveyed on an annual basis or more often if a complaint warrants investigation.

Inspectors, typically a small team of trained nurses and social workers, will observe resident care procedures, staff/resident interaction, and environmental conditions and sanitation. They apply an established protocol, which includes interviews with a sample of patients family members, caregivers, and administrative staff. Clinical records are also closely examined. Fire safety specialists evaluate whether a nursing home meets standards for safe construction and emergency preparedness. When an inspection team finds that a home does not meet a specific standard, it issues a citation for the specific deficiencies, and the facility is required to submit a plan of correction and comply with the requirement. With more than 150 regulatory standards, a wide range of clinical and administrative issues are covered.

Figure 12.2 is a sample "overview" summary from the Medicare Web site NHCompare, which lists health care deficiencies, fire safety deficiencies, and nurse staffing minutes per patient day.

Figure 12.2 **Sample of a Health Care Deficiencies, Fire Safety Deficiencies, and Nurse Staffing Minutes Per Patient Day Report on the Medicare Web Site**

About the Nursing Home	Quality Measures	Total Number of Health Deficiencies Fire Safety Deficiencies	Nursing Staff Hours per Resident per Day	CNA Hours per Resident per Day
FACILITY NAME FACILITY NAME CITY, STATE AND ZIP CODE PHONE NUMBER Mapping/Directions View all information about this nursing home	Information for 19 of the 19 quality measures is available	5 Health Deficiencies 0 Fire Safety Deficiencies	52 minutes	1 hour 49 minutes
			Total Number of Residents: 165	

Source: http://www.medicare.gov/NHCompare

The NHCompare Web site offers further staffing, health care deficiency, and fire safety details. Figure 12.3 shows an example of survey postings citing a specific facility for staffing and health and fire safety deficiencies.

The staffing survey shown in Figure 12.3 indicates that the subject facility provides less than half of the national and statewide averages for registered nursing minutes. One reason the subject may allot fewer RN minutes per patient day may stem from economies of scale that relate to the larger patient census. The subject also has fewer CNA hours per patient day, which may also be attributable in part to economies of scale.

For this facility, the higher census and lower nursing staff ratios have not translated into a higher number of health care deficiencies. Figure 12.4 shows the deficiencies reported in the most recent survey of the same facility along with the severity levels and the amount of patients (residents) affected by each

Figure 12.3 **Sample of a Detailed Nurse Staffing Minutes Per Patient Day Report on the Medicare Web Site**

Nursing Homes and/or Skilled Nursing Facilities for residents needing short or long stay Nursing Staff Hours Per Resident Per Day, is the average hours worked by the licensed nurses or nursing assistants divided by total number of residents. The amount of care given to each resident varies.					
	Number of Residents	**Licensed RN Hours per Resident per Day**	**Licensed LPN/LVN Hours per Resident per Day**	**Total Number of Licensed Nurse Staff Hours per Resident per Day**	**CNA Hours per Resident per Day**
National Average	95.4	30 minutes	48 minutes	1 hour 18 minutes	2 hours 18 minutes
Average in Illinois	106	36 minutes	36 minutes	1 hour 12 minutes	2 hours
FACILITY NAME	165	14 minutes	37 minutes	52 minutes	1 hour 49 minutes

Source: http://www.medicare.gov/NHCompare

deficiency. The quantity and severity of the deficiencies found at the subject facility, measured against the competitors, can provide an objective basis for assessing quality of care differences that can affect occupancy and payor mix as well as private-pay rates and other rates set by market forces.

Other Intangible Factors

The general reputation of the operator may not match survey results and that facility may experience success or failure in a market for reasons unrelated to the care it provides. A facility can promote its reputation through aggressive advertising, marketing, and public relations efforts. Ownership affiliation with a hospital system, a prominent religious institution, or another enterprise may allow a nursing facility to price its private-pay rates more aggressively. On the other hand, relationships with non-profit organizations often reduce incentives to increase private-pay rates. Rates at for-profit facilities may experience lasting competitive pressure if the facility competes with a number of non-profit facilities that set private-pay rates below market levels. If the subject is a non-profit facility with unusually low private-pay rates, the rate forecasting and valuation analysis may need to mark those rates up to market levels.

Using the information gathered through personal interviews and inspections of the competitive properties, coupled with information obtained through public sources, the appraiser can estimate market rates for private-pay beds through a comparison process that is similar to the market rent comparisons made for apartment, office, and retail property. However, because of

Figure 12.4 **Sample of Detailed Health Care and Fire Safety Deficiency Report on the Medicare Web Site**

FACILITY NAME **STREET ADDRESS** **CITY AND STATE** **PHONE NUMBER**			
Date of last standard health inspection:			01/10/08
Quality Indicator Survey			No
Dates of Complaint Investigations:			02/01/2007 - 04/30/2008
Total number of Health deficiencies for this nursing home:			5
Average number of Health Deficiencies in Illinois:			8
Average number of Health Deficiencies in the United States:			9
Range of Health Deficiencies in Illinois:			0 - 82
View Previous Inspection Results			
? Resident Rights Deficiencies			
Inspectors determined that the nursing home failed to:	**Date of Correction**	**Level of Harm (Least -> Most)**	**Residents Affected (Few -> Some -> Many)**
1. Properly hold, secure and manage each resident's personal money which is deposited with the nursing home. (01/10/2008)	01/18/08	2 = Minimal harm or potential for actual harm 1 **2** 3 4	Some
2. Quickly give a resident's personal money to the heads of his or her estate after the resident's death. (01/10/2008)	01/18/08	2 = Minimal harm or potential for actual harm 1 **2** 3 4	Some
? Nutrition and Dietary Deficiencies			
Inspectors determined that the nursing home failed to:	**Date of Correction**	**Level of Harm (Least -> Most)**	**Residents Affected (Few -> Some -> Many)**
3. Make sure that residents are well nourished. (01/10/2008)	01/18/08	2 = Minimal harm or potential for actual harm 1 **2** 3 4	Few
4. Store, cook, and give out food in a safe and clean way. (01/10/2008)	01/18/08	2 = Minimal harm or potential for actual harm 1 **2** 3 4	Some
? Environmental Deficiencies			
Inspectors determined that the nursing home failed to:	**Date of Correction**	**Level of Harm (Least -> Most)**	**Residents Affected (Few -> Some -> Many)**
5. Keep all essential equipment working safely. (01/10/2008)	01/18/08	2 = Minimal harm or potential for actual harm 1 **2** 3 4	Some

↑	↑	↑	↑
This column displays deficiency text and the date the deficiency was found.	Date the inspectors found deficiency corrected.	Level of harm is the assessment of the effect the deficiency has on residents.	Number of residents potentially or actually affected by the deficiency

the many subtle differences between nursing facilities, isolating just one difference between two properties to support a matched pair analysis and specific dollar-amount rate adjustments is nearly impossible Therefore, non-specific adjustment amounts must usually suffice for rate adjustments.

Table 12.1 is a comparison grid that illustrates a suggested process for adjusting private-pay rates. This example compares the semi-private room rates charged at two competitive facilities to the rate charged for a semi-private room at the subject. The subject and the second competitive facility offer private toilet facilities in each patient room while the semi-private rooms in the first competitive facility share toilets with another room. Note that the adjustment comments refer to each competitive facility as being superior or inferior to the subject facility.

In this example, the subject currently charges $170.00 per day for a semi-private room. Comparison with two direct competitors indicates that the current rate for the subject is below market level. If the subject has not implemented a rate increase for some time, increasing the rate to the upper end of the adjusted range, to $180.00, may be justified. That would result in a 5.9% increase, which may be reasonable given the market competition and general inflationary pressures. If the

Table 12.1 **Comparison and Rate Adjustments for Private-Pay Patient in Semi-Private Room With and Without Private Toilet**

		Comparable 1		Comparable 2	
	Subject	**Comment**	**Adjustment**	**Comment**	**Adjustment**
Semi-private room rate	$170.00		$165.00		$190.00
Physical Plant Considerations					
Effective age of building	20	30	+	10	-
Quality and overall appearance	Good	Inferior	+	Superior	-
Common area amenities	Good	Inferior	+	Superior	-
Private room size, privacy	Average	Similar	0	Superior	-
Patient room toilet/bathing	Private	Semi-private	+	Private	0
Location Considerations					
Proximity to medical services	Good	Superior	-	Inferior	+
Accessibility	Average	Similar	0	Similar	0
Surrounding environment	Average	Superior	-	Similar	0
Quality of Care					
Level of care	Typical	Same	0	Same	0
Nurse staffing ratios (total nursing hours PPD)	2.8	2.6	0	3.2	-
Health care survey results	5	11	+	6	0
General reputation of operator	Average	Inferior	+	Average	0
Quality of food and type of food service	Average	Heavy adv./mkt.	-	Average	0
Net difference			+++		---
Indicated market rate for semi-private room with private toilet			$180.00		$175.00

subject recently increased the rate to $170.00, another increase may meet with resistance. Still, a rate of $175.00 is probably justified in the near future.

Using this comparison and adjustment process for each major room type (private, semi-private, etc.) and applying the adjusted rates to the estimated annual private-pay days for each, the appraiser can calculate annual routine private-pay revenues. The private-pay revenue calculations shown in Table 12.2 continue the case study developed in previous chapters.

Case Study

Table 12.2 Forecast Routine Revenue for Private-Pay Patients

Type of Room	Days	Private-Pay Occupancy	Average Daily Rate	Total Revenue
Private-pay, private room	3,785	10.4	$210.00	$794,850
Private-pay semi-private room, with private toilet	4,758	13.0	175.00	832,650
Private-pay semi-private room, with shared toilet	3,721	10.2	170.00	632,570
Total private-pay routine revenue	12,264	33.6	$184.28	$2,260,070

Private-pay revenue for ancillary services and miscellaneous income are estimated separately. These revenues are significantly less than the routine revenues and are treated as separate line items following routine revenues in most operating statements.

Medicare Part A Revenues

Chapter 5 presented a fairly comprehensive overview of the principles of Medicare reimbursement. These revenues are legislated and, other than some possible manipulation of Medicare DRGs, there is no action that a facility or the competitive market can take that will affect Medicare reimbursements. Facilities typically bill the Medicare intermediary at the end of each month and usually receive payment four to six weeks later. A very brief summary of Medicare Part A reimbursement principles is presented below.

Medicare Part A is the federal health insurance program for people 65 years of age or older, and it also covers younger people with certain disabilities and people with permanent kidney failure. Medicare covers the patient's entire cost for the first 20 days of an eligible stay. To receive another 80 days of potential coverage, the patient or his or her secondary insurer must make a co-payment. As of October 1, 2007, the co-payment was $128.00, and that co-payment is typically paid by the patient or by Medicaid. To receive the Medicare coverage, the patient must have spent three consecutive days as an inpatient in a hospital and be discharged to a nursing facility to continue receiving skilled nursing and rehabilitation care. Note that very few patients actually qualify for the full 100 days of Medicare coverage.

Medicare reimburses nursing facilities for Part A services using a flat-rate, case-mix structure known as the prospective payment system (PPS). PPS classifies patients into 53 categories based on nursing and rehabilitation needs known as RUGs III (resource utilization groups). Each category has a specific rate that is adjusted using a regional wage index. There are four components to PPS rates:

1. Nursing
2. Therapy
3. Therapy, non-case mix
4. Non-case mix

The RUG rate for each of the 53 categories consists of three of the four components: nursing, non-case mix, and either therapy or non-therapy case mix. The nursing and therapy components of the rate are adjusted for case mix, while all categories receive the same non-case-mix rate. The rate for the therapy, non-case mix is not adjusted for case mix. Table 12.3 presents the national rates for urban and rural facilities at 1.0 case mix indices for the nursing and therapy components.

Table 12.3 **Federal/PPS Unadjusted Rate Components—Effective October 1, 2008**

	Urban	Rural
1. Nursing @ 1.0 index	$151.74	$144.97
2. Therapy @ 1.0 index	$114.30	$131.80
3. Therapy, non-case mix	$15.05	$16.08
4. Non-case mix	$77.44	$78.87

Note: These rates are adjusted annually, using the federal fiscal year beginning October 1. Consult the *Federal Register* or visit www.gpoaccess.gov/fr/ for updates and further details.

Each of the 53 RUGs only receives *three* of the *four* components. There are 23 RUGs that involve therapy or rehabilitation services, and rates for those RUGs include the sum of (1) nursing, (2) therapy, and (4) non-case-mix. For the other RUGs, the rate is the sum of (1) nursing, (3) therapy, non-case mix, and (4) non-case-mix. The nursing case-mix indices range from 0.50 to 1.90, and the 23 therapy case-mix indices range from 0.43 to 2.25. The national average Medicare nursing and rehabilitation case-mix indices and the average percentages of total Medicare patient days using the 23 RUG categories receiving the rehabilitation rate component for the second quarters of 2006 and 2007 are summarized as follows.[3]

Period	Nursing	Therapy	Percentage of Medicare Days With RUGs Rehab
2nd Quarter 2006	1.29	1.04	91.2%
2nd Quarter 2007	1.31	1.14	85.2%

To estimate Medicare Part A revenue, Medicare patient days and rates need to be established. Several approaches can be taken to arrive at the revenue estimate, depending on the level of detail desired. The simplest way to estimate the Medicare revenue is to multiply the forecast Medicare patient days by the historical average Medicare rate, trended for inflation adjustments and possible changes in case-mix. The approach most often applied, which provides more accuracy and detail, is to estimate the average nursing and therapy case-mix indices and calculate an average Medicare rate to be applied to the total number of Medicare patient days forecast in the competitive market analysis. To estimate the case-mix indices for the nursing and therapy components of the rate, the appraiser must obtain the facility's historical Medicare census distributed to each of the 53 RUGs categories. The operator should be able to provide this level of detail fairly easily through billing statements or management tools. The following example illustrates this process step by step.

Calculation of the Medicare Part A Average Rate

As a first step, the nursing component of the rate is forecast by developing an average nursing case-mix index and multiplying that index by the Medicare nursing rate, which is adjusted for a local wage index. In this case, the prior year, current year, and national average nursing case-mix indices are considered in the development of a forecast index (see Table 12.4).

The next step in the Medicare rate development is to estimate the therapy portion of the rate. The process is the same as the one applied to develop the nursing component above, but with one more adjustment. The therapy component only applies to the 23 "therapy" RUG categories; the days involving "therapy, non-case mix" RUGs should be eliminated. Prior year, current year, and national average "therapy case-mix" indices are considered in the development of a forecast therapy index (see Table 12.5).

The next step is to calculate the "therapy non-case mix." This step involves applying the labor-adjusted "therapy, non-case-mix" rate to that percentage of the Medicare patient days that

3. Centers for Medicare & Medicaid Services.

Table 12.4 **Development of Nursing Component of the Medicare Rate—Nursing Component**

Medicare Revenue Forecasting, Step One			
Historical and forecasted nursing case-mix indices			
Subject, prior year	1.32		
Subject, current YTD	1.38		
National average, 2Q 2007	1.31		
Subject, forecasted	1.36		
Nursing rate, urban		$151.74	
Forecasted nursing case-mix index		1.36	
Labor portion of rate	×	0.69783	
Nursing rate subjected to wage indexing		143.90	
Local wage index	×	0.8695	
Subtotal			$125.12
Nursing rate, urban		$151.74	
Forecasted nursing case-mix index		1.36	
Non-labor portion of rate	×	0.30217	
Nursing rate subjected to wage indexing			62.31
Total average nursing component of the Medicare rate			$187.43

Note: Figures are rounded.

Table 12.5 **Development of Nursing Component of the Medicare Rate—Therapy or Rehab Component**

Medicare Revenue Forecasting, Step Two				
Historical and forecasted therapy case-mix indices and percentage of total Medicare days with therapy RUGs				
	Therapy Index			% Therapy Days
Subject, prior year	1.08			82.2%
Subject, current YTD	1.12			86.1%
National average, 2nd Quarter 2007	1.14			85.2%
Subject, forecasted	1.12			85.0%
Therapy rate, urban			$114.30	
Forecasted therapy case-mix index			1.12	
Labor portion of rate			0.69783	
Therapy rate subjected to wage indexing	×		$89.33	
Local wage index	×		0.8695	
Subtotal				$54.20
Therapy rate, urban			$114.30	
Forecasted therapy case-mix index			1.12	
Non-labor portion of therapy rate	×		0.30217	
Therapy rate subjected to wage indexing				38.68
Total average therapy component of the Medicare rate				$92.89
Percentage of total Medicare patient days with one of the 23 therapy RUGs		×		85.0%
Total weighted-average therapy component of the Medicare rate				$78.95

Note: Figures are rounded.

are classified within the 30 "therapy, non-case-mix" RUGs. This component of the rate is not adjusted for any sort of acuity factor. The rate compensates the operator for medical supplies, prescription drugs, medical equipment, ambulance services, laboratory and x-ray charges, orthotics, certain prosthetics, and a few emergency room treatments (see Table 12.6).

The fourth step involves the "non-case-mix" component. This component of the rate is not adjusted for any sort of acuity factor. It compensates the operator for administration, management, social services, dietary services, housekeeping, laundry, utilities, property maintenance, property insurance, property taxes, and capital-related costs (see Table 12.7).

Table 12.6 Development of Therapy, Non-Case-Mix Component of the Medicare Rate

Medicare Revenue Forecasting, Step Three			
Historical and forecasted therapy non-case-mix utilization			
			% Non-therapy Days
Subject, prior year			17.8%
Subject, current YTD			13.9%
National average, 2nd Quarter 2007			14.8%
Subject, forecasted			15.0%
Therapy, non-case-mix rate, urban		$15.05	
Labor portion of rate	×	0.69783	
Therapy, non-case-mix rate subjected to wage indexing		$10.50	
Local wage index	×	0.8695	
Subtotal			$9.13
Therapy non-case-mix rate, urban		$15.05	
Non-labor portion of therapy rate	×	0.30217	
Therapy rate subjected to wage indexing			4.55
Total average therapy component of the Medicare rate			$13.68
Percentage of total medicare patient days with one of the 30 "therapy, non-case-mix" RUGs		×	15.0%
Total weighted-average "therapy, non-case-mix" component of the Medicare rate			$2.05

Table 12.7 Development of Non-Case-Mix Component of the Medicare Rate

Medicare Revenue Forecasting, Step Four			
Non-case-mix rate, urban		$77.44	
Labor portion of rate	×	0.69783	
Therapy, non-case-mix rate subjected to wage indexing		$54.04	
Local wage index	×	0.8695	
Subtotal			$46.99
Non-case-mix rate, urban		$77.44	
Non-labor portion of the non-case-mix rate	×	0.30217	
Therapy rate subjected to wage indexing			23.40
Total non-case-mix rate			$70.39

The final step in estimating the Medicare Part A revenue is to sum the average rate for the four components and multiply that product by the forecast total Medicare patient days. The calculations shown above will be incorporated into the continuation of the case study in Table 12.8.

Case Study

Table 12.8 Medicare Part A Reimbursement Summary

Medicare Revenue Forecasting, Step Five		
Total average nursing component of the Medicare rate		$187.43
Total weighted-average therapy component of the Medicare rate		78.95
Total weighted-average "therapy, non-case-mix" component of the Medicare rate		2.05
Total non-case-mix rate		70.39
Total average Medicare Part A rate, forecasted		$338.82
Total annual forecasted Medicare patient days	×	4,307
Total forecasted Medicare Part A Revenue		$1,459,302

Note: Figures are rounded.

A third technique for estimating the Medicare Part A revenue is to run a series of rate calculations for each of the 53 RUG rates, adjusted for the wage index, and apply those rates to the estimated annual Medicare patient days for each RUG category. An example of this set of calculations is presented in Table 12.9. These calculations are easily made using any spreadsheet software.

Table 12.9 Sample Medicare Revenue Forecast Using Medicare Patient By RUG Days

RUG-III Category	Labor Portion	Local Wage Index	Labor-Adjusted Portion	Non-Labor Portion	Total Rate	Patient Days	Total Revenue
RUX	$434.70	0.8695	$377.97	$188.23	$566.20	100	$56,620
RUL	381.75	0.8695	331.93	165.31	497.24	150	74,586
RVX	329.57	0.8695	286.56	142.71	429.27	100	42,927
RVL	307.33	0.8695	267.22	133.08	400.30	246	98,475
RHX	279.38	0.8695	242.92	120.97	363.89	0	0
RHL	274.08	0.8695	238.31	118.68	356.99	0	0
RMX	319.82	0.8695	278.08	138.49	416.57	350	145,801
RML	293.35	0.8695	255.07	127.02	382.09	394	150,543
RLX	227.05	0.8695	197.42	98.32	295.74	64	18,927
RUC	369.05	0.8695	320.89	159.80	480.69	56	26,919
RUB	338.34	0.8695	294.19	146.50	440.69	284	125,155
RUA	322.45	0.8695	280.37	139.63	420.00	50	21,000
RVC	296.75	0.8695	258.02	128.49	386.51	125	48,314
RVB	281.92	0.8695	245.13	122.08	367.21	400	146,884
RVA	253.33	0.8695	220.27	109.70	329.97	250	82,493
RHC	258.20	0.8695	224.50	111.80	336.30	300	100,891
RHB	246.55	0.8695	214.38	106.76	321.14	187	60,052

Table 12.9 **Sample Medicare Revenue Forecast Using Medicare Patient By RUG Days *(continued)***

RUG-III Category	Labor Portion	Local Wage Index	Labor-Adjusted Portion	Non-Labor Portion	Total Rate	Patient Days	Total Revenue
RHA	228.55	0.8695	198.72	98.97	297.69	124	36,914
RMC	237.23	0.8695	206.27	102.72	308.99	94	29,045
RMB	230.88	0.8695	200.75	99.97	300.72	250	75,180
RMA	225.58	0.8695	196.14	97.68	293.82	71	20,861
RLB	209.05	0.8695	181.77	90.52	272.29	4	1,089
RLA	178.34	0.8695	155.07	77.23	232.30	4	929
SE3	261.50	0.8695	227.37	113.23	340.60	96	32,698
SE2	222.31	0.8695	193.30	96.27	289.57	200	57,914
SE1	197.96	0.8695	172.13	85.72	257.85	40	10,314
SSC	194.79	0.8695	169.37	84.34	253.71	50	12,685
SSB	184.20	0.8695	160.16	79.76	239.92	40	9,597
SSA	181.02	0.8695	157.40	78.38	235.78	75	17,683
CC2	193.72	0.8695	168.44	83.89	252.33	7	1,766
CC1	176.78	0.8695	153.71	76.55	230.26	20	4,605
CB2	168.32	0.8695	146.35	72.88	219.23	17	3,727
CB1	160.90	0.8695	139.90	69.67	209.57	51	10,688
CA2	159.84	0.8695	138.98	69.22	208.20	15	3,123
CA1	149.25	0.8695	129.77	64.63	194.40	20	3,888
IB2	142.90	0.8695	124.25	61.88	186.13	1	186
IB1	140.78	0.8695	122.41	60.96	183.37	9	1,650
IA2	129.13	0.8695	112.28	55.92	168.20	0	0
IA1	123.84	0.8695	107.68	53.62	161.30	7	1,129
BB2	141.84	0.8695	123.33	61.42	184.75	0	0
BB1	137.61	0.8695	119.65	59.58	179.23	1	179
BA2	128.07	0.8695	111.36	55.46	166.82	0	0
BA1	119.60	0.8695	103.99	51.79	155.78	1	156
PE2	154.55	0.8695	134.38	66.92	201.30	1	201
PE1	151.37	0.8695	131.62	65.55	197.17	6	1,183
PD2	147.14	0.8695	127.94	63.71	191.65	3	575
PD1	145.02	0.8695	126.09	62.79	188.88	15	2,833
PC2	139.73	0.8695	121.50	60.50	182.00	0	0
PC1	137.61	0.8695	119.65	59.58	179.23	14	2,509
PB2	122.78	0.8695	106.76	53.17	159.93	0	0
PB1	121.72	0.8695	105.84	52.71	158.55	6	951
PA2	120.66	0.8695	104.91	52.25	157.16	0	0
PA1	117.49	0.8695	102.16	50.87	153.03	9	1,377
						4,307	$1,545,226

The Medicare Part A revenue is often reported within a detailed profit and loss statement (see Table 12.10).

The contractual allowance corrects the billings to match the actual, nor anticipated, Medicare reimbursement received. The rev-

Table 12.10 Typical Statement of Medicare Part A Revenue

Medicare Part A revenue	
Routine revenue—room and board	$2,763,727
Ancillary revenue	
Medical supplies	59,077
Pharmacy	323,470
Physical therapy	1,460,863
Occupational therapy	1,367,537
Speech therapy	680
IV therapy	39,431
X-ray	14,692
Lab	29,058
Less: contractual adjustment	(2,287,757)
Net Medicare Part A revenue	$3,770,778

enues combine or separate the amounts received from the patient (co-pay) and the Medicare intermediary. The net Part A revenue should equate or closely approximate the PPS rates multiplied by the respective Medicare days under each RUG category.

In restating historical revenues and making a forecast, the appraiser may choose to show both gross revenue and contractual allowances or to display simply the net revenue (gross revenue minus contractual allowances). Given the amount of figures running through the revenue analysis, opting for a single, net revenue figure for each routine revenue source (Medicare, Medicaid, etc.) has advantages. The same principle can be applied to ancillary revenues.

Medicaid Revenues

Chapter 6 provided a substantial amount of background on the Medicaid reimbursement principles for nursing facilities. A brief review of salient rate-setting information from that chapter is presented here.

All or nearly all Medicaid revenue is classified as routine revenue as most Medicaid systems will not pay additional reimbursement for ancillary services. Medicaid patients may be covered partially for ancillary services through a supplemental insurance, most likely through Medicare Part B or a Medicare Advantage (managed care). Any revenue received through these coverages is classified as ancillary revenue.

The state's portion of the Medicaid reimbursements is billed at the end of the month and may be received more than a month later. Some states may take several months to pay. Payments tend to be delayed when a state is having budget or cash flow problems. The patient's share of the Medicaid reimbursement, commonly referred to as the *patient-paid amount*, is often received at the beginning of the month. The payment typically represents most of the patient's Social Security income and/or other retirement pension income. Facilities will often try to prevent family members from somehow intercepting these entitlement payments through admission agreements, to the extent allowed by law. Some facilities incur bad debt expenses because they are unable to collect the Medicaid patient's retirement pensions. Most states will limit or simply not compensate the operator for bad debt and uncollected charges.

Medicaid is a program shared between each state and the federal government. Most states reimburse nursing facilities for Medicaid prospectively, using predetermined Medicaid rates over a prescribed period, and provides no final cost settlement. (A final cost settlement refers to the difference between the final allowable costs and the actual reimbursement.) Retrospective payment systems, which are employed by only a few states, make an interim payment to the providers over a rate period. The interim payment reflects an estimated rate that is typically based on the previous costs of the individual facility. After the actual costs of the provider are reviewed by the state or its intermediary, a final cost settlement is made to reconcile the difference between the amount actually paid through the interim rate and the actual, allowable cost incurred during that same time period. Most Medicaid reimbursements are paid in arrears and several states hold back payments for months because of spending deficits.

Calculation of Medicaid Reimbursement

Payment systems have a variety of rate calculation methods, but they are generally either flat-rate systems or facility-specific systems.

Flat-rate reimbursement systems pay all nursing facilities within a specific group the same daily rate, despite differences in actual, allowable costs and other variations. The flat rate may apply to one or a few categories of expense such as administrations, dietary, and capital, or to all expenses. Other expenses may be reimbursed on a facility-specific basis. Flat rates are typically based on the prior expense history of the entire state or a geographic portion of the state. Some states will adjust flat reimbursement rates for acuity levels.

Facility-specific reimbursements are typically based on the actual annual expenses of the facility as reported in state-standardized Medicaid cost reports. Typically, states will develop cost ceilings for various cost centers, categories, or groupings; often cost centers are divided into these categories:

- Direct patient care (nursing, ancillary, and social services)

- Support services (administrative, management, activities, dietary, housekeeping, laundry, maintenance, and utilities)
- Capital (property tax and insurance, mortgage interest, depreciation, tangible asset rent, and return of equity)

Case Study—Medicaid Rate Calculation

The following section illustrates the development of a Medicaid reimbursement rate (see Tables 12.11 and 12.12). This is a continuation of the case study and makes use of the forecasts of occupancy and payor mix from Chapters 10 and 11 and the operating expenses that are developed in Chapter 13. This Medicaid reimbursement calculation reflects a typical, facility-specific, cost-based, prospective rate. For illustration purposes, the rate period and the cost period from which the rate will be derived occur simultaneously; therefore, no inflationary adjustment or trending is applied.

Assume the following:

- Facility-specific, cost-based reimbursement—i.e., actual allowable cost—will be used to calculate the reimbursement.
- The Medicaid rate has seven components:
  1. Direct care—nursing, social services, and activities
  2. Support cost—dietary, housekeeping, laundry, maintenance, and utilities
  3. Property cost—property insurance, property taxes, interest, depreciation, and rent on building and equipment
  4. Administrative, liability insurance, and management
  5. Provider taxes
  6. Cost-saving incentive payment
  7. Quality-of-care incentive
- Rate ceilings for direct care and support costs are set at 115% of the statewide median allowable expense per patient day.
- Administrative reimbursement is limited to 15.0% of the total allowable direct care, support, property, and provider tax expenses.
- Property cost allows 100% of actual property insurance and taxes; capital reimbursement is based on a fair market rental system that pays a 10.0% rate of return for interest, depreciation, and rent, applied to a $30,000-per-bed value.
- A minimum utilization of 90.0% is applied to the property cost.
- A cost-saving incentive is applied to "support expenses" and equals 50% of the difference between the ceiling and the actual allowable expense of the subject, limited to a maximum of $2.00 per patient day.
- The quality-of-care incentive provides the operator with an additional $1.00 in the final rate if the annual health survey produces fewer than 10 total deficiencies per 100 beds and there are no deficiencies tagged with "actual harm" or "immediate jeopardy" or with "widespread" under "residents affected." The subject facility will qualify for this incentive.

Table 12.11 Medicaid Rate Calculation

Reimbursement Category	Forecasted Stabilized Expense	Forecasted Stabilized Expense PPD	Medicaid Allowable	Medicaid Ceiling	Amount Reimbursable
1. Direct care expenses					
Nursing	$3,012,856	$77.00	$77.00		
Social services and activities	195,640	5.00	5.00		
Ancillary (therapy, drugs & medical equipment)	504,166	12.89	0.30		
Total direct care	$3,712,662	$94.89	$82.30	$88.00	$82.30
2. Support costs					
Dietary	$547,792	$14.00	$14.00		
Laundry	156,512	4.00	4.00		
Housekeeping	195,640	5.00	5.00		
Maintenance	176,076	4.50	4.50		
Utilities	105,646	2.70	2.70		
Total support costs	$1,181,666	$30.20	$30.20	$33.00	$30.20
3. Property cost					
Property insurance	$21,520	$0.55	$0.55		
Property taxes	60,648	1.55	1.55		
Fair market rental	360,000	9.20	9.20		
Total property costs	$442,168	$11.30	$11.30	$11.22	$11.22
Subtotal, used for calculating administrative ceiling (Item #4) at 15.0% of amount to the right				$123.72	
4. Administrative, liability insurance, and management					
General & administrative	$430,408	$11.00	$11.00		
Central office/ management fee	332,588	8.50	8.50		
Liability insurance	71,213	1.82	1.82		
Total administrative, liability insurance, and management	$834,209	$21.32	$21.32	$18.56	$18.56
5. Provider tax ($800.00/bed)	$96,000	$2.45	$2.45		$2.45
6. Cost-savings incentive					
Support cost rate ceiling				$33.00	
Actual allowable support cost for the facility				$30.20	
Difference				$2.80	
Cost saving incentive, 50% of the difference if less than ceiling, maximum incentive is $2.00					$1.40
7. Quality of care incentive					$1.00
Total Medicaid reimbursement rate					$147.13

Table 12.12 Medicaid Rate Calculation—Minimum Utilization and Capital Reimbursement Calculations

		Forecasted Occupancy	Minimum Utilization
Fair Market Rental Determination			
Reimbursement basis for fair market rent (per bed)		$30,000	
Times total licensed and certified beds	×	120	
Times total allowable capital basis		$3,600,000	
Times fair market return factor	×	10.00%	
Fair market rental, capital		$360,000	
Patient days (see below)		39,128	
Fair market rental, capital ppd		$9.20	
Property Cost Minimum Utilization Calculation			
Property insurance		$21,520	$21,520
Property taxes		60,648	60,648
Fair market rental		360,000	360,000
Total property cost		$442,169	$442,169
Divided by patient days, lesser of actual or minimum @ 90% occupancy	/	39,128	39,420
Fair market rental per patient day		$11.30	$11.22
Patient Day Calculations			
Total licensed and certified beds		120	120
Potential annual days		43,800	43,800
Occupancy rate forecasted		89.3%	90.0%
Forecasted annual days occupied per bed		39,128	39,420

Managed Care and Other Insurance Revenues

Managed care and other private insurance payments for routine and ancillary services are typically negotiated between the private insurance company and the nursing facility. The appraiser should investigate the number of managed care contracts in effect. Given the number of possible insurance companies contracting with nursing facilities in a particular market, and the confidential nature of most managed care contracts, competitive market rates for these insured groups are not easy to obtain. Moreover, gathering and analyzing that information in detail is not practical for valuation purposes. Some managed care companies will only approve a limited number of facilities in a given market–usually low bidders with the best patient outcomes–and exclude the other facilities. Other insurance companies will approve any facility willing to accept their rates and terms. Facilities that rely heavily on just one or a few private insurance/managed care contracts take on additional risks, as their revenue is vulnerable to lapsing contracts or difficult rate negotiations.

Historical and current actual average per-diem rates represent a reasonable guideline for estimating private insurance revenues. Management should be queried regarding trends in managed care and private insurance rates. Reviewing the actual rate documents for the facility from private insurance and managed care providers is prudent, especially for those companies that provide a large number of patients to the subject facility. Ultimately, managed care and private insurance revenue forecasts must often rely on historical revenues and guidance from management. The revenue forecast will often not reflect market levels since the rates are difficult to compare to other properties and are not developed from any set of clearly defined calculations.

For purposes of simplicity, no case study application of managed care census and revenues is provided.

Ancillary Revenues

Ancillary revenues are derived from physical, occupational, and speech therapy, other therapy services, examinations, pharmaceutical sales, personal care services, and special food and beverage sales. The vast majority of ancillary revenue is reimbursed through Medicare Parts A and B. Other ancillary revenues can be achieved through direct patient billing (private pay) or private supplemental insurance.

As a review, Medicare Part A combines routine and ancillary reimbursement into a single rate; however, many nursing facility financial statements will separate Medicare routine and ancillary revenues. Medicare Part B provides limited coverage for physical, speech, and occupational therapy and for certain other services to patients who are not covered by Part A. Medicare Part B revenue should be classified as entirely ancillary.

Part B therapy and ancillary reimbursements are based on a fee schedule with caps on therapy services. As of October 1, 2008, the Part B annual therapy caps were $1,810 on combined physical and speech therapy and $1,810 on occupational therapy per patient.

It is important to segregate all Medicare Part A from Part B net revenues when reviewing and analyzing historical revenues.

Since Medicare Part A PPS combines routine and ancillary reimbursement into a single rate, all Medicare Part A revenue can be forecast as part of routine revenue. Using the total Part A Medicare average PPS rate in the revenue forecast is much simpler than drilling down into the next level of analysis. Many financial statements will itemize Part A routine and ancillary revenues in separate revenue accounts. In detailed financial or operating statements, the routine and ancillary revenue may be reported in extreme detail, showing a single ancillary service, say gross revenue for physical therapy alone, with a separate line adjusting the gross revenue for the contractual allowance. (The contractual allowance is the difference between the billed amount for the service and the estimated collectible amount under Medicare.) Care should be exercised to ensure that all contractual adjustments are correctly treated in analyzing historical revenues and applying revenue forecasts.

Historical ancillary revenues should provide a solid starting point for estimating future ancillary revenues once a proper statement of net ancillary revenues is developed. Medicare Part B revenue will typically be less than the total "therapy caps" of $3,620 per year per non-Medicare patient using the facility. For example, if there are 100 patients using the facility under Medicaid and private-pay who have Part B coverage, the *maximum* ancillary therapy revenues paid under Part B will be $362,000 annually.

Ancillary revenues are also achieved from charges for therapies, medications, medical supplies, etc. provided to patients covered by private insurance and self-pay patients. These revenues are typically itemized clearly in a revenue statement. Contractual allowances may be associated with these revenues. It may be advantageous to display "net ancillary revenues" when restating historical revenues and making ancillary revenue forecasts. Separating Medicare Part B ancillary revenues from other sources of ancillary revenue may be splitting hairs given that these revenues often represent a very small percentage of the total net revenues of the facility. However, in a few circumstances where there is substantial ancillary revenue, segregating the revenue by source may be prudent.

Miscellaneous Revenues

Miscellaneous revenue can be earned from personal services not included in the routine rate (such as barber and beauty shop services and laundry of patients' personal clothing), employee and guest meal sales, transportation services, equipment rentals, telephone and cable/satellite television subscriptions, rental income from surplus building or parking space, and other service or product sales. These revenues are typically small in proportion to routine and ancillary revenues. Historical revenues are the best guide for forecasting future miscellaneous revenue. Unless these revenues appear to be unusually low or high, comparing miscellaneous revenues to comparable facilities may overemphasize the obvious.

Other Revenue Issues

Interest and financial income are usually reported in the income and expense statement, however, these revenues are not normally included in revenue forecasts seen by purchasers.

Bed hold revenue is achieved when a patient is temporarily absent from the nursing facility. For example, many Medicaid systems will pay a nursing facility a specific fraction of the normal routine rate for Medicaid patients that have been sent to a hospital. Private-pay patients may be required, under the admissions agreement, to pay a portion or all of the standard daily rate when they are absent in order to hold the bed. A patient's overnight absence is typically excluded from the inpatient or in-house census, but will be counted as bed-hold census. The customary charge and accounting for bed holds should be discussed with management. Ideally, the revenue and bed-hold census will appear as separate line items in the operating statement. Historical bed-hold census and revenue provide a reasonable basis for forecasting future revenue when the treatment of the bed holds remains consistent. States have been known to reduce or eliminate bed-hold reimbursements temporarily to help balance their budgets.

Bad debt represents the difference between the amount actually collected and the amount expected to be collected based on actual reimbursement and private-pay charges. Bad debt is typically associated with the inability or unwillingness of the patient, or the responsible party, to pay the facility. Bad debt may occur when a patient transitions from Medicare to private-pay or Medicaid or the patient shifts from private-pay to Medicaid and the patient has exhausted all his or her money prior to being approved for Medicaid; thus, the patient is "uncovered" for a period. Some operators report that they will occasionally have difficulty collecting the patient's share, or co-pay, when the primary payor is Medicaid or Medicare. A number of other circumstances will lead to bad debt and uncollected revenues. Bad debt can be treated as an adjustment to revenue or as an expense. Treating bad debt above the net revenue line limits the management fee and/or other expenses that may be measured as a percentage of revenue. If bad debt is an allowable expense for Medicaid reimbursement, then treating it as an expense may be more appropriate.

Prior year revenue adjustments, which may be positive or negative in the current-year revenue statement, should be redistributed to the period(s) in which the revenue was initially booked. Sometimes these revenues can be substantial and the management of the facility must explain and account for that revenue adjustment. As an example, in 2005 the state of Indiana paid large lump sums to nearly every Medicaid-certified nursing facility for a provider-tax rate enhancement from 2004. Many operators reported that income in 2005 and, as a result, the 2005 earnings appeared dramatically overstated and the 2004 earnings seemed very depressed. The revenues received later in 2005 should have been adjusted back to 2004.

Income from surplus building space rented to third parties may need to be treated differently than rent from related parties. In any case, contract rent should be measured against market rent levels. Rental income could be achieved by leasing surplus space to tenants who will use the space for offices, outpatient therapy, adult day care, and specialty inpatient or outpatient services. However, vacancy levels may be substantial because third-parties will generally prefer freestanding or conventional settings. Occasionally, a portion of a building that is not necessary for the operations of the nursing facility may be used by management for corporate or central office purposes. While the actual rental income may be based on a lease, market rent and market vacancy levels should be applied in revenue forecasting. Depending on the extent of rental income, special consideration of this revenue may be required when adjusting prices in the sales comparison approach and considering the selection of an overall capitalization rate and discount rate in the income capitalization approach.

A key consideration in analyzing various sources of non-nursing facility rental or business income is the original design intent for the space being utilized for the extra functions. For instance, the earnings from an outpatient therapy business or an adult day care center operated as an adjunct to the nursing facility is probably more sustainable if the building was designed specifically for outpatient therapy or day care use, rather than created by adapting space that was designed and originally used for traditional nursing home functions. Ideally, outpatient therapy and adult day care units would include separate, distinct parking and entrance areas that minimize interactions with the residents and staff of the nursing facility.

Revenue from adult day care, outpatient therapy, or other medical-related services provided to non-facility residents can become a tricky valuation issue. First, if a facility, through the same entity that owns the nursing facility operations, is providing any of these "additional" services, it is probably necessary to segregate the revenues and operating expenses related to the activity. Medicare and Medicaid cost reporting requires that all non-nursing-facility-related expenses be separated. If these activities are being performed by a related party, which warrants separate accounting, the problem of allocating the revenue and expenses goes away. In either case, a determination by the appraiser or the client as to whether or not the additional "business" activities are to be included in the valuation will be essential. This determination may necessitate the employment of an extraordinary assumption or a hypothetical condition to the appraisal or consulting assignment.

In determining if these revenues and their impact on value are to be included, several questions must be asked. First, has the activity been profitable and, if so, is the profitability sustainable? If it is not profitable, then eliminating that business from the valuation may be appropriate. Eliminating the business could open up building areas for other pursuits or for expansion of the nursing facility–with direct or indirect revenue benefits. Second, would the typical buyer (or new tenant) be interested in continuing that business activity? If the answer is no, then can the space used for the activity be converted to another, more profitable use? If the typical buyer would be willing to continue operating the additional business, then the valuation becomes complicated. One easy way around the problem of a "secondary" business is to assign a market rent to that space, eliminate any revenue and operating expenses associated with the business activity, and apply an extraordinary assumption that circumvents the valuation of the intangible aspects of that business. If the earnings from the business activity are melded into the nursing facility earnings, then special considerations may be necessary in the development of the sales comparison and income capitalization approaches.

Conclusion

The development of a revenue forecast involves considerable arithmetic. It brings together occupancy and payor mix estimates that were developed through the competitive market analysis and routine daily rate, ancillary, and other revenue measures developed through historical and market comparisons and technical reimbursement analyses. Table 12.13 continues the case study and summarizes salient revenue concepts. The figures tie back to earlier census forecasts and will be carried forward to subsequent chapters, which present important operating expense, capitalization, and sales comparison principles.

Summary

Revenues are primarily achieved from routine services and, to a lesser extent, from ancillary services and miscellaneous, other-care charges. Routine revenue covers room and board, nursing and personal care, social services, activities, and administrative services. Ancillary services include revenues

Table 12.13 Revenue Forecast, Including All Routine, Ancillary and Other Revenue

Calculation of Annual Resident Days:				
Number of beds	120			
Potential resident days	43,800			
Occupancy rate	89.3%			
Estimated resident days	39,128			
Revenue Source	**Resident Days**	**Census Mix**	**Daily Rates**	**Revenues**
Private, VA & other	12,264	31.3%	$184.28	$2,260,070
Medicare Part A	4,307	11.0%	338.82	1,459,302
Managed care	0	0.0%	-	-
Medicaid	22,557	57.6%	147.13	3,318,741
Assisted living	0	0.0%	-	-
Totals	39,128	100.0%	$244.83	$7,038,113
Ancillary (Medicare Part B and other)	39,128		$1.75	$68,474
Other revenues	39,128		0.50	19,564
Bad debt	39,128		(0.50)	(19,564)
Total effective gross revenue			$181.62	$7,106,587

derived from therapies, medical supplies, certain medications, and charges for other services. The vast majority of ancillary revenue is reimbursed through Medicare Parts A and B and through managed care and other private insurance. Private-pay and Medicaid rates cover routine revenues. Ancillary revenues from private and Medicaid patients are billed and accounted for separately. Medicare and managed care rates include both routine and ancillary revenues; however financial statements may show these revenues separately.

Private-pay rates are unregulated in most states and subject to competitive market forces. Estimating market private-pay rates involves considering the historical rates achieved by the subject, comparing the rates of competitive facilities, and adjusting those rates for differences between those facilities and the subject in terms of physical plant, location, and quality of care characteristics.

Medicare Part A revenue forecasting involves estimating the number of patient days for each of the 53 RUG categories and then applying the specific rates to each DRG. Consideration should be given to the historical DRG mix of the subject, industry averages, and factors that might cause the DGR mix to change. Accounting systems may separate Medicare Part A routine and ancillary revenues but, for practical purposes, the historical revenues can be combined since forecasting separate routine and ancillary Medicare revenue is not a feasible exercise.

All or nearly all Medicaid revenue is classified as routine revenue, as most Medicaid systems will not pay additional reimbursement for ancillary services. Medicaid patients may be covered partially for ancillary services through a supplemental insurance, most likely Medicare Part B or Medicare Advantage (managed care). The Medicaid revenue is calculated by applying the estimated patient days to the Medicaid rate. As presented in Chapter 6, Medicaid rate determination can be very complicated in states that apply facility-specific, cost-based reimbursements, but fairly simple in flat-rate states. In cost-based systems, operating expenses drive reimbursements, and thus the appraiser should reconcile the projected operating expenses to the Medicaid rate. Medicaid patients will generate ancillary revenues through their Medicare Part B coverage; historical Part B income can be a guide for estimating this revenue.

Managed care revenue will include routine and ancillary services and may be reported separately or combined. Managed care revenues are negotiated between the facility management and insurance companies. The rates are typically not made public or readily shared with the public. It is effective and efficient to forecast this revenue using a combination of current average rates and historical average per-diem rates. Discussions with management can be useful in forecasting managed care revenues.

Ancillary revenue from Medicare Part B and other payors can be based on the historical experience of the subject, comparable facilities, and discussions with management. Other revenue from bed holds and miscellaneous sources can also be referenced to historical levels. Bad debt can be treated as a revenue adjustment. Historical experience and discussions with management should serve as the best guide for making this estimate.

Chapter 13

Operating Expense Analysis

The operating expenses of nursing facilities include the costs of providing patients with nursing, therapy, social, and activity programs; dietary, housekeeping, and laundry support services; administrative and management functions; plant operation; and non-capital property expenses. The non-capital "real estate" expenses (property insurance, property taxes, utilities, and facility maintenance) often make up less than 10% of the total operating expenses of a nursing facility. Because total operating expenses will typically range from 75% to 90% of total net revenue, and thus only 10% to 25% of revenues will translate into earnings, it is critical to use precision in analyzing and developing an expense forecast.

Estimating operating expenses should include analyses of:

- The actual operating expenses of the subject facility for the past few years
- Management's budget and/or a pro forma statement
- Comparison of operating expenses in dollars per patient day ($/PPD) to other facilities that are comparable in size, acuity, wage levels, and geographic factors
- Comparison with Medicaid reimbursement ceilings, particularly if the state employs a facility-specific, cost-based reimbursement system

Data Sources and Standards

Available Operating Expense Data

The management of the subject facility should be able to provide the actual operating expenses for the subject, including internal, unaudited income and expense statements, audited statements, and/or Medicare or Medicaid cost reports. A complete set of financial statements would include the income and expense statements, a balance sheet, a statement of changes in financial position, and any other disclosure documents necessary for compliance with acceptable accounting principles. Reviewing all three data sources (internal, audited, and cost reports) may be beneficial, especially if a great deal of reliance will be placed on the actual results rather than a synthesis of expenses from the subject and comparable facilities. Audited statements will typically exclude some meaningful details and may categorize expenses into accounts that are not consistent with Medicaid rate-setting mechanisms. As a result, reliance on audited statements only often limits the analysis. Relying on unaudited statements can be risky too, but internal, unaudited statements will typical provide sufficient detail to allow the appraiser to match and compare the expenses to relevant Medicaid reimbursement structures and expense comparables.

Obtaining reliable, consistent operating expense data for comparable facilities is relatively easy since the information is available in the Medicaid cost reports. The operator and preparer of the cost report certify under penalty of fraud, with all the financial and legal consequences that a successful prosecution could bring, that the information contained in the report is truthful and accurate. This certification should provide comfort to those relying on the information. Another bonus is that cost report data makes use of consistent definitions and classifications for operating expenses. Typically, the state will not make the cost reports available to the public until a desk audit has been performed. During that audit, some expenses may need to be reclassified to fit the narrowly defined categories required for the reimbursement calculations.

Complete cost reports for any and all Medicaid-certified facilities can be obtained by making a Freedom of Information Act (FOIA) request to the agency that administers the Medicaid program for that state. Medicare cost reports are available through the Medicare intermediary or by requesting the entire cost report database from CMS. The Medicare cost report data comes in a huge file that must be managed using a database program. Many states will provide cost report data in an electronic file for all Medicaid-certified facilities in that state. These files can be managed with most spreadsheet software programs.

Units of Measurement and Standard Chart of Expense Accounts

Some insights can be gained from examining expenses as a percentage of revenue or as total departmental expenses, but *the primary unit of comparison for analyzing and forecasting operat-*

ing expenses is per patient day. Classifying operating expenses in the same way they are classified in the Medicaid cost report for that state provides an efficient basis for analysis. For the most part, expense classifications in Medicaid cost reports are fairly uniform from state to state and within the industry's standard system of accounts. The process of analyzing and comparing the subject expenses to comparable facilities and forecasting Medicaid reimbursements is facilitated by matching the subject expenses with the classifications in the Medicaid cost reports.

Table 13.1 provides a brief overview of the standardized expense categories, which form the primary basis for comparing

Table 13.1 **Typical SNF Operating Expenses and Best Units of Comparisons for Each Expense Category**

Departmental Expenses	Best Unit of Comparison	25th Percentile		75th Percentile
Patient Care				
Nursing	Per patient day	$40.00	to	$100.00
Total nursing wages and benefits				
Supplies and non-prescription drugs				
Medical records				
Medical director and consultants				
Other				
Social Services and Activities	Per patient day	$3.00	to	$7.50
Total wages & benefits				
Other				
Therapy and Ancillary	% of Medicare & managed care revenue	25.0%	to	40.0%
Total physical, speech, and occupational therapy				
Prescription drugs				
Medical supplies, equipment, and other				
Support Costs				
Dietary	Per patient day	$11.00	to	$16.00
Wages & benefits				
Food cost				
Other				
Laundry and Housekeeping	Per patient day	$6.00	to	$9.00
Total wages & benefits				
Other				
Property Cost–Non-Capital				
Plant Maintenance and Repairs	Per patient day	$3.00	to	$5.00
Total wages & benefits				
Other				
Utilities	Per square foot	$1.50	to	$3.00
Electric				
Natural gas				
Water & sewer				
Cable/satellite TV service				
Other				
Property Insurance	Per square foot	$0.20	to	$0.50
Reserves for Replacements	$/bed/year	$300	to	$600
Property Taxes	$/bed or $/square foot	Location specific		
Other				
General & administrative	Per patient day	$10.00	to	$20.00
Administrator salary				
Other salaries				
Employee benefits				
Other				
Central Office / Management Fee	% of net revenue	3.5%	to	6.0%
Liability Insurance	$/per bed/year	$300	to	$1,500
Provider Tax	$/licensed bed or % of non-Medicare revenue			

Note: Using the best unit of comparison should not preclude the use of other units of measure as well.

Source: Tellatin, Short, Hansen & Clark, Inc, 2008 survey based on Medicaid and Medicare cost report data and proprietary information, figures are rounded.

and forecasting expenses and typical cost ranges. The ranges are broad and reflect significant cost differences across the country.

Fixed and Variable Expenses

Variable operating expenses are those expenses that can be easily adjusted in response to fluctuations in the census and acuity level. The expense categories that have the greatest degree of flexibility include ancillaries (therapy, prescription drugs, etc.), nursing staff (particularly nurse aides), dietary, and laundry. Management expense, if measured as a percentage of revenue, would be completely variable. Property-related expenses, including housekeeping, maintenance and repairs, utilities, property insurance, replacement reserves, and property taxes, are substantially fixed. Other expenses are moderately fixed, but can be affected by census changes.

A long-term change in the average daily census of just one or two patients may have little impact on staffing ratios or supplies. Sensitivity to census threshold levels that cause staffing changes is an important consideration and may warrant discussion with the management of the facility if a significant change in occupancy is expected. The impact on cash flows caused by fixed and variable expenses may be relatively mild for facilities with substantial Medicaid census that receive annually rebased, facility-specific, cost-based reimbursements, provided the facility's costs remain below reimbursement ceilings. On the other hand, if a facility is substantially dependent on Medicare and private-pay patients, a change in the census level may have a substantial impact on earnings, as the daily rates are less sensitive to expense variations.

Labor Costs

Salaries, wages, and benefits make up more than half of the total operating costs of the typical nursing facility; in fact, Medicare reimbursements tie approximately 70% of the total reimbursement to wage and benefit expenses. Local labor costs, wage inflation trends, and employment levels combined with staffing ratios form the nucleus of variable and some fixed expenses. The management of the subject should be able to provide a report that shows staffing and wage statistics, including hours paid and wages sorted by department and position.

Staffing data may be expressed in several units of measurement. The most common unit is full-time equivalent (FTE). One FTE represents a 40-hour work week, which equates to a total weighted-average of 2,080 hours per year. Staffing levels are also measured by the number of minutes or hours of staff per patient day. In either case, these measurements are typically grouped and analyzed by department–e.g., nursing, dietary, etc.

Staff hours and wage statistics for comparable properties are available in the Medicaid cost reports for many, but not all, states. If this data is available, a fairly comprehensive comparative analysis can be performed. Staffing data for nursing services only is available through the On-Line Survey Certification and Reporting System (OSCAR) and accessed through the Medicare Web site: www.NHCompare.com. If staffing data for comparable facilities is not available from Medicaid cost reports or has not been obtained from surveys or proprietary sources, then any staffing forecast for the subject cannot be validated through market comparison. In these cases, wage and benefit comparisons may be restricted to per-patient-day expenses, without added insights from staffing analysis. The absence of staffing and wage data does not preclude the development of a well-substantiated salary, wage, and benefit analysis and forecast. The case study will show several levels of labor cost analyses, which can lead to solidly supported conclusions.

For comparison purposes, occupational wage data is available from the U.S. Department of Labor, Bureau of Labor Statistics (BLS), Occupational Employment Web site: www.bls.gov. Table 13.2 profiles national average wage levels for various positions that closely match the job descriptions in skilled nursing facilities. The BLS Web site also provides wage data for the various standard occupational classification (SOC) system codes organized by geographic markets to account for differences in wage levels.

Note that the wage data in the table does not reflect employee benefits and payroll taxes, which include the employer's share of Social Security and Medicare tax withholdings, worker's compensation insurance, employer-paid health insurance premiums, sick and vacation pay, and other benefits. Operating statements and cost report figures may include or exclude some or all of the employer's share of Social Security, Medicare, and other employer-paid benefits. These expenses may be grouped under each department or they may be consolidated into a separate category and not allocated to nursing, dietary, administrative, and the other departments. For consistency, it may be necessary to group or allocate the employee benefits of the subject and expense comparables into the categories used for Medicaid reimbursement calculations.

The historical expenses of the subject and comparable facilities provide a solid basis for estimating labor costs. Typical employee benefit expenses, including the employer's share of Medicare and Social Security, will approximate 15% to 25% of total salaries and wages.

Table 13.2 Wage Levels for Job Descriptions That Match Positions Required in Skilled Nursing Facilities

		Percentiles				
SOC Code	**Number and Occupation**	**10%**	**25%**	**(Median)**	**75%**	**90%**
29-1111	Registered nurses	$20.20	$23.95	$28.85	$35.18	$41.97
29-1122	Occupational therapists	20.35	25.46	30.67	37.36	45.28
29-1123	Physical therapists	23.33	27.83	33.54	39.49	48.12
29-1125	Recreational therapists	10.43	13.60	17.76	22.75	27.90
29-1127	Speech-language pathologists	19.33	23.45	29.18	36.63	45.55
29-2061	Licensed practical and licensed vocational nurses	13.16	15.53	18.24	21.78	25.08
29-2071	Medical records and health information technicians	9.46	11.24	14.08	18.09	22.81
21-1022	Medical and public health social workers	13.54	16.95	21.48	26.80	31.90
31-1012	Nursing aides, orderlies, and attendants	8.10	9.45	11.14	13.36	15.52
31-2011	Occupational therapist assistants	13.40	17.45	21.66	26.03	29.95
31-2012	Occupational therapist aides	8.73	10.34	12.54	15.73	21.96
31-2021	Physical therapist assistants	13.36	17.27	21.22	25.16	29.49
31-2022	Physical therapist aides	8.05	9.31	11.05	13.33	15.78
35-1011	Chefs and head cooks	10.37	13.47	17.87	23.94	31.04
35-1012	First-line supervisors of food preparation and serving workers	8.61	10.48	13.48	17.43	21.88
35-2012	Cooks, institution and cafeteria	6.88	8.21	10.26	12.72	15.38
37-1011	First-line supervisors of housekeeping and janitorial workers	9.93	12.29	15.79	20.45	25.67
37-2012	Maids and housekeeping cleaners	6.73	7.59	8.82	10.74	13.24
43-3031	Bookkeeping, accounting, and auditing clerks	9.77	12.25	15.17	18.78	22.87
49-9042	Maintenance and repair workers, general	9.42	11.96	15.66	20.34	24.97

Source: *The Occupational Employment Statistics (OES) May 2007 Survey*, U.S. Bureau of Labor Statistics, Division of Occupational Employment Statistics

Note: OES wage estimates represent the wage and salary component of worker's compensation only, and do not include the employer costs of non-wage benefits or employer contributions to Social Security or Medicare.

Nursing Care

Nursing care expenses are greater than any other costs of a nursing facility. Nursing care includes the salaries, wages, and benefits for the director of nursing, nursing supervisors, staff registered nurses (RNs), licensed practical nurses (LPNs), certified nurse aides (CNAs), and agency nurses; in-service nursing staff training; medical and other related supplies; and non-prescription drugs. For a typical nursing facility with an average census mix and expenses that are consistent with market levels, the nursing component will typically range from 25% to 40% of total operating (non-capital) expenses.

Because the nursing home industry is experiencing increasing levels of acuity, nursing expenses typically are increasing more quickly than inflation. The appraiser should ascertain from management the past, current, and anticipated future staffing situation of the subject. In some markets, shortages of nurses may cause facilities to rely heavily on outside nursing pools for staffing. From a care management perspective, nursing pool staff nurses are generally more costly and less desirable. An unusually high reliance on nursing pools relative to the competitive market could be an indication of poor management or other problems. If nursing staff is represented by a labor union either at the subject or in the local market, the appraiser should consider this when comparing nursing expense data and assess the influence that union representation may impose on value.

Much of the nursing expense is governed by local wage levels, minimum staffing ratios, and patient acuity levels. The historical expenses of the appraised property, comparisons to Medicaid ceilings, and comparisons to facilities that are similar in size, occupancy, mix, and acuity level should provide a solid basis for projecting future costs. Using a top-down approach to analyzing nursing expenses, the appraiser may begin by simply examining total nursing expenses on a per-patient-day basis. The next level of analysis would involve analyzing the salaries, wages, and benefits for each "class" of nursing (RNs, LPNs, and aides) separately in addition to the analysis of other nursing expenses. A deeper level of analysis could include an examination of staffing ratios and hourly wages.

As an alternative, analyzing and forecasting a single, per-patient-day nursing expense provides a fast and easy way to forecast the nursing care expenses. This approach may be sufficient when the total nursing expenses have been steady over the recent past, the census and acuity levels have been consistent and are expected to remain so, the total expenses fall into a tight range for comparable facilities (total census, mix, and acuity), and the expenses fall in line with Medicaid reimbursement ceilings or limits. If the total per-diem nursing expense does not meet these conditions, a deeper examination of the nursing expenses may be appropriate. Questions should be raised, and a more detailed analysis performed, when the expenses are significantly greater or less than the Medicaid reimbursement limit and fall outside the range for comparable properties. More study will also be needed if the facility has been cited for an abnormally high number of patient care deficiencies in recent healthcare surveys.

Using the case study data, Table 13.3 illustrates how total nursing expenses may be compared to comparable data. Delving deeper into nursing expense analysis, a comparison of salaries, wages, and benefit expenses for RNs, LPNs, nurse aides, and contract nursing and other related nursing expenses can be easily conducted using Medicaid cost report data. Table 13.4 expands

The census forecast for the subject facility is less than the census achieved in recent periods because additional competitive supply has entered the market and siphoned off demand from the existing facilities, including the subject. Thus, some reduction in total nursing expenses can be expected. However, the nursing expenses, measured on a per-patient-day basis, are likely to increase since some of the expenses are fixed and some staffing efficiencies will be lost.

Table 13.3 Forecasting Total Nursing Expenses, Total Expense Level

	$/PPD	% of Rev	Total
Subject, two years prior, inflation trended	$72.85	41.6%	$2,967,472
Subject, one year prior, inflation trended	$77.84	39.9%	$3,238,922
Subject, year to date, annualized	$72.18	42.1%	$3,003,410
Comparable mean, inflation trended	$75.50	38.5%	
Comparable low, inflation trended	$68.12	34.7%	
Comparable high, inflation trended	$82.54	43.1%	
Forecasted total nursing expense	$77.00	42.4%	$3,012,856
Forecasted patient days	39,128		
Forecasted total net revenue	$7,106,587		

the analysis of historical and forecast nursing expenses for the subject and a set of expense comparables. The wage figures incorporate the employee benefits contributed by the employer.

An analysis of staffing ratios and wage levels is also useful in estimating nursing expenses since nursing is a labor-intensive cost center. Staffing is typically examined using FTE ratios, with specific estimates for RNs, LPNs, and aides working day, evening, and night shifts. The management of most facilities should be able to provide staffing and payroll information as a part of their standard accounting. Most Medicaid cost reports require staffing and wage information. The OSCAR data provides nursing staffing minutes for RNs, LPNs, and nurse aides.

Minimum nurse staffing levels are imposed at the federal level through the Nursing Home Reform Act (NHRA) as part of the Omnibus Budget Reconciliation Act (OBRA) of 1987. The act requires Medicare- and Medicaid-certified nursing facilities to have: an RN director of nursing (DON), an RN on duty 24 hours every day (or only eight hours a day if the facility is not Medicare-certified), and a licensed nurse (RN or LPN) on duty the rest of the time. Moreover, all nurse aides are required to have a minimum of 75 hours of in-service training. The DON is allowed to serve in the capacity of the RN on duty for facilities with fewer than 60 patients.

Most states require minimum nursing staff ratios. The standards vary widely, not only in absolute amounts, but also in

Table 13.4 **Detailed Comparison of Historical Nursing Expenses of the Subject and Expense Comparables**

	Subject			Comparables*			
	Two Years Prior	One Year Prior	Year to Date	Mean	Low	High	Forecast
Per Patient Day							
RNs (Including DON and ADON)	$15.43	$14.37	$15.31	$13.85	$9.18	$18.98	$17.31
LPNs	19.30	20.84	19.53	21.68	14.75	23.93	17.51
CNAs & aides	28.36	32.65	27.27	29.85	18.24	37.84	31.63
Other nursing staff	2.54	2.37	2.75	3.35	1.01	6.25	2.66
Contracted services (agency staffing)	2.43	3.02	3.19	1.58	0.47	9.55	2.25
Supplies	0.96	1.34	1.23	0.74	0.59	1.41	1.22
Drugs (non-ancillary)	0.71	0.54	0.45	0.71	0.54	0.45	0.46
Professional and consulting fees	0.98	1.17	1.13	1.32	0.44	3.57	1.17
Other–nursing	2.16	1.52	1.32	1.15	0.33	1.89	2.80
Total nursing	$72.85	$77.84	$72.18	$75.50	$68.12	$82.54	$77.00
Percentage of Revenue							
RNs (Including DON and ADON)	8.8%	7.4%	8.9%	8.1%	5.5%	11.0%	9.5%
LPNs	11.0%	10.7%	11.4%	11.8%	8.1%	13.1%	9.6%
CNAs & aides	16.2%	16.7%	15.9%	15.8%	9.5%	20.3%	17.4%
Other nursing staff	1.5%	1.2%	1.6%	1.6%	0.6%	3.1%	1.5%
Contracted services (agency staffing)	1.4%	1.5%	1.9%	0.9%	0.4%	5.5%	1.2%
Supplies	0.5%	0.7%	0.7%	0.5%	0.3%	1.1%	0.7%
Drugs (non-ancillary)	0.4%	0.3%	0.3%	0.3%	0.2%	0.2%	0.3%
Professional and consulting fees	0.6%	0.6%	0.7%	0.8%	0.3%	2.1%	0.6%
Other–nursing	1.2%	0.8%	0.8%	0.7%	0.3%	1.1%	1.5%
Total nursing	41.6%	39.9%	42.1%	38.5%	34.7%	43.1%	42.4%
Percentage of Revenue							
RNs (Including DON and ADON)	$628,423	$597,853	$637,175				$677,306
LPNs	785,987	867,341	812,546				685,147
CNAs & aides	1,155,022	1,358,745	1,134,831				1,237,423
Other nursing staff	103,584	98,758	114,578				104,000
Contracted services (agency staffing)	98,985	125,784	132,578				88,000
Supplies	38,975	55,874	51,248				47,584
Drugs (non-ancillary)	28,754	22,412	18,795				17,887
Professional and consulting fees	39,850	48,750	46,875				45,800
Other–nursing	87,892	63,405	54,784				109,709
Total nursing	$2,967,472	$3,238,922	$3,003,410				$3,012,856

* The figures in the columns below do not add up to the totals because the itemized mean, high, and low expenses for the various facilities are random.

staffing standards or figures. Among the states with minimum nursing staff ratio standards, 20 states express the ratio in hours per patient day (HPPD). These states are California, Colorado, Connecticut, Georgia, Idaho, Illinois, Indiana, Iowa, Massachusetts, Minnesota, Mississippi, Nevada, New Jersey, New Mexico, North Carolina, Tennessee, Vermont, West Virginia, Wisconsin, and Wyoming. For instance, California requires 3.2 HPPDs of direct patient care. Arkansas, Maine, Oregon, and South Carolina express their standard as a staff-to-resident ratio. For example, Maine maintains a direct care staff-to-resident ratio of 1 to 5 during the day, 1 to 10 in the evening, and 1 to 15 at night. There are 10 other states that express standards in both HPPD and staff-to-resident ratio: Delaware, Florida, Kansas, Louisiana, Maryland, Michigan, Ohio, Oklahoma, Pennsylvania, and Texas. Montana's requirement is based on the number of licensed beds, regardless of occupancy, and Alaska expresses the requirement as a staff-to-occupied bed ratio.[1]

Most states mandate minimum staffing levels that exceed federal requirements. Many states limit nursing units to a maximum of 40, 44, 50, or even 60 beds per nurse unit or nurses' station. Typical staffing ratios are often expressed by the number of RN, LPN and CNA full-time equivalents for day, evening, and night shifts. Typical nurse staffing standards using hours per patient day (HPPD) and patient-to-staff ratios by shift are shown in Table 13.5.

Staffing ratios may vary based on facility size, specialty units (memory care, rehabilitation, head injury, ventilator, etc), licensing status (intermediate, developmentally disabled, or skilled), and intensity of care.

RNs may substitute for LPNs and LPNs may substitute for CNAs. Many nursing facilities have difficulty fully staffing 100% of the time. Management will turn to agency or outside nursing

Table 13.5 **Typical Direct Nursing Care Staffing Standards for Skilled Nursing Facilities**

Staff per patient	**RN**	**LPN**	**Aides (CNAs)**	**Totals**
Day (7:00 am to 3:00 pm)	1:30 to 1:60	1:15 to 1:30	1:6 to 1:10	1:4 to 1:7
Evening (3:00 pm to 11:00 pm)	1:60 or Fewer	1:30 to 1:60	1:8 to 1:12	1:6 to 1:10
Night (11:00 pm to 7:00 am)	1:60 to On Call	1:30 to 1:60	1:12 to 1:20	1:8 to 1:15
Hour per patient day				
Minimum	0.13	0.53	1.87	2.53
Maximum	0.53	1.06	3.00	4.59

1. *State Experiences with Minimum Nursing Staff Ratios for Nursing Facilities: Findings from the Research to Date and a Case Study Proposal*, Jane Tilly, Kirsten Black, and Barbara Ormond, The Urban Institute, and Jennie Harvell, U.S. Department of Health and Human Services, February 2003.

pools to fill vacancies when nursing employees are unavailable. Agency nursing is undesirable since the charges are often twice the hourly rates earned by in-house employees and agency nurses will be less familiar with the patients. A history of agency use should be examined. Interviews with the management of the subject and/or some other facilities in the market area will help assess the demand for outside nursing labor pools. A wage and benefit survey or comparison may show that the subject facility is missing the market and that resetting compensation to market levels could eliminate or reduce agency use and bring nursing expenses to normal market levels. Many nursing facility operators will state that they compete harder for nursing staff than they do for patients. With fairly strict economic limits on pay, nursing facilities must sometimes add perks to compete for nursing staff. The location, physical plant, and reputation of the operator are important considerations for nurses being recruited just as they are for patients and their families.

Some local markets may suffer prolonged nurse shortages, which can prevent a facility from operating at full capacity because it is unable to meet required staffing ratios. In these instances, the occupancy, revenue, and expense forecasting is much more complicated.

The case study is continued in Table 13.6, which shows staffing data comparisons and forecasts along with hourly and total salary, wage, and benefit expenses for the nursing department.

Case Study

Table 13.6 **Detailed Nursing Department Staffing and Salary, Wage, and Benefits Analysis and Forecast**

Salaries, Wages & Benefits	Forecast Minutes Per Day	Total Forecast Annual Hours	Forecasted FTEs	Total Average Hourly Compensation*	Total Annual Compensation
RN	30	19,564	9.41	$34.62	$677,306
LPN	48	31,302	15.05	21.89	685,147
Aides	138	89,994	43.27	13.75	1,237,423
Other staff		5,200	2.50	20.00	104,000
Total salaries, wages and benefits	216	146,061	70.22	$18.51	$2,703,876
Agency					$88,000
Supplies					47,584
Drugs (non-ancillary)					17,887
Professional and consulting fees					45,800
Other–nursing					109,709
Total nursing					$3,012,856

* Average hourly compensation includes all salaries, wages, employer's share of FICA, Medicare, and other payroll taxes, and all employer health and other insurance contributions, paid vacation, and personal time.

Table 13.6 Detailed Nursing Department Staffing and Salary, Wage, and Benefits Analysis and Forecast *(continued)*

Nursing Staffing Comparison and Forecast

	Average Census	Minutes Per Patient Per Day: RN	LPN	Aides	Total Annual Hours
Subject, prior year	114.0	28	50	136	148,409
Subject, year to date	114.0	28	47	135	145,635
State average, per NHCompare	106.0	36	36	120	123,808
National average, per NHCompare	95.4	30	48	138	125,356
Projected RN, LPN & aides	107.2	30	48	138	140,861

Nursing Staff Hourly Salaries, Wages, and Benefits Expense Analysis and Forecast

License Status of Nursing Staff	Prior Year	YTD	Forecasted	Prior Year	YTD
RN	19,418	19,418	19,564	$597,853	$637,175
LPN	34,675	32,595	31,302	867,341	812,546
Aides	94,316	93,623	89,994	1,358,745	1,134,831
Totals for nursing staff	148,409	145,635	140,861	$2,823,939	$2,584,552

	Average Hourly Wages & Benefits			National Figure, Per BLS, Without Employer Contributions		
	Prior Year	YTD	Forecasted	25%	(Median)	75%
RN	$30.79	$32.81	$34.62	$23.95	$28.85	$35.18
LPN	25.01	24.93	21.89	15.53	18.24	21.78
Aides	14.41	12.12	13.75	9.45	11.14	13.36

In this case study, the prior and current year's per-patient-day nursing minutes for the subject facility are compared to statewide and national averages obtained from the OSCAR data. In this case, the subject has fewer RN minutes than the state and national average but, since it has a higher-than-average census, it appears to have gained some economies of scale relative to RNs. Although the subject has been staffing LPNs and aides at higher levels than the state average, staffing has been consistent with national averages. Because the forecast census level of the subject will be declining as a result of increased competitive supply, it is reasonable to expect the subject to experience diminished staffing efficiencies.

In the table the salaries, wages, and employer-paid benefits are combined for the subject, but are excluded from the BLS figures. For an apples-to-apples comparison, an additional 15% to 25% should be added to the industry wage levels to account for the employer's share of Medicare and Social Security and other paid benefits. For purposes of this case study, the forecasted combined hourly salaries, wages, and benefits for RNs and LPNs equal 120% of the BLS median figures. The resulting hourly levels are consistent with the historical levels, trended for inflation. The forecasted hourly amount for nurse aides is slightly higher than the national median, plus benefits, and is consistent with actual historical levels, trended for inflation and local wage pressures.

The depth of analysis required should be considered before the appraiser gathers and analyzes data that may prove unnecessary or inadequate. For instance, if the historical nursing wage and benefit expenses for the subject have been fairly consistent and in line with expense comparables, a detailed wage and staffing ratio analysis may be unnecessary. If, however, the total nursing payroll expenses for the subject have been erratic over the recent past and appear to be inconsistent with comparable data, digging deeper into the cost center with FTE and wage analyses is worthwhile. Also, if the forecast occupancy or acuity level of the subject is expected to change substantially, staffing ratios may require alteration, increasing or decreasing the staff ratios or the mix of RNs, LPNs, and CNAs. Heavy dependence on contracted or agency nursing staff is a short-term solution in most cases. Effective recruiting, higher pay, and increased benefits will often minimize use of agency nurses. Detailed FTE and wage forecasts may be necessary to normalize this condition if the market regards extensive use of agency nurses as abnormal.

Other nursing expenses include medical supplies, over-the-counter drugs, a fee for the medical director, consultant services related to nursing, in-service nurse training and continuing education, and other costs related to nursing care. Note that nursing facilities are required to cover most prescription drugs for Medicare Part A patients, but are not liable for drug costs for private-pay and Medicaid patients. Medicare Part D will cover some portion of the drug expenses for private-pay and Medicaid patients, and those expenses and payments are between the patient, the Medicare Part D provider, and the drug supplier, not the nursing facility. Prescription drug expenses are typically classified as ancillary expenses.

In conclusion, nursing expenses are the single largest expense category for most nursing facilities. A comparison of historical per-diem costs and total nursing expenses provides a starting point for forecasting this expense. More detailed analyses are beneficial when census, acuity, and/or staffing levels are expected to change.

Social Services and Activities

Social services and activities provide programs that address the spiritual, social, and recreational needs of patients. This expense category includes the wages of social worker(s) and the activities director and aides, plus supplies for activities. The bulk of this expense is in the form of wages and benefits for full-time and part-time employees.

The social worker typically coordinates patient admissions and discharges with families and local hospitals and provides emotional and psychological support to patients and families. Some facilities will have a separate job position for an admissions director, which is included in this general category. Activities personnel plan, coordinate, and conduct individual and group recreational and social events for patients and seek to involve volunteers from the community. Arts and crafts, readings, religious programs, games, live performances, newsletters, and other enrichment activities are managed through activities personnel. Most nursing facilities will operate with just a few social worker and activities FTEs. This category is a blend of fixed and variable expenses, and only a substantial change in census will affect the number of FTEs.

Therapy and Ancillary

This cost center includes expenses for providing:

- Therapy (physical, speech, and occupational)
- Certain medical supplies
- Certain medical equipment
- Pharmacy products
- X-rays and lab and diagnostic tests
- Limited ambulance transportation

Ancillary services are the backbone of the rehabilitation services at a skilled nursing facility. Rehabilitation involves a greater scope of medical services than simple nursing care. The growing need to provide ancillary services at the nursing facility level to maximize earnings, coupled with the loss of lower-acuity private-pay patients to assisted living, are important factors behind the ownership consolidation trend in the industry. Operators of individual facilities are finding it more difficult to compete for rehabilitation patients because management expertise may be stretched thin. Therapy and prescription drugs constitute the largest expenses within the ancillary expense category.

Therapy

The combination of physical, occupational, and speech therapy is generally the largest component of ancillary expenses and typically represents 60% to 70% of total ancillary expenses. Most ancillary expenses are incurred by Medicare Part A and managed care patients (including Medicare Advantage alternatives) or Part B patients. Medicaid pays for little to no ancillary services, and most private-pay ancillary services are paid through Part B or private insurance.

Most nursing facilities with fewer than 15 to 20 Medicare patients cannot justify employing full-time therapists on staff. Facilities often contract with outside or related-party therapy companies to provide professional staff on an as-needed basis. Contracted therapy charges are often based on one of the following formulas.

1. Percentage of the therapy component of the Medicare rate for the specific resource utilization groupings (RUGs)

   Example: If the wage-adjusted therapy component for the RUG category RVB is $60.00 per day and the therapy service contract is based on a percentage of the DRG rate, say 80% of the rate, the therapy company will provide all the required therapy under that category for $48.00 per day.

2. Per minute of therapy–typically $0.90 to $1.15 per minute

   Medicare time studies indicate that an RVB RUG will average 65 minutes of combined physical, occupational, and speech therapy, and the patient is required to receive a minimum of 60 minutes of therapy daily. Under a contract with a therapy company, the nursing facility could pay the therapy company $0.90 per minute for all therapies, or $54.00 for this specific RUG ($0.90 × 60 minutes).

Many regional and national nursing home operators have established their own therapy companies to provide cost-efficient services to the facilities that they manage and operate and compete to provide third-party therapy services to facilities in which they have no other interest. Many "ownerships" will use related-party therapy companies to sidetrack or shift profits away from the nursing facility entity. Several reasons are cited for this action, but the practice is mainly employed to reduce liabilities and establish higher reportable costs to Medicare. With less perceived profit on the nursing facility level, creditors and plaintiffs may have less reason to pursue judgments against the facility. In the marketplace, buyers and tenants of nursing facilities will evaluate the total assets of the facility by gathering in all the actual and/or potential earnings from the nursing facility and its related parties. The practice of splintering the earnings derived from the nursing facility may also be applied to charges from related-party management and pharmacy businesses and from self-insured liability insurance. When related-party companies are used, it is important to determine if the rates charged to the facility are competitive and represent the best value in the market.

Pharmacy

Medicare Part A requires the nursing facility to provide and pay for all prescription and non-prescription medicines for patients using Medicare. Pharmacy expenses for private-pay and Medicaid patients are typically minimal for the nursing facility since the payment for the drugs will be managed between the patient, the insurance carrier (Medicare Part D), and the supplier. Hospitals discharging Medicare Part A patients with very costly prescription regimes to skilled nursing facilities may have greater difficulty placing these patients than other patients with minimal drug costs. Nursing facilities may need to play a game of "give and take" with hospitals. They can maintain or improve their relationships with hospital discharge planners by accepting these higher-cost patients. Over the long run, and with careful management, the low- and high-cost pharmacy expenses of different patients should average out to normal levels.

Many nursing facilities view pharmacy as a break-even proposition, with expenses equaling reimbursements. Management should be questioned about their pharmacy arrangements and asked if they anticipate any change in the procurement of medicines that may modify the cost levels relative to current and historical expenses.

Other Ancillary Expenses

Other ancillary expenses include certain medical supplies and equipment, x-rays, lab and diagnostic tests, ambulance transportation, and some infrequent costs that nursing facilities are required to cover for Medicare patients.

Developing Ancillary Expense Forecasts

Forecasting ancillary expenses begins with examining the actual historical expenses of the subject. These expenses can be compared with expenses at other facilities on a per-patient-day basis, using total patient days or just the Medicare/managed care days. Or the subject expenses can be compared using the ratio of ancillary expenses to total Medicare Parts A and B and managed care revenues. Keep in mind that ancillary expenses are affected by economies of scale. Evidence shows that when more Medicare and managed care patients receive therapy and/or the Medicare case mix index is higher, the ancillary expense margin and per-diem expense decline.

Ancillary expenses typically run between 25% and 40% of Medicare Parts A and B revenue. A fairly simple method for estimating ancillary expenses is to compare the historical total ancillary expenses as a percentage of Medicare and managed care revenues for the subject to the percentages for comparable facilities that have similar Medicare volume. An example of this comparison is shown in Table 13.7.

A 2006 survey of ancillary expense margins for regional skilled nursing facility operators revealed the total ancillary expense ratios shown in Table 13.8.

Table 13.7 **Ancillary Expense Comparable Data**

	Facility 1	Facility 2	Facility 3	Mean
Total Medicare and managed care revenue	$1,856,137	$1,317,218	$2,994,416	$2,055,924
Total ancillary expenses	$595,820	$442,426	$791,164	609,803
Ancillary expenses as a percentage of total Medicare and managed care revenues	32.1%	33.6%	26.4%	30.7%
Medicare Part A and managed care days	4,793	3,687	7,854	5,445
Ancillary expenses for Medicare Part A & managed care PPD	$124.31	$120.00	$100.73	$115.01

Table 13.8 **Summary of SNF Operator Survey of Medicare and Managed Care Revenue and Ancillary and Therapy (Rehabilitation) Expenses**

Operator Identity	Period Ending	Number of Facilities	Approximate Licensed Beds	Approximate Medicare & Managed Care Mix	In-House or Third-Party Therapy
Great Lakes Region, Private	06/30/05	15 to 20	1,800 - 2,000	16.6%	3rd Party
Great Lakes Region, Private	11/30/05	8 to 10	1,200 - 1,400	14.0%	3rd Party
Missouri-Illinois, Private	11/30/05	12 to 15	1,000 - 1,100	11.0%	3rd Party
Midwest and West, Private	11/30/05	30 to 35	3,300 - 3,600	11.0%	3rd Party
California, Private, Related Party Supply Company	06/30/05	15 to 20	1,750 - 1,900	16.2%	3rd Party
Southeastern U.S.	11/30/05	12 to 15	1,850 - 2,000	21.0%	Mostly 3rd Party
Midwest, Single State	12/31/06	12 to 15	1,400 - 1,500	20.0%	3rd Party
Midwest and Southwest	12/31/06	16 to 20	1,500 - 1,750	8.0%	3rd Party
Northeast, Midwest & South-Central, Private	08/31/05	40 to 45	4,250 to 4,500	15.5%	3rd Party
Southern California, Private Company	12/31/05	12 to 15	1,375 to 1,425	27.7%	3rd Party
Illinois-Missouri, Private	06/30/05	12 to 15	1,850 - 2,000	22.5%	3rd Party

Operator Identity	Total Medicare A & B and Managed Care Net Revenue	Total Therapy and Ancillary Expenses	Therapy-Only Expenses	Therapy & Ancillary Expenses as % of Total Medicare & Managed Care Revenue	Therapy Expenses as % of Total Medicare & Managed Care Revenue
Great Lakes Region, Private	$35,247,633	$10,808,136	$7,226,032	30.7%	20.5%
Great Lakes Region, Private	25,778,991	8,046,334	5,182,140	31.2%	20.1%
Missouri-Illinois, Private	10,656,401	3,324,642	2,257,161	31.2%	21.2%
Midwest and West, Private	19,495,000	7,590,756	4,353,656	38.9%	22.3%
California, Private, Related Party Supply Company	46,442,493	15,710,760	11,839,104	33.8%	25.5%
Southeastern U.S.	57,496,243	15,991,153	9,554,476	27.8%	16.6%
Midwest, Single State	26,367,467	8,762,092	5,209,609	33.2%	19.8%
Midwest and Southwest	11,696,413	4,723,856	2,993,428	40.4%	25.6%
Northeast, Midwest & South-Central, Private	81,867,966	26,005,278	13,698,155	31.8%	16.7%
Southern California, Private Company	59,091,874	11,981,145	7,607,598	20.3%	12.9%
Illinois-Missouri, Private	48,134,000	10,819,000	6,554,000	22.5%	13.6%
Totals	$422,274,479	$123,763,151	$76,475,358	29.3%	18.1%
Standard Deviation				6.0%	4.2%

Source: Survey of operators conducted by Tellatin, Short & Hansen, Inc., in January and February 2006.

As Figure 13.1 illustrates, ancillary expenses as a percentage of total Medicare and managed care revenue decline as the Medicare and managed care census mix increases among the surveyed companies.

Putting these points together in the continuing case study, ancillary expenses are forecast in Table 13.9.

Figure 13.1 **Relationship Between Medicare and Managed Care Census Mix and Ancillary Expense Margin as a Percentage of Medicare and Insurance Revenue from Survey of Regional SNF Operators**

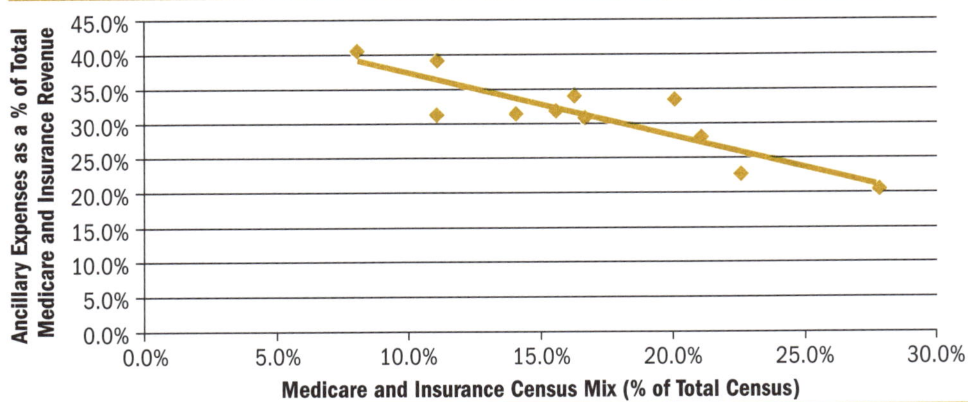

Case Study

Table 13.9 **Forecasting Ancillary Expenses Using Percentage of Medicare and Managed Care Revenue**

Period	Two Years Prior	Prior Year	Current YTD, Annualized	Forecasted
Medicare Part A revenue	$1,647,185	$1,821,952	$1,888,875	$1,459,302
Managed care revenue (none forecasted)	-	-	-	-
Total ancillary revenue, including Part B	39,867	61,785	72,485	68,474
Total Medicare and managed care revenue	$1,687,052	$1,883,737	$1,961,360	$1,527,776
Total ancillary expenses	$487,985	$587,474	$547,893	$504,166
Ancillary expense as a percentage of total Medicare and managed care revenues	28.9%	31.2%	27.9%	33.0%
Medicare and managed care patient days	4,987	5,374	5,475	4,307

In the case study, the forecast Medicare census is less than historical levels because the market will experience significant new competition, which is expected to reduce the Medicare census for the subject and the other, existing facilities in the market. As a result, the ancillary expense margin, or the expenses as a percentage of Medicare revenues, should increase as the ancillary expense survey indicates. The forecast Medicare census mix declines from 13.2% in the current year to 11.0% in the forecast year. Based on the trend line indicated by the surveyed data, the ancillary expense margin with a 13.2% Medicare mix would be approximately 34%, while at an 11.0%

Medicare mix, the margin increases approximately 200 basis points to 36%. Thus, the indicated ancillary expense margin forecast for the subject appears to increase roughly 200 basis points to approximately 33%.

Another valid way to measure therapy and ancillary expenses is to compare per-patient-day expenses. Since these expenses are largely attributable to the Medicare and managed care census, the comparison in more effective when total ancillary expenses are divided by Medicare and managed care days (see Table 13.10).

Table 13.10 Comparison of Total Therapy and Ancillary Expenses Over Three-Year History of the Subject to Expense Comparables and Forecasted Amount for the Subject

Comparable	Medicare and Managed Care Days	Ancillary & Therapy Expense Margin	Ancillary & Therapy Expenses PPD
1	4,793	32.1%	$124.31
2	3,687	33.6%	$120.00
3	7,854	26.4%	$100.73
Averages	5,445	30.7%	$115.01
Subject			
Two years prior	4,987	28.9%	$97.85
Prior year	5,374	31.2%	$109.32
Current	5,475	27.9%	$100.07
Subject forecast	4,307	33.0%	$117.06

Another, more technical approach to forecasting ancillary expenses is to tie therapy and other ancillary expenses to actual reimbursements. As mentioned earlier, a portion of three of the four Medicare PPS rate components include reimbursement for therapy and ancillary expenses. The fourth component of the PPS rate is the "non-case mix" rate, which reimburses the facility for administrative, dietary, housekeeping, laundry, plant operations, and capital costs. The three components that incorporate ancillary expenses are: nursing, therapy, and therapy, non-case mix.

The "therapy" and "therapy, non-case mix" reimbursements are tied almost entirely to therapy expenses. CMS states that non-therapy ancillary comprises 43.4% of the nursing component of the PPS rates for urban areas and 42.7% for rural areas. The ancillary expenses covered under "nursing" include prescription medicines, medical supplies, and certain medical equipment. Finally, an expense margin should be assessed against the projected Part B ancillary revenues.

Table 13.11 presents a suggested method for estimating therapy ancillary expenses using the revenues from the various components of Medicare reimbursement. The calculations tie into the on-going case study.

Table 13.11 Estimating Ancillary Expenses Using Specific PPS Reimbursement Components

Medicare Part A therapy or rehab reimbursement			
Average therapy (rehab) portion of the PPS rate for the 23 rehab RUGs	$78.95		
Number of rehab RUG days for the forecast year	× 3,661		
Total therapy reimbursement for the 23 rehab rugs		$289,046	
Therapy, non-case mix portion of the PPS rate	$13.68		
Number of non-rehab Medicare days	× 646		
Total non-case-mix reimbursement for non-rehab RUGs		8,838	
Medicare Part B therapy reimbursement		68,474	
Total Medicare reimbursement for therapy			$366,357
Projected therapy expense margin			× 68.28%
Total therapy expenses			$250,165
Part A, non-therapy ancillary expense projection (based on nursing component)			
Average nursing portion Medicare Part A reimbursement	$187.43		
Total Medicare days	× 4,307		
Total		$807,250	
% of nursing related to non-therapy ancillary		× 43.40%	
Non-therapy ancillary portion of the rate			$350,347
Projected non-therapy ancillary expense margin			× 72.50%
Projected non-therapy ancillary expense			$254,001
Total forecasted ancillary expense			$504,166
Comparison of Forecast to Surveyed Facilities		**Surveyed Mean**	**Forecasted**
Total therapy expenses per Medicare patient day		$65.69	$58.08
Total forecasted ancillary expense per Medicare patient day		$106.31	$117.06

Note: Figures are rounded.

The deepest level of analysis involves actually calculating specific FTE, productivity, RUGs days, average drug expenses, and detailed line item expenses for therapy and other ancillary expenses. These analyses will typically require fairly complicated software and accurate data. This type of analysis does not lend itself to easy comparison with market data. Unless the analyst is attempting to develop a detailed operating budget, this level of detailed analysis is probably counterproductive.

Therapy and Ancillary Expense Summary

Therapy and ancillary expenses are tied directly to the Medicare and managed care census. Most Medicaid systems will not reimburse for therapies, nor are facilities expected to provide therapies to Medicaid patients. Moreover, while facilities are responsible for providing patients prescription drugs, Medicaid pays the drug supplier directly, bypassing the facility. Private-pay patients typically receive limited therapy beyond Medicare Part B and private insurance coverage. Ancillary expenses can be measured and easily compared to comparable data as percentages of Medicare and managed care revenue, or compared on a per-patient-day basis using Medicare and managed care patient days. Most nursing facilities will contract with related or third-party therapy companies to provide therapists and services because employing in-house therapy staff often proves to be less efficient. Related-party therapy and pharmacy arrangements may be set at rates that exceed or are less than the rates of third-party providers. Excessive related-party therapy charges shift profits from the facility level to other entities. In cases where the related-party therapy charges are below market or below actual cost, a false indication of earnings may be presented for the operating entity of the facility. It is important to capture these related-party earnings or losses at the facility level to fully account for earnings and value.

Dietary

The dietary expense department includes the cost of raw food, staff wages, supplies, nutritional supplements, maintenance, and consulting fees. Raw food costs will typically represent 40% to 50% of the total dietary expense, and wages, salaries, and benefits will make up another 40% to 50%. Dietary expenses are often higher in facilities that attract high proportions of private-pay and Medicare patients because meals tend to be more elaborate. Younger patients using the nursing facility for rehabilitation will require higher food standards. Inflation aside, this expense category should be fairly stable as long as the occupancy level remains stable.

Laundry and Housekeeping

These fairly self-explanatory categories include supplies, salaries, and employee benefits. The level of occupancy and the size and efficiency of the building significantly affect the relatively fixed per-patient-day expenses for laundry and housekeeping. Under stabilized conditions, these expenses should remain constant and keep pace with inflation.

Plant Operations

Plant operations include utilities, wages for maintenance staff, and contract and outside services and supplies. Utility expenses constitute about 40% to 60% of plant operating expenses. Plant operating expenses will vary depending on the age and level of deterioration of the structural and mechanical components, the average number of square feet per bed, the efficiency of the insulation and HVAC systems, and the amount of air-conditioning supplied to the building. These expenses are relatively fixed, and fluctuations in the occupancy should have a minor effect on the total expenses. It may be useful, or required by some underwriters, to break out the various utilities from this expense category, but most Medicaid reimbursement systems group all these costs into a single classification. Since nursing facilities are always open and intensely used, their utility and maintenance expenses may be greater than the expenses for most residential property. These expenses are best measured in comparison with similar nursing facilities on an annual per-square-foot or per-patient-day basis.

Property Taxes and Property Insurance

These fixed expenses are self-explanatory. In most cost-based, facility-specific Medicaid reimbursement systems, property taxes are fully passed through or 100% allowable; the tax reimbursement may be subject to a minimum occupancy calculation.

An argument can be made that property assessments should be tied to an allowable Medicaid capital cost basis for facilities that have a 100% Medicaid census. The basis for this argument is that a state agency is essentially valuing the property at one amount for reimbursement purposes, while a local assessor is setting the value at a different amount for taxation. This argument breaks down when the facility has any significant Medicare and/or private-pay census. It is important to consider the consequences of a sale (actual or hypothetical) on the assessed value and potentially on the Medicaid reimbursement. Property assessment comparisons can be made on the basis of value per bed or value per square foot. Most assessors will rely heavily on the cost approach in their valuations because that approach may exclude intangible asset values. The sales comparison and income capitalization approaches are more complicated to apply and comparable data is difficult to obtain. Many states tax real estate and personal property, so researching and forecasting both forms of taxation will be necessary.

Property insurance is a relatively fixed expense and historical and current insurance premiums usually provide a solid basis for forecasting this expense. Earthquake, flood, and hurricane coverage should be incorporated into the policy and premiums for facilities in areas that are prone to these events and require specific, elective coverage. General and liability insurance premiums are separate from property insurance, and they are usually treated differently in facility-specific, cost-based Medicaid reimbursement systems.

Reserves for Replacement

Reserves for replacing short-lived building components and furniture, fixtures, and equipment (FF&E) are usually established to even out cash flows over the course of the investment and to maintain the competitiveness of the property. This expense is often referred to as *cap-ex* (capital expense). An assessment is made to determine the remaining life, costs, and expected life of short-lived building items and FF&E. The property needs assessment can be made by the appraiser and/or other third parties. Management of the facility may have developed a long-term capital replacement plan. Ultimately, the appraiser will need to conclude a reserve amount that provides for adequate replacement of worn, dated, and obsolete items. Many facilities delay capital expenditures, which places a greater burden on future cash flows and overall competitiveness.

Reserves are often estimated using per-bed amounts developed from surveys or by following market convention. It is certainly acceptable to use a reserve figure developed from market convention; however, that amount should be verified with the approximate cap-ex needs of the property established through personal observation and/or confirmation with management. As with so many valuation judgments, consistency is paramount: Do unto your sales as you do unto your subject. This means that if a conventional reserve amount is being applied to the subject's operating expenses, then it may be prudent to use a similar amount in the calculation of the operating expenses for the comparable sales used in the development of the capitalization rate and earnings multiplier. Cap-ex needs will vary and if there are known differences between the sales and the subject, those differences should certainly be included in the calculations.

Analyzing cap-ex costs further, the cost approach can be applied to determine the replacement costs and lives of the short-lived improvements and FF&E. A typical life for the FF&E is 10 to 15 years, which means that reserves will run between 7% and 10% of the replacement cost of the FF&E. Estimating reserves for short-lived building and site improvement items requires some further calculation. Table 13.12 shows the calculation of replacement reserves for short-lived items.

The table shows two reserve figures, with and without a sinking fund. A sinking fund is defined as "a fund in which periodic deposits of equal amounts are accumulated to pay a debt or replace assets; usually designed to receive equal annual or monthly deposits that will accumulate, with compound interest,

Table 13.12 Calculating Building and Site Improvement Reserves for Replacement Calculations

Replacement item	RCN for Short-Lived Components	Expected Total Life	Annual Reserve Percentage	Reserve w/o Sinking Fund	Reserves with 5.0% Sinking Fund
Roof cover (100%)	$125,000	20	5.0%	$6,250	$3,780
Interior construction (15%)	160,000	20	5.0%	8,000	4,839
Ceilings (50%)	75,000	20	5.0%	3,750	2,268
Plumbing	72,000	20	5.0%	3,600	2,177
HVAC (30%)	60,000	12	8.3%	4,980	3,770
Exterior walls and windows	120,000	25	4.0%	4,800	2,514
Electrical	75,000	25	4.0%	3,000	1,571
FF&E	950,000	20	5.0%	47,500	28,730
Totals	$1,637,000			$81,880	$49,651
Annual reserves per bed				$819	$497

Note: Figures are rounded.

to a predetermined sum at the end of a stated period of time."[2] Typically, a sinking fund reserve is established for a new or newer building; if a building or asset is well into its economic life, a straight-line replacement reserve may be more appropriate.

Administrative and General

The administrative and general category includes the wages of the administrator, the assistant administrator, and the office clerks as well as the cost of business supplies, telephone, postage, legal fees, employee recruiting and in-service training, marketing, advertising, education, travel, license fees, and accounting. The operating statements for this category may include central office, management fees, liability insurance, employee benefits for all departments, and other expenses that may need to be reclassified to match Medicaid classifications and avoid potential double accounting.

Administrative expenses are relatively fixed and not heavily influenced by changes in the census level. Some administrative and general expenses are not allowed for Medicaid reimbursement, including advertising, marketing, and excessive salaries, benefits, and "profits and perks" for management or ownership. Excessive costs that are not essential to the efficient operation of the facility are sometimes charged to administrative and/or management expenses as a way to pull out profits. By analyzing detailed operating statements, which are generally available in the Medicaid cost reports or, better yet, from a highly detailed internal operating statement, the appraiser can identify exces-

2. *The Dictionary of Real Estate Appraisal*, 4th ed. (Chicago: Appraisal Institute, 2002), 266.

sive or even inadequate expenses from these departments. These charges are probably more noticeable in facilities that are owned by the key employees at the facility level.

Central Office/Management Fee

This expense category includes overall supervision, financial services, long-range planning, and government relations. These services are generally conducted off premises at corporate offices. The projected expense reflects competent management, even though the actual management may be more or less capable than is typical. Facilities with steady census and earnings are indicative of good management; irregularities in occupancy and earnings, in an otherwise stable market, may be an indication of inferior management.

The cost for management services is often expressed as a percentage of gross revenue, but many operators charge flat fees and include profit incentives. Typical management costs run between 4.0% and 6.0% of net revenue. Many management companies will charge a base fee, usually a percentage of revenue, or a flat monthly fee plus another fee that allows them to participate in profits. Depending on the treatment of management expenses (percentage of revenue or flat fee), this expense may be completely variable or somewhat fixed.

There is a difference between management expense and management fees. Management expense relates to the real cost of providing the management functions to a facility and exclude those amounts that the market regards as "profits and perks." Just as excessive expenses from a related-party therapy company are placed back to the nursing facility entity, excessive management fees should be adjusted out. For example, the owner of a small chain of nursing facilities may expense the management company's season tickets to entertainment or sports events, even though those seats are not used for business purposes. Similarly, lease payments for a private airplane used primarily for personal travel, or higher-than-market contributions for personal life insurance or a pension plan, should be adjusted from the management expense. These expenses are not allowable for Medicaid reimbursement and fall into a gray area for IRS purposes.

The prices market participants offer for facilities ultimately reflect the real cost of management. In fact, if two buyers are in a bidding war for a facility and both forecast the same revenues, operating expenses (excluding management), and cost of capital, the bidder that is able to realize greater economies of scale within the central office or management expenses will be able to make a higher offer.

General and Professional Liability Insurance

Most skilled nursing facilities carry some type of general and professional liability insurance coverage. Since the market believes having liability insurance is important, the operating expense forecast should include the cost of this insurance. If an operator does not have coverage or the coverage is not at an acceptable market level, it is important to adjust the expenses to include a market-rate liability insurance expense.

Insurance premiums and coverage amounts vary substantially by operator and by state. Most lenders and landlords require the operator to carry liability insurance for $1,000,000 for a single occurrence and $3,000,000 for multiple occurrences. Depending on the type of policy, policy limits, deductibles, claims history, and the state where the facility is located, professional liability insurance with an umbrella might range from $400 to $900 per bed or even higher. The appraiser should request a summary of the coverage amounts and premiums from the management of the facility and discuss this topic. Expense comparable data obtained from Medicaid or Medicare cost reports will disclose the insurance expense, but it will not explain the types and amounts of coverage.

Liability insurance costs rose steeply between 1998 and 2003 as tort liability lawsuits increased dramatically in Florida, Texas, California, Alabama, Mississippi, and Arkansas. Many insurance carriers discontinued liability coverage to nursing facilities entirely. Tort reforms and improved management of incidents that could evolve into litigation matters have slowed the rapid increases in premiums, and in many extremely high-cost states, premiums have actually declined. Some larger operators may self-insure using commercially available off-shore captives to reduce costs. In these cases, it may be more appropriate to forecast the insurance expense using a competitively priced amount from a commercial carrier. Moreover, to the extent possible, the liability insurance coverage and expense should be considered in a consistent manner for the subject and for the comparable sales used in the development of market-derived capitalization rates and internal rates of return.

Provider Taxes

As mentioned in the discussion of Medicaid in Chapter 6, many states place a bed or revenue tax on nursing homes and then use these collections to obtain additional federal matching funds. If the state employs this tax, it is crucial to include it in the operating expense forecast. The appraiser should confirm the amount of the tax with an authority, such as the state health care association or the Medicaid rate-setting division, as these taxes often change.

Other Expenses

A nursing facility may have other expenses that relate to excess land or to non-nursing facility functions of the improvements. Care should be taken to isolate these expenses from the nursing facility operating statement and treat them accordingly.

Case Study

Operating Expenses Summary

Table 13.13 shows a summary of revenue and operating expenses for the 120-bed facility that is the subject of the ongoing case study.

Table 13.13 Forecasted Stabilized Revenue and Operating Expenses

Calculation of Annual Patient Days				
Number of beds	120			
Potential patient days	43,800			
Occupancy rate	89.3%			
Estimated patient days	39,128			
Revenue Source	**Patient Days**	**Census Mix**	**Daily Rates**	**Revenues**
Private, VA & other	12,264	31.3%	$184.28	$2,260,070
Medicare Part A	4,307	11.0%	338.82	1,459,302
Medicaid	22,557	57.6%	147.13	3,318,741
Totals	39,128	100.0%	$179.87	$7,038,113
Ancillary (Medicare Part B and other)	39,128		$1.75	$68,474
Other revenues	39,128		0.50	19,564
Bad debt	39,128		(0.50)	(19,564)
Total effective gross revenue			$181.62	$7,106,587
Operating Expenses		**% of Revenue**	**$/Patient Day**	
Direct care expenses				
Nursing		42.4%	$77.00	$3,012,856
Social services and activities		2.8%	5.00	195,640
Ancillary (therapy, drugs & medical equipment)		7.1%	12.89	504,166
Support costs				
Dietary		7.7%	14.00	547,792
Laundry		2.2%	4.00	156,512
Housekeeping		2.8%	5.00	195,640
Maintenance		2.5%	4.50	176,076
Utilities		1.5%	2.70	105,646
Property costs				
Property insurance		0.3%	0.55	21,520
Property taxes		0.9%	1.55	60,648
Cap-ex, replacement reserves		1.0%	1.84	72,000
Administrative, liability insurance, and management				
General & administrative		6.1%	11.00	430,408
Central office/management		4.7%	8.50	332,588
Liability insurance		1.0%	1.82	71,213
Provider tax ($800.00/bed)		1.4%	2.45	96,000
Total operating expenses		84.1%	$152.80	$5,978,705
Net operating income or earnings before interest, depreciation, amortization, and rent (EBITDAR)				$1,127,881

Summary

Nursing facility operating expenses typically range from 75% to 90% of total net revenue. The forecasting of operating expenses involves analyzing the trailing, current, and budgeted expenses of the subject and comparing those expenses to comparable facilities and possibly to regional statistics and Medicaid reimbursement limits. The operator's financial statements should include census and revenue information that is clearly separated by payor source. The operating expense information should provide sufficient detail so that the expenses can be organized and grouped into categories that match the state's Medicaid reimbursement system. Labor reports are also useful. Comparable expense data can be obtained from Medicaid cost reports in nearly every state. Medicare cost reports are also available from CMS (Centers for Medicare & Medicaid Services) in a large, electronic database format. Since the format of the Medicare cost report often differs from the Medicaid reimbursement expense classification, states' Medicaid cost reports are generally preferred. Expense comparables should ideally be drawn from facilities in the same state as the subject and be located in labor markets that have the same or similar wage index levels. The facilities should also have a comparable number of beds, census, payor mix, and acuity.

Operating expenses are typically reduced to a per-patient-day unit of comparison since reimbursements are generally calculated using this measurement. Other units of measurement include percentage of revenue, per labor unit, and per square foot. These other measurements are appropriate for certain expenses. Management expenses are often measured as a percentage of net revenue. Because nursing and therapy are labor-intensive, these expenses can be analyzed and forecast using staffing ratios and hourly wage levels. Property-related expenses, including maintenance, utilities, property insurance, property taxes, and even housekeeping, can be measured with building square footage figures.

Salaries, wages, and benefits represent the largest portion of the operating expenses. Wage levels and staffing ratios form the nucleus of variable and some fixed expenses. Actual staffing ratios often exceed minimum nursing ratios set by the state. Variable operating expenses can be adjusted relative to fluctuations in the census and acuity level. The expenses that have the greatest degree of flexibility, relative to census changes, include ancillaries (therapy, prescription drugs, etc.), nursing staff (particularly nurse aides), dietary, and laundry. Relatively fixed expenses include property-related expenses (housekeeping, maintenance and repairs, utilities, property insurance, replacement reserves, and property taxes) and administrative expenses, liability insurance, and the salaries for the directors of nursing and dietary services. Therapy and ancillary expenses closely correlate to levels of Medicare and managed care census.

The treatment of replacement reserves and management expenses should be consistent for the subject and the sales used in the development of capitalization and discount rates.

Chapter 14

Highest and Best Use Issues

Any generally accepted definition of market value hinges on the principle of highest and best use. Highest and best use may is defined as:

> The reasonably probable and legal use of vacant land or an improved property, which is physically possible, appropriately supported, financially feasible, and that results in the highest value. The four criteria the highest and best use must meet are legal permissibility, physical possibility, financial feasibility, and maximum productivity.[1]

The Appraisal Institute provides comprehensive instruction on the subject of highest and best use through its classroom courses, seminars, and publications, including *The Appraisal of Real Estate*, and articles in *The Appraisal Journal*. This text does not provide a thorough examination of highest and best use, but a brief review of the key concepts and the issues germane to the valuation of nursing facilities is presented here.

Highest and best use is determined for the vacant site and for the property as improved. In both cases, every use considered must meet four criteria; the use must be

- Legally permissible
- Physically possible
- Financially feasible, and after meeting these three, it must be
- Maximally productive

These criteria are listed sequentially. This is the most efficient processing order for determining highest and best use. Should a physically possible use fail to be legally permissible, then there is no reason to pursue analysis of that use.

---

1. *The Dictionary of Real Estate Appraisal*, 4th ed. (Chicago: Appraisal Institute, 2002), 135.

Highest and Best Use of Land as though Vacant

Most appraisal assignments will require an analysis of the highest and best use of the site as though vacant. Since land is generally valued as though vacant, it is essentially that as-vacant highest and best use is considered in the land valuation. The highest and best use of the site as though vacant must be measured in relation to its existing use and all potential alternative uses. The extent of highest and best use analysis increases as the proportion of land value and transferable intangible personal property value increase relative to the total property value.

In many small markets, just one or a few nursing facilities are needed to satisfy the market demand. In these cases, the chances that a particular, existing nursing facility site represents the highest and best use as though vacant becomes random because there may be many other sites that could fulfill the four criteria of highest and best use for a nursing facility site as well, if not better, than the current site.

The analysis of the highest and best use of the site as though vacant takes on importance when the improvements are approaching the end of their expected economic and useful life. Many nursing facilities developed in the 1960s and 1970s may now suffer high levels of functional and/or external obsolescence. If they also have substantial underlying land value for alternative uses, closure of the facility and sale of the property for new development may be warranted.

In some cases, the development of the site to its highest and best use may be impeded by a long-term lease of the facility that delays the fee ownership from achieving the highest and best use. The tenant may continue to find it profitable to operate the facility, yet a higher return to the landlord could be achieved if the lease were to be terminated. The tenant may be precluded from redeveloping the site because the remaining term of the lease is not long enough to recapture the investment or the lease requires the tenant to return the property to the landlord in its original condition. In such cases, the landlord may need to wait patiently for the lease to expire or offer the tenant an amount that equals or exceeds the value of the tenant's interest as compensation for early termination of the lease.

The value of intangible assets introduces an added dimension to the highest and best use analysis for nursing facilities. The value of the intangible assets of a nursing facility can be substantial when competitive supply is regulated by certificates of need or bed moratoriums. In some states, the certificate of need or license may be transferable to a replacement facility, either on the same site or an alternative site. In this case, it may prove to be economically feasible to abandon the existing improvements and relocate to a new, state-of-the-art replacement facility, using the transferable intangible assets. The abandoned improvements may have little or no value, given the special use design and the difficulty of adapting the improvements to economically viable alternatives.

Highest and Best Use as Improved

The analysis of the highest and best use as improved for nursing facilities usually presents few, if any, alternative uses that could achieve sustained returns that match the quality and quantity of the returns from the present use. The highest and best use as improved analysis should also examine the business or operational aspects of the facility to determine maximum productivity. This analysis could include the following suggestions:

- Increase certification from ICF to SNF, or include Medicare, which could result in a higher census, a better census mix, and higher profits from ancillary business.
- Make capital improvements to enhance occupancy, census mix, and rates (including Medicaid rates).
- Downsize licensed beds to increase the size of more profitable therapy areas, achieve higher certification, or improve Medicaid rates (minimum utilization limitations).
- Replace the existing facility with a new facility that will generate higher rates, a better census mix, and greater profits over a longer period. The value of the new facility should exceed the cost to create the replacement and the loss in value of the existing facility after it is relicensed or vacated.
- Make other physical or operational changes that produce positive economic benefits.

If a nursing facility is no longer profitable, an alternative use could generate a greater economic return. Like schools or motels, nursing facilities can rarely be converted to another use without substantial renovation. Many alternative uses, commercial or residential, may not be legal under current zoning laws, or the location may not be economically viable for a particular use. Sales of closed nursing homes are deeply discounted relative to the replacement cost of the improvements. Because the downside of closing the facility is severe, operators should be vigilant in maintaining their competitive position, making necessary capital improvements and improving operations to remain profitable over the functional life of the improvements. However, many factors affecting the financial performance of a nursing facility, such as reimbursement policies and competitive supply, are beyond the control of the operator.

The ultimate measure of highest and best use is financial, which implies that the property is competing in a market of private ownership pursuing financial profitability. However, there are many instances in which nursing facilities may not represent the highest and best of the property as improved, yet they continue to operate to serve a public need or charitable purpose. Over 30% of all nursing facilities' licensed beds and occupied beds are controlled by non-profit or governmental concerns whose primary motivations are not necessarily economic. When appraising a nursing facility with a highest and best use as improved that differs from the existing use, or when the land value exceeds the value as improved, it may be necessary to arrive at two separate values to address the appraisal problem:

1. A market value based on the highest and best use (either as improved or as though vacant)
2. A value in use that presumes the continuation of the existing nursing facility use

The appraiser must carefully develop and clearly report each value to avoid creating a misleading report and prevent inappropriate use of the appraisal.

Excess land often warrants separate highest and best use consideration in analyzing the highest and best use of the improved site. However, the excess land may be merged with the as-improved site when considering the highest and best use of the total site as though vacant.

Summary

Highest and best use analysis for a vacant nursing facility site must consider all potential uses for the site that are physically possible, legally allowed, and economically feasible. Of those uses, the use that produces the highest return to the land is the highest and best use. Often that use is not for a nursing facility, even though the site is devoted to that use. The analysis of highest and best use as improved may require more focus on operational issues of the building, rather than consideration of alternatives to nursing facility use. Most nursing facilities are specifically designed for that use and are not adaptable to alternative uses. The highest and best use for buildings with functional obsolescence or facilties that have market or reimbursement deficiencies may require consideration of capital improvements to eliminate obsolescence, change the level of certification, and change bed capacity to better fit the market, operating efficiencies, and reimbursements. Occasionally, the property may be worth more dead than alive because the current improvements are no longer the highest and best use.

Chapter 15

Income Capitalization and Discounted Cash Flow Analysis

The process of converting net operating income into value is referred to as *capitalization.* Direct capitalization is peformed in a single step, dividing the estimated income by a capitalization rate or multiplying the income by an earnings multiplier. The capitalization rate is expressed as a percentage. If the capitalization rate is 12.5%, then the earnings or net income multiplier is the reciprocal, or 8.0 (1/0.125). In direct capitalization, value is estimated from a known income and rate. In fact, when two of the three components–income, rate, and value–are known, the third is easily calculated by use of the IRV formula:

Using a capitalization rate, the following formula combinations are available to solve for the unknown.

Value = Income / Rate (capitalization rate)

Income = Value × Rate (capitalization rate)

Rate = Income / Value

Using an earnings multiplier, the following formula combinations are available to solve for the unknown.

Value = Income × Rate (earnings multiplier)

Income = Value / Rate (earnings multiplier)

Rate = Value / Income

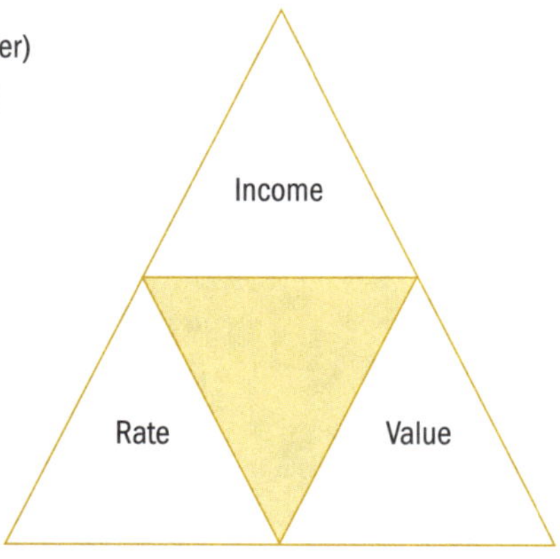

Yield capitalization using discounted cash flow (DCF) analysis is another income capitalization technique. In DCF analysis, the revenues, operating expenses, and net operating income (*NOI*) or *EBITDAR* are forecast for a set of sequential periods or years. The discounted value of those earnings and the discounted value of the property at the termination of the cash flow forecast are totaled to provide an indication of value. This approach is most useful when there are predictable, but irregular, cash flows, which are difficult to treat in direct capitalization. In most instances, the market prefers direct capitalization to DCF analysis. Issues that arise in the application of DCF analysis are addressed later in this chapter.

Irregularities in the cash flow of a facility can result from expected changes in competitive market conditions, changes in reimbursements or operations, or other circumstances that render current cash flow unreliable for valuation benchmarking. DCF analysis is useful in the valuation of new facilities and facilities undergoing market repositioning. After major renovations, market absorption may take some time. However, the market, which consists of operators, landlords, and lenders, prefers direct capitalization over DCF analysis when earnings are expected to be stable. HUD, the nation's largest insurer of nursing facility loans, prohibits any reliance on DCF analysis.

Appraisals of nursing facilities must draw on the disciplines of both real estate valuation and business valuation. In the real estate world, the income that is capitalized into a value indication is generally referred to as *net operating income* (*NOI*), the income before any deductions for the cost of capital. In business valuations, that income is often referred to as *earnings before interest, depreciation, amortization, and rent* (*EBITDAR*). Rather than dividing *EBITDAR* by a capitalization rate, which is expressed as a percentage, it is multiplied by an earnings multiplier. These mathematical operations yield the same results. The expression of income as *EBITDAR* more precisely defines that income. *NOI* and *EBITDAR* are generally considered the same, however, *EBITDAR* clearly implies that management expenses are included as an item of expense and deducted from earnings. Pushing back the management expense into the earnings is expressed as an *EBITDARM* figure. Landlords and tenants of leased facilities often compare *EBITDA* (after rent) and *EBITDAR* (before rent)

Direct Capitalization

The direct capitalization method converts a single year's income expectancy (I) into a value indication (V). The relationship between income and value is expressed in the overall capitalization rate (R_O). Because this method does not distinguish between the return on and the return of capital, the rate is often referred to as the *overall capitalization rate.* Using *IRV*, overall capitalization rates are derived by using this simple formula:

Rate = Income / Value

$$R_O = I / V$$

The overall capitalization rate (R_O) incorporates the following:

- A return on the equity investment
- Debt service
- Principal build-up
- Anticipated changes in income and value
- Recapture of depreciating components of the property
- The physical quality of the property
- Other economic factors

The following direct capitalization techniques are typically applied in the valuation of nursing facilities:

1. Direct overall capitalization–based on comparable sales data
2. Band of investment–applying mortgage and equity rates derived from market data
3. Debt service coverage method–applying the debt coverage ratio

Developing Capitalization Rates from Comparable Sales

As applied in commercial real estate appraising, overall capitalization rates derived from comparable sales data can be conclusive evidence used to estimate value through the capitalization process. The technique is most effective when the net operating income (*NOI*) estimates for the subject and the comparable sale properties are stabilized. Under stabilized market and operating conditions, the capitalization rate of a sale is most appropriately derived from the expected net operating income for the first year of ownership.

The *NOI*s of the comparable sales may be influenced by the same short- and long-term changes in the competitive market and reimbursement structures as the income of the subject. Close examination of the competitive market and reimbursement issues for each sale is important. Since *NOI*s fluctuate widely from year to year and operating margins are narrow, the overall capitalization rates for a group of sales may fall into a wide range. To compensate for these fluctuations, the appraiser should focus on the average overall rate derived from a group of sales, rather than comparing a few isolated sales.

Obtaining data to develop overall capitalization rates from sale transactions requires an investment of time and effort. Fortunately, in most states a substantial amount of revenue and operating expense information is available from Medicaid cost reports, which are available to the public through a FOIA request. The cost reports provide detailed census and operating expense characteristics and usually comprehensive revenue data as well. Since the buyer's cost reports are often filed six to 15 months after the change of ownership or sale, that information may not be available for review during the period when the appraisal is being developed. However, the seller's final cost report or most recent past report is more likely to be available. In any case, the cost report serves as a solid basis for estimating stabilized revenues and operating expenses for the comparable sales.

The appraiser will need to forecast stabilized *NOI* using a combination of the seller's actual census, revenue, and expenses; actual figures from the buyer's first reporting period; pro forma figures developed from an offering memorandum or other marketing materials; the underwriting documents for the financing; the buyer's forecast; and other sources. A synthesis of information from various sources may be necessary to arrive at an appropriate *NOI* or *EBITDAR* figure. The appraiser should take every opportunity to interview the buyers and receive their perspectives on the *NOI* and capitalization rate. Interviewing the principals to the sale transactions is critical when no other resources to develop *NOI* are available. Interviews with buyers and sellers should include their definitions of *NOI* to ensure consistency. Interview questions may include the following:

- Does the *NOI/EBITDAR* reflect trailing or forecasted figures?
- Does the revenue include anticipated adjustments to revenue that are expected to occur as a result of changes in occupancy and census mix as well as changes in private and government reimbursement rates?
- Does the buyer expect to improve earnings through increased census, a change in payor mix, rate adjustments, and/or reductions in operating expenses?
- Do the expenses include all appropriate costs, including market levels of management, cap-ex, and adjustments for differences in operations?
- Will the facility be repositioned in the market through substantial renovations?

Consistency in Capitalization Rates

The revenue and operating expenses used to derive an *NOI* for the comparable sales should be treated in the same manner as the revenue and expenses used to develop the *NOI* for the subject. For consistency, the appraiser should investigate:

- Trailing vs. pro forma *NOI*

- Consistent treatment of management fees and reserves for replacement for the sales and the subject.
- Leased fee vs. fee simple capitalization rates
- Individual sale vs. portfolio sale transaction capitalization rates
- Medicaid rate rebasing due to changes in ownership or other changes affecting Medicaid reimbursement

The need for consistent comparisons is universal in all appraisal disciplines.

In Table 15.1, the trailing (seller's) *NOI* is compared with the forecasted (buyer's) *NOI*, and resulting differences in the capitalization rate are shown. The forecasted revenues increase

Table 15.1 **Seller vs. Buyer *NOI* and Capitalization Rate**

	Seller/Trailing	Buyer/Forecast
Revenues		
Gross potential revenue	$6,000,000	$6,300,000
Vacancy rate	10.0%	7.9%
Net revenue	$5,400,000	$5,800,000
Operating expenses		
Direct care expenses		
Nursing	$2,400,000	$2,480,000
Social services and activities	160,000	180,000
Ancillary (therapy, drugs & medical equipment)	400,000	420,000
Support costs		
Dietary	450,000	465,000
Laundry	120,000	130,000
Housekeeping	160,000	170,000
Maintenance	140,000	150,000
Utilities	80,000	85,000
Property costs		
Property insurance	20,000	25,000
Property taxes	50,000	50,000
Cap-ex, replacement reserves	40,000	40,000
Administrative and general		
Administrative	350,000	360,000
Liability insurance	200,000	210,000
Provider tax ($800.00/bed)	80,000	80,000
Subtotal	$4,650,000	$4,845,000
NOI before management, or *EBITDARM*	$750,000	$955,000
Central office/management fee	$270,000	$290,000
NOI after management, or *EBITDAR*	$480,000	$665,000
Sale price	$5,000,000	$5,000,000
Capitalization rate (*NOI* after management–*EBITDAR*)	9.6%	13.3%
Capitalization rate (*NOI* before management–*EBITDARM*)	15.0%	19.1%

because of inflation and a slight step up in the Medicaid capital reimbursement. The buyer is forecasting an increase in occupancy resulting from various management adjustments and simple market realities. Operating expenses are expected to increase slightly because of inflationary pressures. However, the increased occupancy is expected to result in only a very small increase in variable expenses and essentially no change in fixed expenses, beyond inflation trending.

Using this capitalization rate extraction example, now assume that the subject and the sale have identical *NOI*s of $665,000 and similar investment risks. If the 9.6% capitalization rate developed from the trailing *NOI* of the sale is applied to the subject's forecasted *NOI* of $665,000, the value indication is $6,927,000, or 26% greater than the sale price of an identical property that sold for $5,500,000 recently. While this problem may seem elementary to most appraisers, it is a critical point that is misunderstood or simply not considered by some market participants.

The *NOI* of a comparable sale should be developed with expenses that include market levels of management and capital replacement reserves if the expense forecasted for the subject includes these expense items. Conversely, overstating expenses by using the excessive management and ancillary expenses charged to a facility through related-party management and therapy entities will understate the *NOI* and the capitalization rate.

Developing Capitalization Rates for Facilities in Inactive Markets

Often overall capitalization rates cannot be developed from recent comparable sales data because the market is inactive. In these situations, the direct capitalization rate must be supported using sales data from other regions, surveys, and interviews with market participants.

Rates derived from sales data from other states may present unique challenges. State regulations, such as differences in certificate of need policies, may exert significantly greater or less control on competitive supply. Also, different Medicaid reimbursement systems present different levels of risks, even though the "real estate" and census characteristics of the facilities may appear very similar. States that have a history of rebasing rates erratically or fall behind on paying operators may cause nursing facilities in those states to sell at higher capitalization rates, when all else is equal.

Conducting interviews with active market participants can be beneficial if those interviewed have no bias and use clearly understood definitions of *NOI* or *EBITDAR* that are consistent with the definition being applied to the subject property. However, there is no assurance that respondents will be unbiased or relate an opinion consistent with the definition. Knowing these limitations, the appraiser can proceed with market interviews and be on guard for inconsistencies and biases.

Capitalization rates developed from published surveys have the advantage of representing current market conditions rather than older sales data. The problem of dated information increases in importance when the market is experiencing rapid valuation changes caused by changes in the cost of capital (interest rates), government policies, and Medicare reimbursements.

However, there are concerns about placing too much reliance on surveyed rates. First, most survey publishers, such as the National Investment Center for Long Term Care Financing (NIC), provide national data for all nursing facilities without regard to location, facility age, payor mix, and other significant elements of comparison. The surveys cover many types of long-term care properties (independent, assisted living, skilled nursing, etc.) and those interviewed include owners, lenders, and others. The respondents may be involved in just one or a few property types, but they will often weigh in on all the property types, even though they do not actively participate in all these market segments. Moreover, the surveys may not establish a clear definition of *NOI* or *EBITDAR*, and some respondents make not understand the significance of using consistent definitions. For example, if half the surveyed respondents report capitalization rates using trailing *NOI* and half report forecasted *NOI* capitalization rates, then the survey will have a significant bias toward the low side.

Equity Capitalization—Band of Investment

The band of investment is a technique for deriving an overall capitalization rate by weighing market proportions of debt and equity and estimating the market rates for each component.

The band of investment formula is:

$$R_O = (M \times R_M) + [(1 - M) \times R_E]$$

Where:

M = the ratio of mortgage value to property value (loan-to-value ratio)

R_M = the annual mortgage constant, or mortgage capitalization rate

R_E = the equity capitalization rate

The mortgage constant is the ratio of the annual debt service (interest plus principal amortization) to the amount borrowed; the rate provides a return on, and of, the borrowed funds or lender's position. The equity capitalization rate is the first-year cash throw-off to the equity position divided by the amount of equity cash invested. It is also referred to as the *equity dividend rate*, the *cash-on-cash rate of return*, or the *current yield* expected by the equity position.

Mortgage or Debt Rate and Ratio

In selecting the appropriate mortgage rate and terms, consideration is given to the typical mortgage rates and terms available in the debt market. Locations, physical plants, and earnings characteristics dictate the type of financing available. Newer, higher-quality facilities and well-established facilities located in stable or improving markets show the least operational risk and command superior financing terms–lower interest rates, lengthier amortization periods, and other favorable terms. Older facilities with average to below-average locations and/or economic prospects will be offered higher interest rates and shorter amortization periods. Even for the same facility and loan amount, rates and terms will vary widely among different lenders. In addition to a mortgage on the real estate assets, the lender may require guarantees from the parent corporation or personal guarantees from principal stakeholders, cross collateralization with other real estate or business assets, and/or a tie-in to accounts receivable.

As mentioned in Chapter 4, the ownership of a nursing facility is often fragmented. Some mortgage lenders will require the mortgage to be secured by not only the mortgaged real estate assets, with guarantees and other controls on the assets of the real estate entity, but they will also reach into the collateral of related-party entities, such as the licensed operator, if the operator is not the real estate holder. The license and operating rights that are conveyed through Medicare and Medicaid certifications and certificates of need are critical assets to the value of the business and real estate. Many lenders (and landlords) take appropriate precautions in loan or lease agreements with the borrower or tenant to be protected from the severing of these various assets. The severing of the real estate from the intangible assets of a nursing facility could be compared to a neutron bomb explosion–the property stays, but the people are gone. These issues deserve consideration when examining the debt structures of actual sale transactions from which equity capitalization rates are being extracted.

Extraordinary financing concessions may result in borrowers obtaining greater debt leverage (loan-to-value ratios), lower interest rates, and extended amortization periods that would not typically be available in the market. As long as the purchase price is unaffected by special financing terms, an argument can be made that applying "market" mortgage terms rather than the actual terms that a borrower has achieved through conceding other collateral is a better measure of market levels in the derivation of equity capitalization rates.

Like commercial real estate, nursing facilities are financed through a large array of competitive financing options, including short-term lending through banks and investment banking arrangements and longer-term loans through small and large private lenders, bond offerings, and FHA-insured loans offered through several HUD programs. These different loan options tend to be highly competitive.

Equity Rate and Ratio

The equity capitalization rate is best determined by extraction from comparable sales data. However, equity rates may also be obtained through interviews with nursing facility investors and through surveys. Equity capitalization rates can be easily extracted from comparable sales data if the price, *NOI*, and mortgage terms are known. If the mortgage terms are unknown or atypical, then typical market financing can be substituted.

The following algebraic expression and subsequent case study example shows the extraction of an equity capitalization rate.

$$R_E = [R_O - (R_M - M)] / (1 - M)$$

Where:

R_E = the equity capitalization rate

R_M = the annual mortgage constant, or mortgage capitalization rate

M = the ratio of mortgage value to property value (loan-to-value ratio)

The principles of extracting equity capitalization rates are the same regardless of the source(s) of the overall rate–i.e., market sales, surveys, or interviews. All that is needed is the overall capitalization rate and the market rate and terms for the debt.

Case Study—Equity Capitalization Rate Extraction

A comparable nursing facility was recently sold with a capitalization rate of 12.0%. The transaction was conventionally financed with a 75% mortgage and the interest rate and amortization term produce an .0800 annual mortgage constant. The terms are consistent with current market conditions. Algebraically, the equity capitalization rate is calculated as follows:

$$R_E = [(.120 - (.0800 \times .75)] / (1 - .75)$$
$$= (.120 - .060) / .25$$
$$= .060 / .25$$
$$= .24$$

The equity capitalization rate is expressed without algebra as follows:

Step 1:	Sale price (*V*):		$10,000,000
	Mortgage ratio (*M*) – consistent with market	×	75%
	Mortgage amount	=	$7,500,000
	Sale price		$10,000,000
	Mortgage amount	–	7,500,000
	Equity	=	$2,500,000
Step 2:	Mortgage amount		$7,500,000
	Annual mortgage constant (R_M)	×	.0800
	Annual debt service	=	$600,000
Step 3:	*NOI* or *EBITDAR* (R_0)		$1,200,000
	Annual debt service	–	600,000
	Return to equity (*EBTD*)	=	$600,000
Step 4:	Return to equity (*EBTD*)		$600,000
	Equity	/	$2,500,000
	Equity capitalization rate	=	24.0%

Since overall capitalization rates and mortgage terms are generally known in the market, there is no reason not to extract equity capitalization rates from market data. Equity capitalization rates developed by interviewing market participants often result in incongruent indications, as many market participants have little or no understanding of the relationships between overall and equity capitalization rates. For example, an operator being interviewed by an appraiser states that he anticipates a 15.0% equity capitalization rate and an overall rate of 12.0%. Competitive market debt is available with a mortgage equal to 70% of the purchase price at a mortgage constant of .0800. This math does not make sense. If the capitalization rate and mortgage terms are accurate, the equity capitalization rate should be 21.3% [(.120 – (.0800 × .70)} / (1 – .70)]. The appraiser would be presenting misleading information if he relies on the 15.0% equity capitalization rate. The buyer seemed certain about the overall rate and mortgage terms, but was clearly less confident in stating the equity rate.

Debt Coverage Ratio

The debt coverage method involves the calculation of an overall capitalization rate from the annual mortgage constant, the loan-to-value ratio, and the debt coverage ratio (DCR) indicated by the market. The debt coverage ratio is calculated as the net operating income divided by the annual debt service.

The derivation of an overall capitalization rate employing the debt service coverage method is presented as follows.

$$R_O = R_M \times M \times DCR$$

Most lenders in the long-term care market sector impose a minimum debt service coverage ratio on a loan in addition to a maximum loan-to-value ratio. The appraiser may be instructed by the client to use a DCR procedure with a specific debt coverage ratio. Because many mortgage amounts are constrained by loan-to-value ratios, using the lender's specific DCR or a typical ratio obtained from surveying competitive lenders' minimum debt coverage ratios may produce an unrealistically low overall capitalization rate and a value indication that is more akin to investment value than market value.

By restating the DCR formula above, the DCR extracted from a sale transaction can be computed as follows:

$$DCR = R_O / (R_M \times M)$$

Case Study—Debt Coverage Ratio

Using the information applied to develop the equity capitalization rate in the previous case study application, an implied DCR can be developed.

$$R_O = 12.0\%$$

$$R_M = .0800$$

$$M = 75\%$$

$$\text{DCR} = .12 / (.080 \times .75) = 2.0$$

Using the lender's minimum DCR to develop the capitalization rate may produce a non-market overall rate that would translate into an investment value conclusion. Assume that a lender wants the overall capitalization rate to be based on a minimum required DCR of 1.5, a loan-to-value ratio (M) of 75%, and a mortgage constant (R_M) of .0800. Using these figures in the DCR equation produces an overall capitalization rate of 9.0% (.0800 × .75 × 1.5). Clearly, that capitalization rate is inconsistent with rates developed from market-extracted data. Placing any significance on this rate in reconciling the overall rate selection would skew the valuation upwards.

Reconciliation and Selection of the Overall Capitalization Rate

The appraiser must consider the quality and quantity of the data applied in each of the three primary techniques for developing an overall capitalization rate. The direct overall rate is based on sales data where price and *NOI* are known, or the rate may be derived from surveys and/or interviews. The band-of-investment technique, which applies weighted proportions of mortgage and equity and their market-appropriate rates, presents more variables and can require market assumptions made by the appraiser; the assumptions may reduce the reliability of this technique. The debt coverage ratio usually is associated with a specific lender's minimum coverage ratio and, as such, the development of the capitalization rate is more detached from "market" evidence. In all three cases, if the rates are calculated using figures that are tied back to substantial, direct market evidence, the rate indications produced should be similar and carry considerable weight.

The technique or techniques that are rooted in the most substantial market data warrant the greatest weight in the reconciliation process. Usually, the direct overall rate extracted from market sales data has the greatest significance. However, overall rates from a small group of sales may produce a wide range of rate indications and the rate variances may appear to have little or no logical correlation with the differences. Overall and equity capitalization rate outliers may need to be culled out. Rate averages may warrant consideration, with the selected rate falling below, at, or above the average depending on the relative risk characteristics of the subject compared to the characteristics typical of the sales group.

The equity capitalization rate, if extracted from comparable market sales data, is a product of the direct overall rate. The band-of-investment technique may be subordinated if the equity capitalization rate and/or the mortgage terms are developed from figures that are not tied to direct, market-extracted data. The debt coverage ratio technique may prove significant if the other techniques rely on older sale transactions and there has been a measurable change in the capital markets (interest rates and/or debt coverage ratios) subsequent to those sale dates. However, if the capital markets have been fairly stable between the dates of the comparable sales and the effective date of the appraisal, then the DCR technique may be less appropriate. Certainly, if the debt coverage ratio relies on a specific or minimum coverage ratio mandated by a client or lender, the indicated overall rate could have little connection to the market.

Case Study—Capitalization Rate Conclusion and Value Indication

Continuing the case study, a 12.0% overall capitalization rate is applied to the stabilized net operating income for the subject facility, which was developed in Chapter 13.

Net operating income or earnings before interest, depreciation, amortization, and rent (EBITDAR)	$1,127,881
Overall capitalization rate	12.0%
Indicated market value of the total assets of the business, rounded	$9,400,000

Other Capitalization Rate Issues

SNF Risk Premiums

Nursing home capitalization rates tend to be several hundred basis points higher than the rates for apartments, offices, and retail properties. The higher capitalization rates are attributable to:

- Greater risks from business or intangible components
- Higher return (recapture) of short-lived tangible personal property assets
- Narrower *NOI* margins, introducing greater operating risk
- Investor reluctance to invest in a specialized business
- Government regulations, possible loss of license, and complicated reimbursement issues
- Special-purpose construction with severely reduced value for alternative use

To demonstrate why nursing facility capitalization rates tend to be higher than rates for most commercial real estate, the value of the various assets of the business enterprise can be paired to fair returns for the respective components. The example that follows assumes a $4,000,000 market value, with an allocation to the real estate and personal property based on depreciated replacement costs. The returns to these components include a return on the assets equal to the weighted-average cost of capital (debt and equity) and recapture rates based on straight-line depreciation. The residual value and *NOI* are attributed to the intangible assets. Considering the risk associated with the intangible component, its return factor is expected to be significantly greater than the total return to the tangible assets (see Table 15.2).

Table 15.3 presents a second perspective on the overall rate and estimated asset returns.

Certainly, differences in building age and location have significant impacts on nursing facility capitalization rates. But, perhaps just as importantly, the payor mix and profit sources affect capitalization rates. Two nearly identical facilities located in very similar locations may command prices in the market that have different capitalization rates as the result of a difference in payor mix or profit sources.

For instance, the earnings for one facility may be heavily dependent on extensive therapy activities, with substantial profits generated from Medicare reimbursements. The therapy services involve greater amounts of human endeavor, which tend to be associated with greater risks. Also, if the facility is very profitable, additional competition may be developed in

Table 15.2 **Example of Capitalization Rate Residual Using Asset Value Allocation**

	Allocated Value	Return	*NOI*
Market value of business enterprise	$4,000,000		
Overall capitalization rate			$540,000
Less return to building and site improvements			
Allocated improvement value per cost approach	($2,700,000)		
Fair return on realty		9.0%	
Recapture of improvements (50-year life)		2.0%	
Fair return to improvements		11.0%	($297,000)
Less return to land			
Allocated land value per cost approach	($250,000)		
Fair return to land		9.0%	($22,500)
Less return to FF&E			
Allocated FF&E value per cost approach	($300,000)		
Fair return on FF&E		9.0%	
Recapture of FF&E (10-year life)		10.0%	
Total return to FF&E		19.0%	($57,000)
Equal allocated intangible asset value	$750,000		
Return to intangible assets		21.8%	$163,500

Table 15.3 **Overall Rate and Asset Returns**

Asset	Allocated Value	% Allocation	% Asset Return	% Weighted Return
Improvements	$2,700,000	67.5	11.0	7.4
Land	250,000	6.3	9.0	0.6
FF&E	300,000	7.5	19.0	1.4
Intangibles	750,000	18.7		4.1
Totals	$4,000,000	100.0		13.6

the foreseeable future. This competition may employ state-of-the-art design and features that cause a substantial shift in Medicare demand to the new property. Just as the recapture period of a building affects the capitalization rate, so can the expected life of extraordinary earnings from therapy services. The $500,000 of *EBITDAR* achieved from therapy and other ancillary services may be capitalized at a higher rate than the $500,000 of *EBITDAR* achieved from private-pay rate premiums and Medicaid capital reimbursements. Of course, the appraiser needs to look to the market for evidence to support the capitalization rate variance attributable to any perceived risk issue, whether it relates to the real estate or the business activities of the nursing facility. Perceived risk might be detected through analysis of sales data or through interviews with operators, investors, and lenders.

Leased Fee vs. Fee Simple Capitalization Rates

Chapter 19 will address issues relating to the valuation of partial interests. Applying a capitalization rate developed from leased fee interest sales data to the valuation of the total assets of the business, or going concern, violates the principle of consistency.

Briefly, nursing facilities are often leased to a third-party investor on a long-term, absolute net lease basis, creating a leased fee interest. Typically, lease rent is set at a substantial fraction of *EBITDAR* or *NOI*. Sales of a leased fee interest are typically priced based on the rental income, with *EBITDAR* used as an indication of the durability and quality of the lease rent. In a financially healthy SNF lease, *EBITDAR* exceeds contract rent, creating a positive position for the tenant or leasehold interest. Generally, in these situations, the leased fee capitalization rate will be less than the capitalization rate for the fee simple interest in an otherwise identical property.

Rates Derived From Portfolio Transactions

The overall capitalization rates derived from portfolio sale transactions may not be appropriate in the valuation of an individual facility. In active markets where there is plenty of equity and debt capital available, portfolio transactions tend to reflect premium pricing and lower capitalization rates than an individual sale with otherwise identical or comparable elements of comparison. Conversely, in markets where capital is scarce, portfolio transactions may trade at a discount compared to an otherwise comparable individual facility sale. Premium pricing is often created by spreading risk over more facilities, as equity investors and lenders are willing to accepted lower returns in return for increased safety. If more appropriate capitalization rates extracted from individual comparable sales are available, the use of a portfolio rate should be avoided. In the event that there is a dearth of recent single-property transactions, rates from portfolio sales may be applied with cautious judgment and adjustment.

A client may request that a portfolio valuation be conducted on a group of properties. Such a valuation may require adjustments to operating expenses and necessitate the use of comparable portfolio sales to develop market-derived capitalization rate indications and apply the sales comparison approach. The allocation of a portion of the "portfolio" value back to an individual facility will require the use of an extraordinary assumption and/or hypothetical condition. The resulting valuation may be misleading if the appraisal does not include an opinion of the "one-off" market value.

Discounted Cash Flow (DCF) Analysis or Yield Capitalization

Yield capitalization is the process of discounting annual cash flows, or streams of *NOI*, and the terminal property value into present value. Revenues, operating expenses, and *NOI* or *EBITDAR* are forecast for a set of sequential periods, or years, using the best available information to predict future conditions. The discounted value of those future earnings plus the discounted value of the property at the termination of the cash flow forecast provide an indication of value. DCF analysis is especially applicable when there is a reasonable probability that the *NOI* will be irregular over the foreseeable future or when the facility is expected to reach stabilized occupancy and earnings several years out that differ from current occupancy and earnings levels. Irregular *NOI* could be the result of changes in occupancy and mix resulting from competitive market forces, reimbursement rate changes, or initial absorption.

The length of the cash flow analysis is a topic of debate. Often forecasts are made to match the loan period or to extend slightly beyond it. Conventional cash flow analyses for nursing facilities seldom extend beyond 10 years and are typically shorter. The final year of the cash flow, which will be used to estimate the terminal value, reflects long-term occupancy, mix, and *NOI* expectations for the period beyond the cash flow forecasts.

The DCF analysis should be sensitive to changes in:

- Occupancy, caused by changes in supply and demand in the market
- Payor mix
- Private-pay rates
- Medicaid and Medicare rates–reconciling these payments with allowable operating expense estimates
- Acuity levels and any impact on rates and ancillary revenue
- Operating expenses caused by any of these factors

Development of Future Occupancy, Payor Mix, and Revenues

The conclusions developed in the competitive market analysis set the stage for forecasting future occupancy and payor mix for the subject. The occupancy or census level is subject to changes in supply and demand. Changes in demand may correspond with changes in population forecasts. However, simply relying on population trends may miss other factors that can drive changes in demand. Assisted living and home health care alternatives may continue to siphon off lower-acuity nursing facility demand. If assisted living facilities are already well established in the market, then little further erosion in traditional nursing demand may be expected. If the state is considering increasing Medicaid waivers for assisted living as an alternative to nursing facilities, however, Medicaid demand will be diverted to assisted living and occupancy rates for nursing facilities will come under pressure.

These same considerations affect payor mix. With respect to payor mix, there is a trend towards greater percentages of Medicare (and managed care) patients in nursing facilities and lower percentages of private-pay census. (For more on payor or census mix analysis, see Chapter 11.)

Revenue forecasting is based on forecasted patient days multiplied by average per-diem rates for that period. All rates will be influenced by inflationary pressures. The private-pay and managed care rates will also be influenced by competitive market conditions. In markets where there is vacancy, competition typically places enough pressure on rates so that they will generally increase by percentages that approximate inflation. Additional rate increases, beyond inflationary trending, can be achieved through increased acuity (which comes with additional expenses), market repositioning of the facility through a capital improvement program, a supply shortage, or improved management.

Medicaid rates will be subject to the reimbursement mechanisms applied by the state. In states that use facility-specific, cost-based reimbursement, it may be necessary to estimate the reimbursement from a previous-year expense forecast so that the rate and reimbursement correspond. The capital portion of the Medicaid rate may trend very differently than the operating expense components of the rate, so the appraiser may be wise to make an effort to reflect the capital component of the reimbursement separately. Known changes in Medicaid trending factors, i.e., rebasing or other foreseeable rate changes, should be incorporated into the forecast. Many states have a history of erratic reimbursement, which will make forecasting this revenue difficult. In these situations, the DCF analysis may prove to be less reliable.

Medicare PPS rates for Part A have historically increased at the beginning of each federal fiscal year, on October 1, and the increases tend to be slightly less than the recognized inflation rate. Next-year rates are generally known three months earlier. Consideration should be given to pending changes and proposals that will affect future PPS rates. Medicare is entering a long period of probable deficits, and some type of reduction in program costs may be forced onto nursing facilities. A consensus of market participants and information from industry trade groups can be used to forecast future Medicare reimbursement changes.

Table 15.4 presents a forecast of revenue for the subject of the case study. The census and payor mix forecast for the 120-bed facility were developed in earlier chapters. The final year cash flow occupancy rate is based on a perceived, sustainable long-term occupancy level, normalized for any short-run imbalances in supply and demand. The census mix forecast reflects the industry trends of declining private-pay mix and increasing Medicare census.

In the forecast, private-pay rates are increased annually by the same rate generally applied to expense inflation, as the market is expected to place no extraordinary pressure on rates in either direction. The Medicaid rate increases relative to the increase in allowable operating expenses. Medicare Part A is forecast to increase at an amount that is slightly less than inflation to hedge against growing budgetary pressures to reduce program expenses.

Table 15.4 DCF Application—Revenue Forecasting

	Year 1	Year 2	Year 3	Year 4	Year 5	Year 6
Occupancy forecast						
Number of beds	120	120	120	120	120	120
Potential patient days	43,800	43,800	43,800	43,800	43,800	43,800
Occupancy rate	89.3%	91.1%	92.9%	94.8%	92.5%	92.5%
Total patient days	39,128	39,902	40,690	41,522	40,515	40,515
Census mix						
Private pay	31.3%	30.7%	30.1%	29.5%	28.9%	28.3%
Medicare	11.0%	11.1%	11.2%	11.3%	11.4%	11.5%
Medicaid	57.6%	58.2%	58.7%	59.2%	59.7%	60.2%
Total	100.0%	100.0%	100.0%	100.0%	100.0%	100.0%
Census mix by days						
Private pay	12,264	12,250	12,248	12,249	11,709	11,466
Medicare	4,307	4,429	4,557	4,692	4,619	4,659
Medicaid	22,557	23,223	23,885	24,581	24,187	24,390
Total	39,128	39,902	40,690	41,522	40,515	40,515

Table 15.4 **DCF Application—Revenue Forecasting *(continued)***

	Inflation Rate	Year 1	Year 2	Year 3	Year 4	Year 5	Year 6
Revenue per patient day							
Private (average)	3.00%	$184.28	$189.81	$195.50	$201.37	$207.41	$213.63
Medicare	2.90%	338.82	348.65	358.76	369.16	379.87	390.89
Medicaid							
Variable portion	3.00%	135.91	139.99	143.65	147.42	151.28	157.44
Capital	1.00%	11.22	11.33	11.44	11.55	11.67	11.79
Medicare Part B and private ancillary	3.00%	1.75	1.80	1.85	1.91	1.97	2.03
Other revenue	3.00%	0.50	0.52	0.54	0.56	0.58	0.60
Bad debt	3.00%	-0.50	-0.52	-0.54	-0.56	-0.58	-0.60
Revenue							
Private (average)		$2,260,070	$2,325,156	$2,394,423	$2,466,579	$2,428,529	$2,449,427
Medicare		1,459,302	1,544,213	1,634,970	1,732,094	1,754,509	1,821,244
Medicaid		3,318,741	3,514,099	3,704,329	3,907,645	3,941,346	4,127,525
Medicare Part B and private ancillary		68,474	71,824	75,277	79,307	79,815	82,245
Other revenue		19,564	20,749	21,973	23,252	23,499	24,309
Bad debt		-19,564	-20,749	-21,973	-23,252	-23,499	-24,309
Total net revenue		$7,106,587	$7,455,292	$7,808,999	$8,185,625	$8,204,199	$8,480,442

Development of Future Operating Expenses and Net Operating Income (*EBITDAR*)

Future operating expenses are impacted by changes in total census, census mix, acuity levels, and inflationary factors. Because of the upward trending in acuity levels, operating expenses for nursing facilities will tend to increase at rates that exceed inflation over the long run, assuming stable census levels.

The modeling of future operating expenses will typically include separate calculations for fixed and variable components. Fixed expenses generally do not fluctuate with occupancy, and prudent management will have to pay these expenses whether the facility is well occupied or not. Variable expenses generally do fluctuate with the level of occupancy or the extent of services. Since nursing facilities are labor-intensive enterprises, management constantly monitors the relationship between occupancy and labor. Within most of the expense categories, the expenses are a combination of fixed and variable expenses.

Reversion Value and Terminal Capitalization Rate

To estimate the reversion value at the end of the forecast period, the net operating income for the year following the last year of the forecast is capitalized by a terminal overall capitalization rate (R_N). Calculating the reversion value usually involves making a deduction for selling or financial restructuring costs. The cash flow for the final year used to calculate the terminal value reflects normalized, long-term levels of occupancy, revenue, operating expenses, and *NOI*; short-term market and/or operating imbalances are avoided in the cash flow forecast for the terminal year as those abnormalities would be unnecessarily capitalized in perpetuity. Some Medicaid reimbursement systems adjust reimbursements as a result of a sale, and the adjustment may impact earnings in the terminal year.

Inflation aside, it is logical that an investor would expect to pay less for a stabilized nursing facility when the reversion occurs since the building will have a shorter recapture period and it may have less market appeal. As a result, the terminal capitalization rate is loaded to account for these additional risk considerations. If the going-in capitalization rate reflected an abnormally high *NOI* used in the direct capitalization, it is conceivable that the terminal capitalization rate may be less than the going-in rate.

Seeking market evidence for terminal capitalization rates for nursing facilities may prove fruitless because few nursing facility investors/operators ever ponder the differences between going-in and terminal rates. In the absence of empirical evidence, the appraiser may simply need to rely on experience

Table 15.5 presents a forecast of operating expenses for the subject nursing facility. The first-year operating expenses were developed in an earlier chapter and an allocation of variable and fixed expenses was estimated. The per-patient-day expenses for the variable portions are trended for inflation and then multiplied by the total patient days for the respective year. The total amount of each fixed expense is simply trended for inflation. The nursing, ancillary (therapy and drugs), and dietary expenses are most sensitive to changes in occupancy and acuity. The management expense is entirely variable in this case. Inflation is forecast at 3.0%, but given the expectation of increasing acuity with higher percentages of Medicare and other lower-acuity patients moving toward alternatives, the nursing and ancillary expenses are forecast to increase at 3.5%.

Table 15.5 DCF Application—Operating Expense Forecasting

	Trending	% Variable	Year 1	Year 2	Year 3	Year 4	Year 5	Year 6
Total net revenue			$7,106,587	$7,455,292	$7,808,999	$8,185,625	$8,204,199	$8,480,442
Operating expenses								
Direct care expenses								
Nursing	3.5%	80%	$3,012,856	$3,167,653	$3,330,519	$3,503,910	$3,555,365	$3,679,803
Social services and activities	3.0%	50%	195,640	203,502	211,697	220,321	224,097	230,820
Ancillaries	3.0%	90%	504,166	528,536	554,087	581,252	585,546	603,113
Dietary	3.0%	75%	547,792	572,597	598,552	626,055	632,936	651,924
Laundry	3.0%	50%	156,512	162,802	169,358	176,257	179,278	184,656
Housekeeping	3.0%	25%	195,640	202,506	209,626	217,051	222,146	228,810
Maintenance	3.0%	25%	176,076	182,255	188,663	195,346	199,931	205,929
Utilities	3.0%	25%	105,646	109,353	113,198	117,208	119,959	123,558
Property insurance	3.0%	0%	21,520	22,166	22,831	23,516	24,221	24,948
Property taxes	2.0%	0%	60,648	61,861	63,099	64,361	65,648	66,961
Cap-ex, replacement reserves	3.0%	0%	72,000	74,160	76,385	78,676	81,037	83,468
General & administrative	3.0%	40%	430,408	446,828	463,911	481,829	491,297	506,036
Central office/management	3.0%	100%	332,588	349,342	366,928	385,664	387,600	399,228
Liability insurance	3.0%	0%	71,213	73,349	75,550	77,816	80,151	82,555
Provider tax	3.0%	0%	96,000	98,880	101,846	104,902	108,049	111,290
Total operating expenses			$5,978,705	$6,255,790	$6,546,250	$6,854,164	$6,957,261	$7,183,099
Net operating income or earnings before interest, depreciation, amortization, and rent (EBITDAR)			$1,127,881	$1,199,502	$1,262,749	$1,331,461	$1,246,938	$1,297,343

and judgment. There is little evidence to suggest that nursing facility investors will behave any differently than commercial property investors in this regard. Secondary evidence will normally support the application of a terminal capitalization rate premium. Commercial real estate investor surveys of capitalization and yield rates often show meaningful premiums for average terminal capitalization rates compared to average going-in rates for the same property type and class. Bond markets nearly always accord higher yields to same-rated investments as maturity dates extend out in time; the same is generally true for certificates of deposits and other timed cash investments. For this if for no other reason, the terminal capitalization rate premium may simply be represented by the difference in the mortgage constant between, say, a 20- or 30-year amortization period and a 10-year DCF analysis.

Development and Application of the Yield Rate

The cash flows from the *NOI* and reversion are discounted to present value at a market-appropriate yield rate (Y_O). The actual yield rate cannot be calculated until the investment is sold; however, the investor may target a yield prior to or during the ownership. The development of an appropriate yield rate requires the appraiser to verify and interpret the expectations and targeted rates of nursing home operators active in the market. The appraiser can verify the forecast census, revenue, and operating expense assumptions of the buyer as part of the process of verifying comparable sales.

Like capitalization rates, nursing facility yield rates are influenced by the physical plant, location, competitive market, reimbursement, and other risks characteristics. Current conditions in the financial, real estate, and healthcare markets should be blended together in the rate selection process, as current perceptions may differ from perceptions in the periods in which the yield rates and other market data were developed or transactions were conducted. Ultimately, all the available information is measured and weighed to guide the judgment of the appraiser in rate selection. In some instances, it may be appropriate to estimate and apply one yield rate to the *NOI* portion of the cash flow and another rate to the reversion value.

Development of a market-supported yield rate normally involves at least one of the following methods:

- Market extraction (cash flows from sales and formulas)
- Market survey
- Property model

Extracting Yield Rates from the Market

Extracting yield rates from comparable nursing facility sales requires clear insight into the physical and operational aspects of the sale properties as well as their competitive markets. The census, revenue, and operating expenses are estimated in much the same manner for the sales as the subject. A terminal value is also developed. For consistency, the cash flow period considered is similar to that used in the DCF analysis for the subject. Once the sale price and cash flows are estimated, the internal rate of return, or yield rate, is calculated.

A sample yield rate extraction for a nursing facility is presented in Table 15.6. In this example, it is assumed that the appraiser has obtained a Medicaid cost report or other fairly detailed operating statement of the sale property and has interviewed the buyer regarding key future cash flow assumptions. The buyer may or may not have a targeted yield rate. Based on the interview, a review of the operating statement, and knowledge of other generally perceived industry and financial conditions, the following assumptions are made.

- Occupancy and total census increase at a rate that is slightly lower than the population growth forecast for the 75-plus age cohort.
- Occupancy in the terminal year considers long-term expectations, resulting in a slightly lower rate than applied in the prior year.
- Private-pay mix and census decline in tandem with the market's perceived and actual trend towards fewer private-pay patients.
- Medicare census increases, keeping step with the general trend of greater Medicare volume.
- Routine rates increase at, or slightly below, the generally anticipated inflation rate, as pressure on Medicare and Medicaid spending continues to force cost-cutting measures.
- Variable and fixed operating expenses increase at anticipated inflation levels, but variable costs, which include much of the patient care expense, increase at a slightly greater rate to reflect anticipated increases in acuity levels.
- The terminal capitalization rate is 50 basis points higher than the going-in rate, reflecting greater risk in the future and a shorter remaining economic life.

Building a Fee Simple Yield Rate from Leased Fee Data

Yield rate calculations for fee simple interests, including the total assets of the business, involve a number of critical assumptions and judgments and, as a result, yield rate indications

Table 15.6 Extraction of an Internal Rate of Return from a Nursing Facility Sale

Occupancy forecast		Year 1	Year 2	Year 3	Year 4	Year 5	Year 6
Number of beds		100	100	100	100	100	100
Occupancy rate		89.0%	90.3%	91.7%	93.1%	94.5%	93.0%
Census mix by days							
Private pay		6,497	6,432	6,368	6,304	6,241	6,179
Medicare		4,873	4,970	5,070	5,171	5,274	5,380
Medicaid		21,115	21,570	22,030	22,494	22,963	22,387
Total		32,485	32,972	33,467	33,969	34,478	33,945
Revenue per patient day	**Trending**						
Private (average)	3.0%	$180.00	$185.40	$190.96	$196.69	$202.59	$208.67
Medicare	2.9%	400.00	411.60	423.54	435.82	448.46	461.46
Medicaid	2.9%	145.00	149.21	153.53	157.98	162.57	167.28
Medicare Part B and private ancillary	3.0%	2.50	2.58	2.65	2.73	2.81	2.90
Other revenue	3.0%	0.50	0.52	0.53	0.55	0.56	0.58
Bad debt	3.0%	(0.25)	(0.26)	(0.27)	(0.27)	(0.28)	(0.29)
Total revenue		$6,269,605	$6,549,945	$6,843,054	$7,149,338	$7,469,376	$7,624,949
Operating expenses							
Variable expense PPD	3.1%	$98.42	$101.47	$104.61	$107.86	$111.20	$114.65
Variable		$3,197,060	$3,345,583	$3,501,080	$3,663,757	$3,833,934	$3,891,679
Fixed	3.0%	1,758,624	1,811,383	1,865,724	1,921,696	1,979,347	2,038,727
Management		313,480	327,497	342,153	357,467	373,469	381,247
Cap-ex, replacement reserves	3.0%	60,000	61,800	63,654	65,564	67,531	69,556
Total operating expenses		$5,329,164	$5,546,263	$5,772,611	$6,008,484	$6,254,280	$6,381,210
NOI—EBITDAR		$940,441	$1,003,681	$1,070,443	$1,140,854	$1,215,096	$1,243,739
Gross reversion (based on a 12.5% going-in cap rate, plus approximately 50 basis points)							$9,567,220
Less selling/restructuring expenses							(287,017)
Net reversion value						$9,280,203	
Sale price and cash flows	$7,500,000	$940,441	$1,003,681	$1,070,443	$1,140,854	$10,495,299	
Implied yield rate, or internal rate of return		17.4%					

among a group of analyzed sales may display an unacceptable rate spread. Yield rates developed from net leased nursing facilities typically require fewer assumptions and judgments, and those decisions are often considered with terminal valuation issues. Leased fee interests typically involve absolute net leases, with rents increasing annually at a specific amount. Purchase options or first rights of refusal to purchase the facility provide fairly precise parameters for calculating the yield rate. The leased fee rates can be used as a test of reasonableness for the fee simple yield rate. Assume the following.

- The *EBITDAR*-to-rent coverage ratio is 1.25:1 (80.0% of *EBITDAR*).
- The leased fee capitalization rate is 10.0%.
- Annual rental increases are 2.5%.
- The purchase option is set at the current-year rent capitalized at 10.0%.
- The leased fee yield rate is 12.0%.
- The fee simple capitalization rate is 12.0%.

As a rule of thumb, the spread between the leased fee going-in capitalization rate and the discount rate (*IRR*) is generally 200 basis points. Since the lease rent has adequate coverage, the rental income is more secure for the leased fee investor than the *NOI* or *EBITDAR* is for an investor in the fee simple interest. Therefore, it is reasonable to expect the yield rate for the fee simple interest to be at least 200 basis points higher than the 12.0% going-in capitalization rate for that same fee interest. Thus, a yield rate of more than 14.0% is indicated.

Similar rate relationships are evidenced by other property types. These rate spreads between fee simple and leased fee interests can be easily identified and are widely accepted in the market. Such rate spreads could be studied and loosely applied to the going-in capitalization rate of a nursing facility. For instance, the average overall rate for full-service hotels may be 10.0%, and the average *IRR* or yield rate may be 13.0%, suggesting a 300-basis-point spread. If an average overall capitalization rate for a nursing facility is 12.5%, the appraiser may interpret an *IRR* of 15.5% for the nursing facility, reflecting the 300-basis-point spread found in the hotel properties.

Note that these suggestions are general rules of thumb, which represent fall-back support in the absence of rate data convincingly developed from comparable sales data, market surveys, or property modeling.

Yield Rates Developed from Market Surveys

Published yield rate surveys for skilled nursing facilities are scarce, whether the facilities are fee simple or leased fee. Surveys conducted by others are considered secondary data, which does not directly pertain to the subject or comparable data. One problem with yield rate data developed from secondary sources is that the assumptions applied and the comprehension of the interviewees may be varied and inconsistent.

Appraisers may elect to conduct their own surveys of market participants. Surveys may be conducted orally or in written form. Written surveys have many advantages as the respondents may take the time to develop more considered responses and the surveyor will have a more tangible audit trail. Interviews may include questions that ask for a range or a specific yield rate. A more substantial survey can follow up on the answers, asking about various components of yield rate development, such as going-in rates; *NOI* growth; property appreciation rates; occupancy, mix, and rate changes; operating expense growth; and terminal capitalization rates. A combination of questions may allow the respondent to reconsider earlier responses in light of later questions that may be designed in a leading manner, setting up a set of sequential, easily followed steps. The survey should also define the terminology used and establish other ground rules to ensure consistency.

A yield rate survey could include the following questions:

Level 1

- What, in your opinion, is the current market average and range for *IRR*s or yield rates?

Level 2

(A rate or a range in *IRR*s can be deduced from responses to these questions.)

- What, in your opinion, is the current market average and range in overall capitalization rates–going-in rates, based on pro forma, or forecasted stabilized earnings?
- Are normal management expenses and reserves for capital replacement considered in the expenses included in your capitalization and yield rates?
- What is the anticipated annual increase or decrease in *NOI* or *EBITDAR* over the holding period?
- What is the anticipated annual change in the overall value of the property?
- How many years are there in an appropriate holding period?
- What is an appropriate terminal capitalization rate?

Level 3–pertains to changes in cash flows

(A rate or a range in *IRR*s can be deduced from responses to these questions and the questions above.)

- What is the anticipated annual change in total occupancy?
- What, if any, is the annual change in private-pay mix?
- What, if any, is the change in Medicare mix?
- What is the expected annual change in private-pay revenue?
- What is the expected annual change in the average Medicare rate?
- What is the expected annual change in the average Medicaid rate?
- What is the expected annual change in operating expenses, measured in patient days?

Gathering a sizable sample of completed surveys from market participants can help the appraiser reach a meaningful indication of market yield rates or internal rates of return.

Yield Rates Developed from the Property Model

The property model produces a yield rate that should not exceed the sum of the going-in capitalization rate and the compounded annual rate of change in property value over the life of the forecast. The formula for the property model is:

$$Y_O = R_O + CR$$

Where:

Y_O = yield rate

R_O = overall capitalization rate (going-in rate)

CR = compounded rate of change in the property value

The equation expresses a direct relationship between the overall capitalization rate and the discount rate. Annual change pertains to change in the depreciation or appreciation between the going-in value and the terminal, or going-out, value.

If the overall capitalization (going-in) rate is 13.0% and the anticipated annual compounded rate of property value appreciation is 2.5%, then the indicated yield rate will not exceed 15.5%.

Reconciliation of Yield Rate Techniques

If multiple approaches are used to develop the yield rate, the appraiser must consider the strengths and weaknesses of each in arriving at an appropriate rate for the subject. Ranking analysis may be used to sort the rate indications developed from the various techniques. Greater weight is placed on the rates developed from the most reliable information.

Case Study

The present value of the cash flow forecast for the subject facility is calculated in Table 15.7.

Table 15.7 Calculating Present Value of the Forecasted Cash Flows

		Year 1	Year 2	Year 3	Year 4	Year 5	Year 6
NOI or *EBITDAR*		$1,127,881	$1,199,502	$1,262,749	$1,331,461	$1,246,938	$1,297,343
Reversion value capitalized going-in rate, plus 50 basis points		12.50%					$10,378,743
Less 3.0% selling and/or restructuring costs							($311,362)
Net reversion						$10,067,381	
Total cash flow		$1,127,881	$1,199,502	$1,262,749	$1,331,461	$11,314,320	
Discount factor	14.5%	0.873362	0.762762	0.666168	0.581806	0.508127	
Present value		$985,049	$914,934	$841,202	$774,652	$5,749,115	
Total present value		$9,264,953					
Rounded to		$9,260,000					

Yield capitalization can be applied to mortgage and equity portions of a nursing facility. Equity yield rates are important decision-making tools and benchmarks for passive equity investors. Generally, the appraiser will not need to go into this much depth in the development of a discounted cash flow analysis. Separate consideration of debt and equity yield rates becomes important when low-interest debt is incorporated into the valuation.

Income Capitalization Approach Reconciliation

When direct capitalization and discounted cash flow analysis are both applied, a reconciliation of the values will be necessary. More often than not, the two value indications will differ. The quality and quantity of the comparable market data may recommend one approach over the other. The direct capitalization approach is generally preferred by the market. It is most reliable when a steady earnings pattern is expected. Typically, overall capitalization rates are easier to extract from market data than yield rates. Predictable, but irregular, cash flows, resulting from foreseeable changes in competitive market conditions, reimbursement changes, or other factors, may require that the appraiser place more importance on yield capitalization or DCF analysis.

Case Study—Concluding a Value Indication Using the Income Capitalization Approach

Direct capitalization and discounted cash flow analysis produced different value indications, however, the difference is considered to be within a reasonable margin of error. Because the market favors direct capitalization, greater weight is placed on that value indication. The value indications, all single-point estimates of value, are

Direct capitalization	$9,400,000
Discounted cash flow	$9,260,000
Concluded value from the income approach	$9,325,000

Summary

There are two generally accepted techniques applied in the income capitalization approach: direct capitalization and discounted cash flow analysis. Direct capitalization is most frequently applied in appraising nursing facilities and it involves converting a single year's net operating income into value. Discounted cash flow analysis involves discounting several years of net operating income and the property value at the end of the cash flow period to present value using an internal rate of return. In estimating market value, capitalization and internal rates of return are tied to market evidence. Such evidence may include rate indications from recent comparable sale transactions and information from investor surveys. Direct capitalization is most applicable when the net operating income is expected to be fairly stable. Discounted cash flow analysis is more useful for properties that are expected to experience irregularities in earnings. Changes in competitive market conditions, reimbursements, or operations are salient factors affecting revenue and expense stability.

An overall capitalization rate is typically obtained from sale data and calculated by dividing net operating income by price. Other direct capitalization techniques include the band-of-investment technique, various residual techniques, and the debt service coverage ratio. To apply the band-of-investment technique, the appraiser weighs the market levels of debt and equity and their respective costs of capital or rates of return. Residual techniques, which isolate rates for the different assets of the going concern, can be applied, but they generally require the use of a number of assumptions that are difficult to support with market data. Applying the debt coverage ratio involves developing estimates of market loan-to-value ratios, interest rates, and coverage ratios. Rather than applying the lender's advertised ratio, the appraiser should develop the debt coverage ratio from actual transactions. Lenders will often underwrite based on conservative, trailing figures. Conducting capitalization rate surveys by interviewing market participants is another technique that can be employed. Rate development using any of these techniques should be tied closely to market evidence.

Consistency is critical in the development of market-derived and surveyed capitalization rates. It is inconsistent and misleading to develop capitalization rates using trailing or prior revenue and expense figures for the comparables if the rates developed from those analyses are to be applied to forecasted earnings for the subject. Some other areas in which inconsistencies may occur include the use of a management expense, reserves for replacement, and Medicaid rate rebasing. Using partial interest sales to reflect a fee simple interest would also be inconsistent. Portfolio sale transaction capitalization rates have the advantage of averaging out highs and lows, but they also can reflect pricing discounts or premiums that may not be appropriate for a single property. Medicaid rate rebasing due to changes in ownership should be considered in the development of capitalization rates from comparable sales.

Discounted cash flow analysis is especially applicable when a facility's earnings will be irregular, but predictable. The internal rates of return or yield rates required in the development of the DCF analysis can be suppported using traditional methods such as surveying investors, developing formulas using market capitalization rates and forecasted changes in value and *NOI*, and abstracting implied yield rates from comparable sales data.

Chapter 16

Sales Comparison Approach

The sales comparison approach relies on analysis of similar properties that have recently been sold, are under contract to be sold, or are listed for sale, and comparing those properties to the subject property. The sales comparison approach is most meaningful in the appraisal of nursing facilities when the value conclusion is developed independently from the income capitalization and cost approaches. Ideally, the approach makes use of contemporary, well-researched, verified sales data that require few price adjustments to account for differences between the subject and the sale comparables.

The principles of supply and demand, substitution, and balance underlie the basic concepts of the sales comparison approach. Buyers represent market demand and properties for sale constitute supply. Although market equilibrium is rarely sustained, the forces of supply and demand tend to gravitate towards balance over the long run. The principle of substitution states that the value of a property is set at the price that it would cost to acquire a substitute property within a reasonable time that has similar utility and desirability. Based on this principle, some credence can be given to the notion that the value of a nursing facility cannot substantially exceed the replacement cost of the tangible assets plus all the costs of assembling the intangible assets, permits, and certifications.

The sales comparison approach is most persuasive in the valuation of nursing facilities when there are sufficient recent sale transactions that are comparable to the subject in as many of ways as possible–i.e., similar in terms of location, physical plant age, quality, size, and economic factors such as occupancy, census mix, reimbursement levels, and earnings. One of the greatest disadvantages of this approach, especially in a market where values are perceived to be changing, is that the approach lags behind the market because sales reflect value at points in the past. One critical observation is that using the sales comparison approach is like driving forward using the rearview mirror. If values in the market are perceived to be generally flat, then this problem is not significant. However, changes in the cost of capital, reimbursements, competitive market conditions, and other factors that steer earnings reduce the reliability of older sales.

Same-state data best reflects the profound influence of Medicaid and CON policies, which vary from state to state. Often there is a dearth of recent nursing facility sales that have similar locations, physical plant characteristics, and economic qualities from which to produce a convincing value indication, even with well-supported price adjustments. Despite the absence of a significant number of recent comparable sales, the sales comparison approach is essential to the valuation process. At times, properties under contract, offers, refusals, options, and listings may be better market indicators than actual sales of nursing facilities if the sale properties are exceedingly dissimilar to the subject.

Identifying and Researching Sales

Potential sources for data on nursing facility sales include, but are not limited to, the following.

- State health planning, licensing, and certificate of need divisions
- Medicaid offices, which list changes in provider numbers, suggesting that ownership of the operation has changed
- State healthcare associations, which provide general knowledge
- Active owner/operators in the market (It's a small world.)
- Brokers specializing in healthcare properties, who typically work in one region of the country or nationally
- Public disclosures from press releases and quarterly or annual financial statements from publicly traded operating companies and healthcare REITs
- Local assessors and deed recorders
- Publications such as *SeniorCare Investor* and *Contemporary Long Term Care*
- Private, fee-based comparable sales data services
- Other appraisers

When there is a change in the ownership or the licensed operator of a nursing facility, states require the proposed new operating entity to apply for a new license. Many states will conduct a buyer suitability investigation to determine if the operator is ethical and financially suitable. Many state healthcare licensing divisions will publish lists of applications and approvals for change of ownership (CHoW) in quarterly or monthly reports. The CHoW reports will identify the names of new operators and the type of transaction–sale of the real estate and/or license, lease of the facility, change in management, or a simple name change for the operator resulting from a corporate or partnership restructuring. While much of the information in the CHoW application is kept confidential, many states will make certain information available for review by the public. Depending on the state, information that may be made available to the public under the Freedom of Information Act may include a copy of the sale contract or lease, the buyer's operating and financial forecast, and/or proposed or actual debt financing. Note that some states may list a price, when the amount actually represents the total rent over the full term of the lease. Confirmation with a principal to the transaction is crucial. In states where CHoW lists are available, the list could be the first stop in the process of gathering sales information.

Nursing facilities are given a Medicare and Medicaid provider number when they receive certification to participate in these programs. In a CHoW, a new provider number is often assigned to the new operator. A list of changes in provider numbers may be available from the state Medicaid division or the Medicare intermediary. While there is often a lag period, the seller's final Medicaid cost report and the buyer's initial Medicaid cost report will prove extremely valuable to the appraiser. The cost reports will not only provide an in-depth look at the operations of the facility (census, revenue, and operating expenses), these reports also generally contain capital cost, financial, and ownership information. Detailed census, revenue, and operating expenses will be clearly stated in a manner consistent with the accounts used in the Medicaid reimbursement system. The reports typically require the disclosure of the purchase price, debt financing amounts and interest rates, and lease payments in addition to the parties involved. Note that each state has its own, unique cost report, which may include 10 to more than 50 pages of information. The cost reports contain a wealth of information, and it is recommended that a copy or copies of the reports be obtained, analyzed, and retained in the appraiser's files.

Officers in state healthcare associations generally know most operators in their state as membership in these non-profit organizations is high. The healthcare associations represent their members on matters of government policy and other issues that affect operators in the nursing home industry. Generally, the associations employ a full-time director plus administrative, research, and other staff. The officers are typically elected from within the membership pool and serve multi-year terms on a volunteer basis. Because these organizations represent a large percentage of nursing home operators, the association director and officers are often aware of completed sales, pending transactions, and properties currently being marketed for sale.

Many nursing home operators are also aware of facilities that have sold or are for sale in their own markets. In fact, these operators may have been solicited, reviewed offering materials, and even visited these properties. Since most nursing facilities are marketed under confidential arrangements, they may not be able to share marketing information with an inquiring appraiser. Probably the best information that other operators can provide is the news that a facility has been sold and possibly some insight into the motivations of the parties to the transaction. Details of the sale will need to be investigated by contacting the parties directly and researching public records (assessment information, Medicaid cost reports, etc.).

While most nursing facilities are marketed without the assistance of brokers, there are many transactions that involve brokers. Because of the specialized nature of the property type, the need for confidentiality when marketing the property, and the knowledge and experience of typical buyers, most owners using brokerage services will contract with a firm that specializes in the senior housing and long-term care industry. Many of the larger firms publish newsletters and will cooperate to varying degrees by sharing transaction information. Often brokers are bound by confidentiality agreements and may be unable to provide specific details, but they should be able to discuss the motivations of the buyers, the marketing time, and any unusual conditions of the sale.

Publicly traded nursing facilities and healthcare REITs make up a fairly significant proportion of the market. Many of these companies will disclose limited amounts of transaction information in press releases on specific transactions and in quarterly and annual statements. Generally, these companies will not issue a press release for smaller transactions, such as a single property or a small portfolio; often information on those deals can be found in their regularly issued financial statements. Appraisers should be aware that public companies tend to buy and sell portfolios or groups of facilities in several states with varied asset qualities in a single transaction. Moreover, when these companies sell facilities, the facilities are often substandard or operationally distressed and the transaction takes on the characteristics of a liquidation sale.[1] REIT sales and other sales may involve the tenant exercising a purchase option. In these situations, the sale price may have been established years ago when the lease was written and that price does not reflect the current market.

Local property assessment records can be used to gather physical plant information and sometimes sale price information too. In states that require public disclosure of real estate prices, the recorded amount may represent the buyer's allocation of the total price for the real estate assets.

Publications such as *SeniorCare Investors* and *Contemporary Long Term Care* provide varying amounts of detail on sale transactions that fall into their purview. Information on transactions is typically mined from publicly announced deals, provided by brokers and investors who want publicity, and uncovered through working with well-established networks.

Private, fee-based comparable sales data services are another source of nursing facility sales. These services provide information that is typically available through courthouse records–deed location, buyer and seller names, some physical and legal information, a plat map, and maybe a photograph. Note that these services will often report transactions that involve the recapitalization of a property, situations in which the seller and buyer are related and the property was not actually placed on the market.

Other appraisers may be a source of sales data but receiving data from other appraisers does not eliminate the need to verify the information. Simply relying on another appraiser's data, without searching for other sales, may cause the appraiser to overlook important, critical sales information that should be included or recognized in the appraisal.

Confirming and Analyzing the Sales

Once a comparable sale is identified and researched by reviewing public information, the next step is to confirm as much critical information as possible with parties to the transaction–the buyer, seller, broker, and attorneys. Although interviewing a party to the transaction may be somewhat tense, an appraiser who speaks with a confident tone may get more information. Moreover, experience demonstrates that appraisers will receive

1. *Liquidation*, as defined in *The Dictionary of Real Estate Appraisal*, 4th ed., is: 1. Forced or voluntary cash realization; the selling of real estate, stocks, bonds, or other investments, either to take profits and limit losses or in anticipation of declining prices. 2. The termination or conclusion of a business or real estate operation by converting its assets into cash. The proceeds from liquidation are distributed first to creditors in order of preference, and the remainder, if any, is allocated to the owners in proportion to their holdings.

more cooperation and success if they have researched the available public information first. Usually, property information can be easily obtained from assessor records. Requesting cost reports from the state may take time, but having some financial and operator data before interviewing one or more parties to the transaction is very useful.

Once an interview with a party to a sale is underway, the appraiser needs to confirm a number of items. It may be necessary to ask questions in the order of their relative importance as time may be limited. A comprehensive interview with a party to a sale will include the following topics:

- Motivations of the buyer and seller
- Extent of market exposure and amount of interest among potential buyers
- Property rights conveyed–fee simple, leased fee, or leasehold
- Asset or stock purchase–i.e., does the sale include current assets and liabilities such as accounts receivable, cash, short-term operating debts, assumption of seller liabilities, and unused employee vacation and personal leave days?
- Purchase price
- Special financing or other concessions that may have affected the price, including seller financing, concessions made with the lender for extreme leverage, or other extraordinary financing that may impact the price or equity rates
- Date of contract (sale or option) versus date of closing
- Is the sale the result of a purchase option established in the lease or management contract?
- Expenditures made immediately after the purchase
- Future capital improvement plans
- Anticipated occupancy, census mix, per-diem rates, and reimbursement changes
- Anticipated revenue, operating expenses, and earnings
- Comparison of trailing revenues, expenses, and earnings to forecasted or pro forma figures, and reasons for differences
- Improvement and site information not obtained from other sources, including perceived strengths and weaknesses of the specific property
- Regulatory issues, survey issues, or physical plant waivers
- Excess land or underutilized assets (which could provide an opportunity for financial gain) that were included in the sale price, requiring price adjustment
- Other information

The appraiser may need to piece together information collected from various parties to the transaction as well as information obtained from public sources. Complete or comprehensive information is seldom achieved, but often enough information is gained from these various sources that a fairly clear and credible account of the sale emerges. Then, meaningful insights into the value of the subject can be gained through the comparison process.

Organizing and Presenting the Sales Data

Once the sales data has been researched and confirmed, the information should be described and presented in the report and maintained in a database. The appraiser should also maintain a file for each sale, incorporating all the information gathered about the sale and the information sources. Table 16.1 illustrates one method of organizing and presenting nursing facility sales research.

Units of Comparison

The price per bed is the most appropriate unit of comparison for nursing facility sales. Effective gross revenue multipliers, overall capitalization rates, and per-square-foot prices are used as tests of reasonableness. While the *NOI* per bed may be used as a valuation benchmark, any method that primarily involves adjusting prices for the difference in the *NOI* per bed is tantamount to a direct income capitalization approach. A value indication derived that way is not independent from the income approach and would produce a second, misleading value indication if the *NOI* of the subject or the sales are incorrect for whatever reason.

Price adjustments are typically made to the price-per-bed amount once the total price is adjusted for property rights conveyed, financing, conditions of sale, capital expenditures made immediately after purchase, and market conditions. While per-square-foot price adjustments may be useful in analyzing the real estate component of the nursing facility, this price indicator is not a primary concern in the valuation of the going concern. The Square-foot prices can be used as a measurement in a test of reasonableness. Effective gross revenue multipliers are not adjusted either, but these figures are very useful in qualitative comparisons such as sensitivity analysis and trend analysis.

Elements of Comparison

Elements of comparison are the characteristics or attributes of properties and transactions that cause the prices for real estate

Table 16.1 Nursing Facility Sale #1

Identification and transaction facts		
Facility name:	Care Home of Middletown	
Property address:	2222 Spring Road Middletown, Any State	
Sale date:	July 1, 20XX	
Seller:	Generally recognized name, but real estate and operations held in separate entities	
Buyer:	Public Company	
Confirmation:	Assessor records, Medicaid cost report and interview with Director of Acquisition for Public Company	
Exposure time:	Three months	
Property rights conveyed:	Fee simple, includes license, operating rights, and business assets; seller retains current assets and liabilities and retires all debt obligations	
Physical property facts		
Number of beds:	100 beds, licensed as SNF beds	
Gross building area:	38,075 square feet	
Gross building area per bed:	381 square feet	
Building description:	One-story, wood frame with brick veneer exterior, gabled roof, PTAC and package HVAC, full sprinkler protection,	
Overall condition:	Average, relative to age	
Deferred maintenance or building waivers:	New information system, signage & some FF&E replacement	
Year(s) built:	1989	
Effective building age as of the sale date:	XX years	
Number of beds in private rooms:	14	
Number of beds in ward rooms (3 or 4 beds):	0	
Land area:	4.89 acres	
Other significant physical plant issues	Seller replaced a boiler and dishwasher and removed underground fuel tank	
Medicare provider number:	36XXXX - reference source	
Price and top-line adjustment		
Total sale price:	$7,700,000	
Minus: special financing (cash equivalency)	0	
Plus/minus: conditions of the sale	0	
Plus: expenditures made immediately after sale	200,000	
Net adjusted price:	$7,900,000	
Operating data	**Forecast**	**Historical**
Occupancy rate:	88.0g%	86.0%
Private-pay mix:	29.0%	28.0%
Medicare mix:	17.0%	16.1%
Quality mix (private & Medicare):	46.0%	44.1%
Medicaid capital rate PPD (net of taxes & insurance):	$12.00	$12.00
Effective gross revenue (EGR):	$7,050,000	$6,656,785
Operating expenses (5.0% mgmt., $300/bed reserves):	-5,985,450	-5,755,240
Net operating income (*NOI* aka *EBITDAR*):	$1,064,550	$901,545
NOI or *EBITDAR* PPD:	$33.14	$28.72
NOI or *EBITDAR* per bed/year:	$10,646	$9,015
Expense margin:	84.9%	86.5%
Net operating income margin:	15.1%	13.5%
Units of comparison		
Base adjusted price per bed:	$79,000	
Price per square foot:	$207.49	
Effective gross revenue multiplier:	1.12	1.19
Overall capitalization rate:	13.5%	11.4%
Equity capital rate (based on market financing):	29.9%	21.6%

to vary.[2] Since nursing facilities have tangible and intangible personal property assets imbedded in the price and value, this definition can be expanded to include those assets. To develop a meaningful and comprehensive value indication using the sales comparison approach, all pertinent elements of comparison should be considered. Double adjusting, or applying adjustments for the same difference more than once, must be avoided.

The elements of comparison considered for nursing facilities are essentially the same elements of comparison used for most other types of real estate:

- Property rights and assets conveyed
- Financing terms
- Conditions of sale
- Capital expenditures made immediately after purchase
- Market conditions
- Location
- Physical characteristics
- Economic characteristics
- Use (zoning)
- Non-realty components of value (used for real-estate-only valuations)

Property Rights and Assets Conveyed

Before the price of a comparable nursing facility can be used in the sales comparison process, the appraiser must adjust the price of the comparable sale for differences between the rights and assets of the subject and the sale.

There are two general transaction types: asset sales and stock sales. Asset sales typical include the traditional real estate rights and the tangible and intangible personal property assets of the nursing facility. Stock sales will typically include the aforementioned assets plus the assumption of current assets and current and long-term liabilities. Current assets may include accounts receivable, working capital, pre-paid expenses, etc. Current liabilities will include accounts payable, deferred employee compensation (bonuses, vacation, sick leave, etc.), deferred taxes, mortgages, short-term and unsecured debts, and other known and unknown liabilities. Generally, seller liabilities stay with the seller, and the buyer or successor in the business typically gains indemnity for the seller's liabilities. The appraiser should confirm the type of sale (asset or stock) and the assets and liabilities that were conveyed in the sale transaction. If the price of any of the comparables includes any assets and/or

2. *The Dictionary of Real Estate Appraisal*, 4th ed., (Chicago: Appraisal Institute, 2002).

liabilities that differ from those being appraised, adjustments will be necessary to equate the sale with the rights appraised for the subject.

The property rights or real estate assets being appraised will typically be the fee simple, leased fee, or leasehold. Chapter 19 examines leased fee and leasehold interests. The typical appraisal assignment will involve the valuation of the total assets of the business, or going concern, including the fee simple interest in the real estate. Most nursing facilities are sold under the same conditions. This chapter will focus on the total assets of the business, including the fee simple interest in the real estate. As discussed in Chapter 4, the intangible assets typically include licenses, certifications, and approvals from government agencies, a work force of trained and licensed staff, patient records, goodwill, management, trade name(s), and other intangibles. Often the ownership of these assets will be fragmented between various entities substantially controlled by the same principals. Many sale transactions will use a "transfer operating agreement" to convey certain intangible rights.

Financing Adjustments

Non-market financing terms can affect prices and warrant an adjustment to reflect the typical financing available in the market. A nursing facility may be sold subject to the assumption of an existing mortgage with a below-market interest rate or with a mortgage amount that exceeds typically available loan-to-value ratios. Occasionally, a seller will create a wraparound loan, which is superimposed on the existing mortgage to preserve a below-market interest rate and/or other favorable loan terms. If the buyer and seller intended the price to be affected by the non-market financing rates and/or terms, then the sale price may require a cash equivalency adjustment.

A cash equivalency adjustment may be calculated by discounting the difference between the actual payment for a favorable mortgage and the payment for the same mortgage amount at a market interest rate over the expected term of the loan.

An example of a cash equivalency adjustment follows. In this example, the buyer assumes an existing mortgage with a $10,000,000, 30-year, amortizing original loan at an interest rate of 5.50%, which has amortized down to a principal balance of $9,246,060.35 after 60 months. The mortgage balloons in five years, or 60 months from this sale date, which means the unpaid principal is due then. The purchase price was $12,000,000, with the buyer paying the seller the difference in cash at the closing. The loan-to-value ratio is roughly 77%, which is consistent with the market ($9,246,000 / $12,000,000). The current mortgage market is competitive and, despite this, the best rate available in the market for the same loan amount and terms is 7.0% with a 30-year amortization and a five-year balloon.

Example of Cash Equivalency Calculation

Current mortgage balance	$9,246,060	
Original amortization term	30	
Interest rate	5.50%	
Monthly mortgage payment	$56,779	
Mortgage balance in 60 months	$8,254,099	
Present value of monthly payments, discounted at 7.0%		$2,867,448
Present value of mortgage balance in 5 years, discounted at 7.0%		5,822,482
Plus cash down payment		2,753,940
Cash-equivalent price (sale price adjusted for financing)		$11,443,870

There are some differences between the market loan terms and rate at the time of the sale and the actual terms and rate assumed or created for a sale that cannot be quantified in a cash equivalency adjustment. These differences include mortgages with imbalances between the market interest rate relative to the credit quality, the loan-to-value ratio, or other collateral. In these cases, the appraiser may need to rely on qualitative analysis. Given the uniqueness of each nursing facility and the infrequency of sales, it is very unlikely that two highly similar sales will have occurred at the same time, one financed with conventional, market financing terms and the other with non-market terms, which would suggest the need for, or the amount of, the price adjustment.

Conditions of Sale

The conditions of sale adjustment considers any abnormal market circumstances in the sale. If the buyer or seller is unusually compelled or motivated to make the transaction, then an adjustment is required. A seller facing imminent decertification, foreclosure, or delicensure could be excessively compelled to sell. A hospital seeking to relieve DRG pressures by purchasing a nearby SNF might be willing to pay substantially more than typical SNF operators since its economic justification is largely tethered to the hospital's economic conditions. The price of a transaction between related parties (family members and partnerships or corporations with common principals) may not represent market value. Sales involving special motivations and conditions are often alien to the definition of market value.

Using such sales as comparables should be avoided, unless the influence on the price can be determined and an adjustment can be quantified. An appraiser may be lured into using a non-market sale because the property may have a number of critical similarities to the subject and the other available sales may be few and less comparable. Using comparables with non-market sale conditions requires additional research, confirmation, and care. The appraiser should clearly disclose the conditions of the sale and make efforts to adjust the price to reflect the market. Note that non-market sales may be rejected when used in expert testimony in litigation.

Portfolio sales often sell at a significant premium in bull markets and at a discount in bear markets. Portfolio transactions may involve price allocations to the individual facilities that may not represent the market values because the allocated prices may serve various tax, reimbursement, and other business interests. If a portfolio sale represents one of the best indicators of value among the available sales, then it may be best to analyze the aggregated data (e.g., overall price per bed, combined overall capitalization rate, net revenue multiplier) and attempt to support a quantifiable adjustment for the portfolio price premium or discount.

Expenditures Made Immediately After Purchase

In the view of many buyers, nursing facilities are often sold with considerable deferred maintenance and pricing is usually adjusted accordingly. An interview with the buyers should include learning of their plans and the estimated cost of immediate capital improvements. The improvement plan may include simply replacing worn and obsolete items (interior finishes, mechanical systems, site improvements, and tangible personal property), or it may involve making substantial renovations and building expansions.

The appraiser should be aware that the buyer's improvements may have had a significant impact, immediately and over the long run, on some or all of these factors: reimbursements, private-pay rates, occupancy and census mix levels, operating expenses, and earnings. It may be necessary to calculate the costs of the buyer's improvements and combine those expenses with the purchase price. The price may require additional adjusting for extensive capital improvement campaigns to reposition the property in the market. The on-going operations and earnings of the facility may have suffered during the construction and the facility may have experienced delays in reaching stabilized earnings because of absorption. The ownership may have invested significant opportunity costs during the repositioning campaign. The stabilized, post-improvement *NOI* or *EBITDAR* may need to be used to calculate the capitalization rate, yield rate, and revenue multiplier. Needless to say, properties that required substantial expenditures immediately after purchase may prove problematic for use in the sales comparison approach and/or for capitalization rate extraction.

Often, expenditures made immediately after purchase will include a substantial amount spent on restructuring the business operations. Much of that cost may result from recruitment expenses. With the change of ownership, some operators may need to purge substantial numbers of employees, incur significant training expense, break contracts with established vendors, and replace those vendors with new suppliers. Most buyers are aware of the costs they will incur in transitioning the operations and have adjusted the price accordingly. Generally, if the buyer assumes the employee vacation and personal leave days from the seller, that adjustment is made independently of the asset purchase.

Market Conditions

Comparable sales that occurred under market conditions that differ from the conditions that exist on the effective date of the appraisal will require adjustments for any differences that affect their value. This adjustment is often referred to as a *time adjustment*, but the passage of time does not cause value changes. It is market conditions, which change over time, that cause value fluctuations.

Changes in Medicare and Medicaid reimbursement, certificate of need requirements, licensing laws, tax laws, inflation, and the cost of capital (equity and debt) are some of the important external forces that affect values. Major changes in any of these external forces can have a broad effect on the value of all facilities, so any major change warrants examination.

Changes in the cost of capital tend to have a universal impact on valuations. Changes in interest rates and equity returns may not have a one-to-one relationship with value. Simply adjusting a sale price to reflect the difference in the cost of capital between the date of the comparable sale and the effective date of the appraisal may not accurately characterize the change in value. However, if other significant factors in the market have remained fairly stable over this time span, then the change in the cost of capital should provide some indication of the general trend in value.

Similarly, a universal and quantifiable change in Medicare or Medicaid reimbursements, or a change in certificate of need laws that may generally affect supply and demand in the market and thus earnings, may not translate directly into a change in value. However, these types of changes may suggest general valuation trends.

The appraiser looks at matched pair sales, grouped sales comparisons, trends in measurable economic factors that broadly impact values, market surveys, and statistical analyses of sale data to develop an appropriate adjustment for market conditions. An adjustment for market conditions that is supported by just a few references may be unreliable. The nursing home market is too independent of general economic price indices (inflation), construction costs, and residential and commercial real estate price trends to rely on those indexes as indicators of changes in price levels in the nursing home market.

Matched pair analysis is an ideal method to support time adjustments, but opportunities to analyze paired sales are rare. Surveys of market participants can be conducted to determine general price trends.

An examination of equity share prices and earnings multipliers for public nursing home companies and healthcare REITs may provide some general guidance on the direction of value change. However, stock prices represent equity-only positions and, therefore, these values will not portray total asset value. Adding the company's debt to the equity value provides a more meaningful indication of the total value and trend. Note that many of the facilities controlled by public nursing home companies are either leased or managed, in which case the real estate interest is minimized. Moreover, the companies are usually not purely nursing home operators; they operate other types of long-term care properties and service businesses. Healthcare REITs tend to diversify their assets between different health care property types, including senior housing, hospitals, surgical centers, and medical offices, and thus their pricing is not a reflection of pure nursing facilities. Also, the income for a REIT is based on lease rents, not the more volatile earnings from operations.

The graph in Figure 16.1 profiles the adjusted quarterly closing equity share prices for five public companies since January 2005. These companies, which are active in operating skilled nursing facilities, include Advocate (AVCA), Kindred Healthcare (KND), National HealthCare (NHC), Skilled Health Care (SKH), and Sun Healthcare (SUNH). SKH is a newer public company, so its history is limited. Since January 2005, several of the largest public companies in the nursing facility sector, including Beverly Enterprises, Manor Care-HCR, Mariner, and Genesis, became private through large, leverage buyouts.

The graph suggests that there was a general upward trend in nursing home equity values between the beginning of the first quarter of 2005 and the third quarter of 2008. This trend may be interpreted many ways, but one conclusion may be that nursing facility valuations generally increased during that period.

Published data can depict general price trends for the industry, but these surveys typically span the entire nation and are not sensitive to local or state factors. Also, the data may be skewed or overweighted by irregular regional concentrations from year to year. An example of price trend data for skilled nursing facilities is shown in Figure 16.2.This information comes from *Senior Care Acquisition Report*, 13th edition, 2008, published

Figure 16.1 **Share Price Trends for Public Companies With Substantial Skilled Nursing Facility Activities**

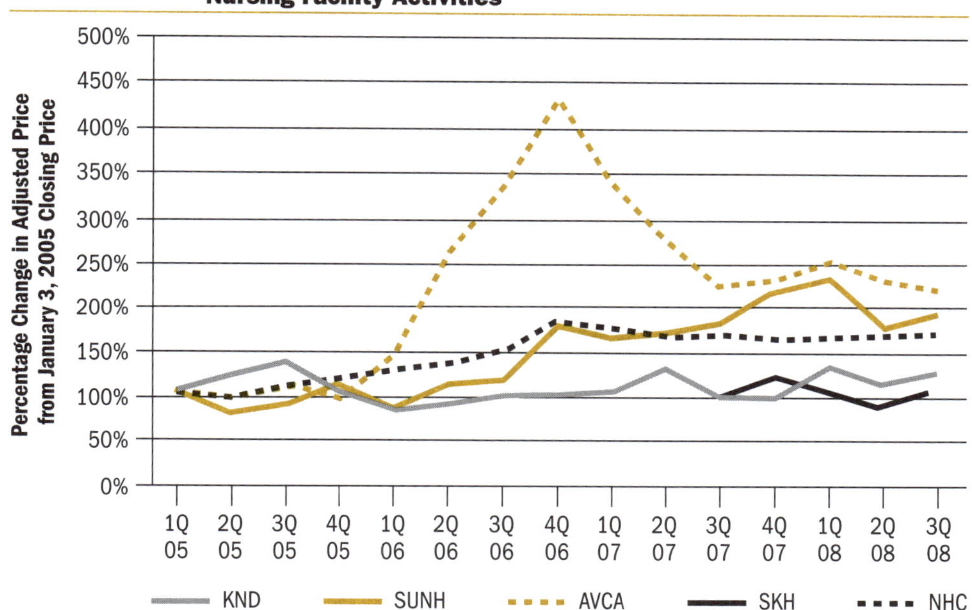

Figure 16.2 **Mean and Median Per-Bed Prices for Skilled Nursing Facility Transactions, Annually 2003 to 2007**

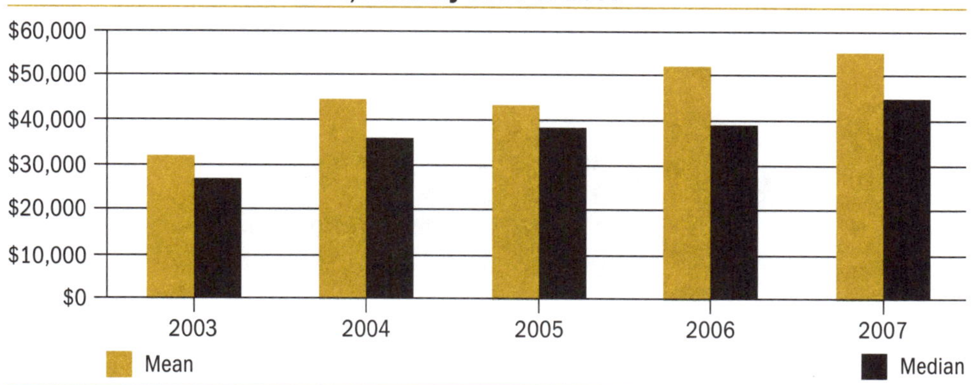

Source: *Senior Care Acquisition Report*, 13th Edition, 2008

by Levin and Associates, a prominent industry researcher and publisher of acquisition data. This survey of actual sale transactions shows that there was a steady increase in per-bed nursing facility values on a national basis between 2003 and 2007.

Changes or pending changes in reimbursement levels can profoundly affect values. A significant change in Medicare reimbursements can affect prices across the country. Substantial changes in Medicaid reimbursement levels, caused by a new rate-setting system, employment or removal of a revenue-enhancing scheme by the state, or rate cuts caused by state budget difficulties, can affect price levels on a statewide basis. For example, say that a state increases Medicaid rates for all facilities by $10.00 more than the general rate of inflation to make up for inadequate reimbursements in prior years. Assume also that the rate increase just became known to the market and the news came as a surprise. The appraiser could attempt to quantify the general increase in value by estimating the typical increase in per-bed *NOI* and applying a market-derived capitalization rate to reflect the increased value. Now, say the average occupancy rate is roughly 90%, the average Medicaid mix is 60%, and the market-derived capitalization rate for the $10.00 marginal increase in the *NOI* is 25%. Given these facts, the average value has increased by $13,140 per bed:

(365 days × 90% occupancy
× $10.00 rate increase)
/ 25% overall capitalization rate = $13,140 per bed value increase

Location

Like most commercial real estate, a nursing facility's location profoundly affects factors that drive value. Private-pay rates, occupancy levels, and payor mixes are susceptible to the influences of location. Neighborhood surroundings, income levels, residential property values, and the economic growth trends of the neighborhood and market area are factors that must be assessed in the regional, neighborhood, and site analyses. These and other factors are intertwined with the success of a nursing facility. Rather than applying potentially large adjustments for location, the influence of this factor can be more objectively measured through adjustments for differences in occupancy, census mix, and private-pay rates.

An unusual locational consideration relates to Medicare and Medicaid reimbursements. A facility may be located on the edge of one geographic reimbursement rate region, but have actual operating expense levels that are more similar to an adjacent area where costs are significantly different (higher or lower) than the costs allowed in its own rate area. This difference may not be noticeable to the casual investor or lender, but most knowledgeable operators will be aware of this anomaly and use it in marketing a facility when the effect is favorable

Location directly affects remaining economic life. Two physically similar nursing facilities may have different remaining economic lives because of location factors. Price adjustments for differences in value attributable to the remaining economic life associated with the location may be treated as a location, physical property, or economic adjustment.

The appraiser must be careful not to double count or adjust twice for this element of comparison. If an adjustment is made for economic differences (payor mix and occupancy) that results from location differences, then the location adjustment, if any, should exclude further location adjustments for these considerations. Generally, the market is more attuned to thinking about valuation problems through a matrix of economic factors (payor mix and occupancy) rather than isolated difference based almost exclusively on location and physical plant factors.

Physical Characteristics

Differences in age, physical condition, and functional design directly impact private-pay rates, payor mix, the Medicaid capital reimbursement rate, the occupancy rate, and the overall economic performance of nursing facilities. Like location adjustments, adjustments for physical differences can be largely covered in adjustments for economic characteristics, including payor mix, Medicaid capital payment, and occupancy, which lend themselves to efficient quantitative adjustments.

The adjustments for economic differences do not necessarily measure the full effect that physical differences have on value. To the extent that differences in the remaining economic life, deferred maintenance, building efficiencies, and quality are not measured by economic criteria, some additional adjustments might be needed for physical differences.

The *Senior Care Acquisition Report*, 13th Edition, March 2008 surveyed a large group of nursing facility sales that occurred in 2007. The report found that SNFs built in the past 10 years sold for an average price of $79,400 per bed, facilities built 10 to 20 years ago commanded an average price of $65,900 per bed, and facilities erected over 20 years ago sold for $43,000 per bed (see Figure 16.3).

Economic Characteristics

Distinguishable economic factors that drive nursing facility values include payor mix, Medicaid capital reimbursement, and occupancy rates. Occasionally, differences in just one of the economic factors can be isolated through matched pair

Figure 16.3 **Mean Per-Bed Prices for Skilled Nursing Facilities Grouped by Building Age, 2007 Sales**

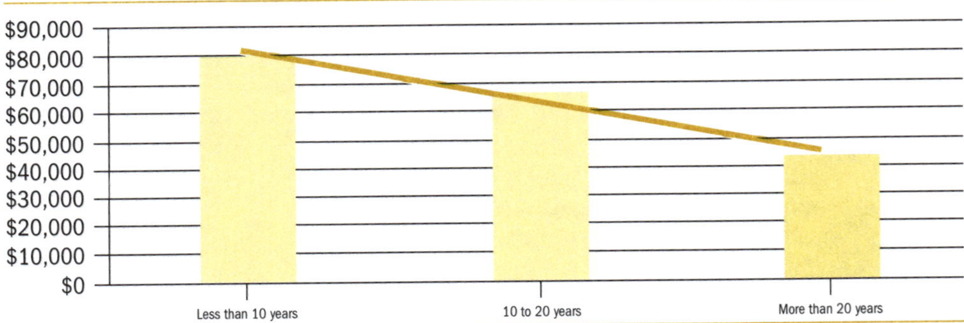

Source: *Senior Care Acquisition Report*, 13th Edition, March 2008

analysis. However, the complex matrix of economic, physical, and location differences undermine most opportunities to apply matched pair analysis. Nevertheless, it is very possible to isolate differences in value by comparing differences in earnings caused by these economic measures.

Medicaid Capital Rates

In a balanced, facility-specific, cost-based reimbursement system, the Medicaid capital rate represents a substantial component of the *NOI* or *EBITDAR* derived from the Medicaid census. Since this figure is easily obtained and simply measured, adjusting for Medicaid capital rate differences is appropriate, provided the market considers differences in capital reimbursement important, either in the comparison process or the development of an operating pro forma. Theoretically, the value of each $1.00 of capital cost rate reimbursement should translate into an approximate value of $2,200 to $2,900 per bed. To support this range, consider capitalizing the marginal $1.00 rate as shown in Table 16.2.

The example assumes that the capitalization rates approximate the return on and of the tangible assets, since the income from the capital payment is derived from realty and FF&E. If the adjustments made for physical plant differences largely account

Table 16.2 **Capitalizing a Marginal Rate**

	Example 1	Example 2
Medicaid capital payment	$1.00	$1.00
Days per year	365	365
Occupancy rate	95%	85%
Annual *NOI* per $1 of capital payment	$346.75	$310.25
Capitalization rates	12.0%	14.0%
Value for $1 of capital payment	$2,890	$2,216

for differences in Medicaid capital reimbursement, no further consideration of the Medicaid capital rate is necessary.

Table 16.3 illustrates an adjustment for differences in the Medicaid capital rates. The technique shown is akin to capitalizing a rental difference in apartment and commercial real estate appraising.

Supporting the capitalization rate for the marginal earnings differences resulting from differences in Medicaid capital, payor, and occupancy is problematic. This type of capitalization rate cannot be derived readily through direct analysis of comparable sales or from surveying the market. It requires judgment and tests of reasonableness. In estimating the capitalization rate for the marginal income differences, the durability of the income difference and the risk are used as a guide. There is greater certainty that the difference in earnings resulted from Medicaid capital reimbursement rather than occupancy levels as occupancy levels tend to vary over time.

In states in which the Medicaid capital rate is the same for all facilities or cannot be distinguished from other components of the rate, there is no basis for applying an adjustment for the capital rate.

In some states, where Medicaid rates are facility-specific but rates or regional rate ceilings have not been reset for years, the current rate may not match the current or future expected operating expenses and no rate rebasing is expected in the future. In this case, an adjustment may be appropriate to reflect the relatively permanent inequity in reimbursement. For instance, assume a facility is receiving a Medicaid rate of $150.00, based on current actual allowable cost and subject to a rate ceiling set 10 years ago, which is only adjusted for inflation trending. If the ceilings were rebased to current cost levels, the revised rate for this facility would be reduced to $140.00. Since no

Table 16.3 **Medicaid Capital Sale Price Adjustment Calculation, with Sensitivity to Occupancy and Mix**

		Subject	Sale	Difference
Medicaid capital payment		$8.50	$6.50	$2.00
Potential patient days		365	365	
Potential capital revenue	=	$3,103	$2,373	
Multiplied by occupancy rate	×	90%	90%	
Medicaid mix	×	70%	80%	
NOI derived from Title 19 capital reimbursement		$1,955	$1,708	$247
Capitalization rate for Medicaid capital payment	/	12.50%	12.50%	
Contribution to overall value	=	$15,640	$13,664	
Difference in value contribution (per-bed adjustment)				$1,976

rebasing is expected in the foreseeable future, this facility will continue to benefit by roughly $10.00 per Medicaid day from the imbalance and command a price premium. On the other hand, a sale property may be receiving a rate of $130.00 based on its costs, but the rate is limited to a trended ceiling from 10 years ago. The current total allowable cost for this facility is $140.00. If the ceilings were rebased to current expense levels for this region, the reimbursement rate for this sale would increase to $140.00. This sale is essentially losing $10.00 per patient day because of inequitable regional ceilings and its price has been negatively impacted.

This situation has occurred in Illinois and New York, where rate ceilings have been high relative to costs in Chicago and New York City and relatively low in Downstate Illinois and Upstate New York. The adjustment is economic in nature, but has a location component. Determining the rate inequity will require confirmation from the buyer or seller and a review of the rate-setting statement and Medicaid cost report. One way to avoid making an adjustment for this potentially significant value factor is to use sales that are located in the same reimbursement region or regions that share similar degrees of rate inequity.

Private-Pay/Medicare (Quality) Mix

NOI derived from private-pay and Medicare patient revenue is almost always greater than *NOI* derived from Medicaid patient revenue. As a consequence, nursing facilities with relatively high private-pay and Medicare percentages tend to have higher incomes and values. Newer facilities and facilities located in markets with high household incomes and residential property values have greater appeal to private-pay patients. Older facilities have greater difficulty competing for private-pay patients. If the location and physical characteristics adjustments fully account for differences in quality mix, no further adjustment is necessary.

The income approach may indicate that the expected *EBITDAR* from a Medicare patient day is $75.00; the expected average *EBITDAR* for a private-pay day is $25.00 and the rate for Medicaid is limited to the capital reimbursement. Capitalizing the *EBITDAR* difference of the subject and sale can produce a sale price adjustment amount (see Table 16.4).

The sales data in Table 16.5 illustrates the relationship between price and payor mix.

The sales data in Table 16.5 was developed from single-facility transactions occurring between 2005 and 2008, confirmed and analyzed by Tellatin, Short, Hansen & Clark, Inc. Sale prices have been adjusted for property rights conveyed, abnormal financing, unusual conditions of sale, and expenditures made

Table 16.4 **Quality Mix Adjustment Based on the Capitalization of Difference in Marginal *EBITDAR***

	Subject	Subject $/PPD	Sale	Sale $/PD
Medicare & managed care mix (MC)	20.00%		8.00%	
EBITDAR per patient day	$75.00		$75.00	
Weighted Medicare & MC *EBITDAR*		$15.00		$6.00
Private-pay mix	20.00%		8.00%	
EBITDAR per patient day	$25.00		$25.00	
Weighted private-pay *EBITDAR*		5.00		2.00
Total weighted *EBITDAR* from quality mix		$20.00	-	$8.00
Difference in weighted quality mix *EBITDAR*				$12.00
Occupancy rate of the subject				90.0%
Annual difference in weighted *EBITDAR* attributable to quality mix (365 × 90% × $12.00)				$3,942
Capitalization rate for marginal income difference				15.0%
Indicated per-bed adjustment				$26,280

Table 16.5 **Comparison of Average Nursing Facility Sale Prices Grouped by Quality Mix**

		Quality Mix Groupings			
	Total Sample	0 to 20%	20% to 35%	35% to 50%	50% to 100%
Effective building age	26	27	29	21	23
Price per bed	$50,663	$36,934	$44,431	$57,830	$70,572
Economic indicators					
Occupancy rate	84.6%	80.4%	82.9%	88.0%	87.7%
Medicare and managed care mix	20.9%	8.1%	12.1%	15.2%	16.7%
Private-pay mix	13.0%	6.2%	15.7%	26.0%	42.4%
Total quality mix	35.9%	14.2%	27.9%	41.2%	59.1%
Sample size	82	13	35	22	12

Source: Tellatin, Short, Hansen & Clark, Inc. 2008

immediately after purchase. The economic data was developed from actual operating data derived from the sales and obtained from sellers, buyers, and Medicare and Medicaid cost reports. The revenues and expenses were based on forecast results for the 12 months subsequent to the sale, adjusted for possible Medicaid rebasing and anticipated operational improvements. The figures do not reflect trailing results. The expenses include management expenses of approximately 4.0% and capital reserves of $300 to $400 per bed per year. The sale data was obtained from 21 states, with a preponderance of sales from Midwestern and Western states.

This same grouped sales data is shown graphically in Figure 16.4. Linear regression demonstrates the significance of the interplay between price and quality mix. It is interesting to note that the average effective building age for each group of sales is fairly consistent, but the two groups with the lower quality mixes have slightly higher effective building ages. Similarly, the groups with the higher average effective building ages and lower quality mixes have slightly lower average occupancy rates. This presentation provides empirical data to support the rationale for applying economic adjustments to nursing facility sale prices. The data will begin to lose contemporary significance after it is published, but continues to support the principles it illustrates here.

Figure 16.4 **Average Per-Bed Sale Price for SNFs Grouped by Quality Mix, 2005 to 2008 Transaction Dates**

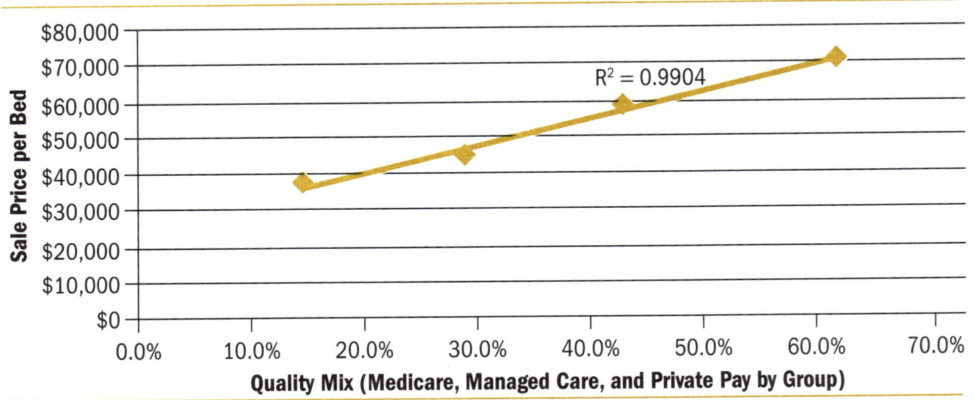

Price Tendencies

The following observations about price tendencies can be made from analyzing the sales data:

- Per-bed prices increase with quality mix.
- Facilities with higher quality mixes typically achieve higher occupancy rates and other performance benchmarks.
- Newly constructed facilities command higher quality mixes, profits, and prices.

Occupancy

The level of occupancy is important to the financial performance of any property. Vacancy rates are influenced by local supply and demand, facility reputation, and physical qualities. Matched pair analysis, regression analysis, or an economic benefit calculation can be useful in determining adjustments for occupancy rate differences. The importance of analyzing occupancy levels is illustrated with an example.

- Assume that a comparable sale and the subject property both have 80 occupied beds. Each occupied bed produces an *NOI* of $25.00 PPD and the facilities are equal except for their licensed capacities and gross building area.
- The sale has 80 licensed beds and is likely to remain full indefinitely. It sold for $5,200,000, or $65,000 per bed.

- The subject has 100 licensed beds and is likely to remain at 80% occupancy in the future.

If everything else is equal (e.g., age, condition, payor mix), the indicated value of the subject would be $5,200,000 (80 occupied beds @ $65,000). However, since value is measured on a per-bed basis, the subject licensed beds are worth $52,000 each, or 20% less than the per-bed price of the sale.

This example illustrates a one-to-one relationship between occupancy and value and assumes that occupancy levels will remain fixed. In practice, occupancy levels are not constant, and the *NOI* per occupied bed can be different because of the minimum utilization aspects of the rate-setting process and economies of scale. One-to-one relationships between occupancy rate differences might not equate to one-to-one value differences.

The appraiser should be mindful that buyers often anticipate improving occupancy levels after acquiring a property through better management and/or capital improvements.

Use

For a nursing facility to qualify as a comparable, it must have the same highest and best use as the subject. If the highest and best of the subject is for continued use as a skilled nursing facility, but a sale property is acquired for the purpose of converting the building to an alternative use, the sale may not be comparable. Typically, this situation arises when a property is on the brink of obsolescence or loss of licensure or has greater value as vacant land.

Non-Realty Components of Value (Used for Real-Estate-Only Valuations)

There are many non-realty items in nursing facilities. Most nursing facilities are sold as going concerns with the tangible and intangible personal property assets intact. If the appraisal assignment is to value the total assets of the business, then sales involving something less than the total assets should be excluded or the price should be adjusted for the value of the missing assets. Allocation of the total assets of the business will be treated in Chapter 18.

The Price Adjustment Process

The sale price adjustments are typically processed in order, following the sequence in which the elements of comparison are discussed here. The first five elements of comparison are generally made to the sale prices of the comparables without regard to the attributes of the subject property. Those adjustments are made for property rights conveyed, financing, conditions of sale, capital expenditures made immediately after purchase, and market conditions (time). The adjustments for location, physical characteristics, and economic differences involve comparing those attributes of the sales with the subject.

It is preferable that adjustments be developed from market evidence, using matched pair sales, grouped sale analysis (including regression analysis), economic-based adjustments, market surveys, and other concrete evidence. However, quantitative adjustments cannot always be made, and the appraiser will often need to rely on subjective judgments based on personal experience and knowledge.

Quantitative and Qualitative Methods of Comparison

Quantitative analysis involves applying adjustments to the comparable sale prices, using either percentages of the sale price or dollar amounts. For example, the appraiser may determine that nursing facility values have increased 5% between the date of a sale and the effective date of the appraisal; that adjustment may be expressed as a percentage by multiplying the prior adjusted price by 105%. Another quantitative price adjustment for quality mix may be expressed as a per-bed amount, say $10,000.

Qualitative analysis involves non-mathematical adjustments. A sale may be considered superior and will command a greater per-bed price than the subject because it is a newer building, with a superior location and quality mix. A mixture of quantitative and qualitative adjustments may be reasonable.

Nursing facility transactions occur in an imperfect market and differences between the subject and the sales are not precisely measured by buyers and sellers. Qualitative differences may be analyzed by ranking sales by their relative degree of similarity to the subject. Each sale is determined to be equal, superior, or inferior to the subject, and a bracketed value indication emerges. Varying degrees of relative adjustment provide greater precision. For instance, the price of one comparable sale that requires downward adjustments for five elements of comparison may be less indicative of the value of the subject than the price of another sale that requires just one adjustment. Although the adjustments applied in qualitative analysis are easier to defend than those applied in a quantitative analysis, the appraiser must justify all the adjustments. Qualitative adjustments often require considerable narrative explanation. Qualitative analysis is difficult to apply when the subject is superior or inferior to all the comparable sales and the value is believed to fall outside

Case Study—Quantitative Price Adjustment

The following application illustrates the use of both percentage and dollar amounts in the processing of sale price adjustments. The subject property is the 120-bed facility used throughout the book.

Based on various comparative analysis techniques, the appraiser determines that there is a $2,500 value difference for each $1.00 of Medicaid capital reimbursement, and a $750 per-bed difference in value for every 1% difference in quality mix. Using these two adjustments, the adjustment process shown in Table 16.6 can be performed. For this example, assume that the sale occurred one year ago at a price of $60,000 per bed. Assume also that the comparable sale receives a $12.50 Medicaid capital reimbursement, while the subject receives a $9.20 reimbursement (with no change in the rate if the property is sold). The subject has a 42.4% quality mix, while the sale has a 30% quality mix.

Table 16.6 Example of Quantitative Price Adjustment

		Sale
Sale price		$70,000
Property rights and assets conveyed		100%
Financing terms		100%
Conditions of sale		100%
Capital expenditures made immediately after purchase		100%
Time and market conditions		105%
Net adjusted price		$73,500
Dollar adjustments applied to the net adjusted price		
Location		$0
Physical characteristics		0
Economic characteristics		0
Medicaid capital reimbursement	[$2,500 × ($12.50 – $9.20)]	8,250
Quality mix	[((42.4% – 30.0) × 100) × $750]	9,300
Occupancy		0
Total currency adjustment		$17,550
Indicated per-bed value		$91,050

the price range of those comparables. In these instances, some application of quantitative analysis should be employed. From a practical perspective, many appraisal assignments will involve a subject that is superior to all the available sales since nursing facilities that are operated profitably are not sold and facilities that experience some difficulties are.

Quantitative adjustments are typical applied first. Elements of comparison that elude specific mathematical measurement are subsequently considered in qualitative analysis. The appraiser may even consider applying both types of analysis to the sale comparables.

Application of the Sales Comparison Approach

The elements of comparison, sequencing of adjustments, techniques for analyzing and adjusting sale prices, and appropriateness of quantitative and qualitative adjustments have been discussed. In the following section, the application of quantitative and qualitative adjustments will be illustrated through a continuation of the case study.

Case Study—Quantitative Sales Analysis

The same three sales are used in the quantitative and qualitative analyses that follow. In both applications of the sales comparison approach, the first five elements of comparison are adjusted quantitatively. The adjustments are applied sequentially and, when no adjustment is applied, the price is multiplied by 100%, resulting in no change to the price. The adjustments are described below.

- **Property rights and assets conveyed.** All the comparable sales are asset-based transactions and involved the conveyance of a fee simple interest in the real estate, plus the tangible and intangible assets of the business. The buyer of Sale 2 also purchased the private-pay receivables. The receivables only involve private-pay patients with co-payments for Medicare Parts A and B. The gross receivables amount to $500,000, and the buyer, who is experienced at pursuing these revenues, expects to net $200,000 after all collection expenses, factoring, and discounting is applied. The sale price is adjusted downward by $200,000, or 2.0% ($200,000 / $10,800,000), or 98.0% of the total price. With the exception of the purchase of one specific set of receivables, there was no transfer of current or long-term liabilities from the seller to the buyer.
- **Financing terms.** None of the sales involved financing outside normal market rates or other terms that would influence the price. Therefore, no adjustments for financing are applied.
- **Conditions of sale.** Sale 1 was sold by a real estate investment trust, whose tenant was in default on the lease and failed to achieve a positive *EBITDAR*-to-rent coverage. The contract rent exceeded market rent. The REIT agreed to let the tenant out of the lease in exchange for the tenant's cooperation in securing a new operator. While the tenant was cooperative throughout the sale process, the price was believed to be discounted slightly to reflect the operating risks that the buyer was likely to assume. Since the prior operator (the tenant) was not normally motivated, like an owner would be, the market and the buyer discounted the price slightly to cover potential transitional expenses, such as the replacement of key staff. Under the terms of the lease, the tenant was required to return the property, including the building and FF&E, in good condition. Moreover, all licenses, certifications, and the existing staff and patients were to be conveyed to the landlord or the landlord's appointed successor. The buyer believed the price was discounted roughly 5%. No adjustments for conditions of sale were necessary for the other sales.

- **Capital expenditures made immediately after purchase.** The buyers of Sales 1 and 3 were able to take control of their facilities without incurring any immediate capital expenditures. However, Sale 2 required $500,000 for the immediate capital replacement of items including a new roof cover, emergency generator, and nurse call system, and for the conversion of all patient and financial records to a computer system. The percentage adjustment is calculated as follows: $1 + [(\$500,000 / (10,080,000 \times 98.0\%)]$. Remember, this sale was previously adjusted for the net value of the purchased receivables.
- **Time and market conditions.** Market evidence shows that there has been upward pressure on nursing facility values. While there are no matched pair sales available for analysis, secondary data shows that values are trending upward. Prices for public nursing homes and healthcare REIT equity shares increased between the sale dates and the effective date of the appraisal. According to a published acquisition report, the national mean per-bed price for skilled nursing facilities increased 5% between the prior and current year surveys. Interviews with several investors shows that prices have trended higher. From an economic perspective, the state's tight certificate of need policy, coupled with modest demand growth and a stable reimbursement environment, have contributed to higher values. Taking all these considerations into account, it is concluded that nursing facility values have increased 5.0% over the past 12 months.
- **Location.** Sales 2 and 3 are located in areas similar to the suburban setting of the subject. The housing characteristics and values and household income levels in the primary market areas of these two sales are comparable to the subject. These two sales possess no measurable location advantages or disadvantages over the subject. The remaining economic lives of the two sale properties are not adversely impacted by location. Given these comparisons, no adjustments for location are applied to Sales 2 and 3.

  Sale 1 is located in an inferior setting and market area, where property values are not keeping pace with the market and housing values and household income levels fall below regional and state levels. The declining nature of the area is expected to adversely affect the property and the remaining economic life. While the substantially lower quality mix is a reflection of the inferior location of this sale, the economic price adjustment applied accounts for a substantial portion of the difference in value attributed to the location difference. However, the economic adjustment does not consider the difference that the location has on remaining economic life and the smaller market appeal the property has because of the location. There is no available data or analysis that will precisely determine the appropriate adjustment, so the appraiser relies on subjective experience in applying the adjustment.
- **Physical characteristics.** The competitiveness of a nursing facility is profoundly affected by the physical plant characteristics. Similar to location adjustments, economic adjustments are applied to reflect much of the difference in the physical qualities of the sales and the subject. The adjustments applied to the sales for physical characteristics relate primarily to remaining economic life and abnormal plant operating expenses. The economic adjustments will account for the physical differences that generate variances in occupancy, quality mix, and revenue rates.

The adjustment factor is based in large part on recapturing the wasting assets of the nursing facility over the expected economic life of the building and tangible personal property assets. However, over the lifespan of the property, additional capital costs will be incurred, beyond the normal amounts accumulated and covered by capital replacement reserves, to reposition the property in the changing competitive market. Using a sinking fund factor of 5.0% and a replacement cost of $90,000 per bed, the annual installment is $429. An additional amount is considered for the capital expenditures needed for future competitive repositioning. Again, other issues involving physical plant differences are captured in the economic adjustments. Therefore, it is concluded that an adjustment factor equal to $500 per bed for each year of difference in the effective building ages will be applied to the sales. The adjustment calculations are shown below.

Physical Adjustment Calculations—Based on Effective Building Age

	Sale 1	Sale 2	Sale 3
Effective building age of sale	28	22	8
Less subject effective building age	14	14	14
Age difference	14	8	-6
Adjustment factor ($500/year)	$500	$500	$500
Net price adjustment	$7,000	$4,000	-$3,000

- **Economic characteristics**

  Medicaid capital reimbursement. An adjustment is applied for the perceived difference in value caused by variations in the Medicaid capital reimbursement rate. Based on market evidence derived from paired sales and group sales analysis, market surveys, and/or economic calculations, it is determined that for each $1 of capital reimbursement, there is a $2,500-per-bed value difference. Using this adjustment factor, the following adjustment calculations are applied to the sales.

Medicaid Capital Reimbursement Adjustment Calculations

	Sale 1	Sale 2	Sale 3
Subject Medicaid capital rate	$9.20	$9.20	$9.20
Less Medicaid capital rate of sale	$6.00	$10.00	$14.00
Rate difference	$3.20	-$0.80	-$4.80
Adjustment factor ($2,500/$1.00)	$2,500	$2,500	$2,500
Net price adjustment	$8,000	-$2,000	-$12,000

Occupancy rate. In this case the occupancy rate of the subject and the rates of the sales are reasonably comparable. All the facilities are set up to operate at their licensed capacity, so there are no beds permanently taken out of service. There is no basis in the market to adjust the sale prices for the slight variations in occupancy rates.

Quality mix. Economic and sales analyses both support adjusting the comparables for differences in quality mix. Adjustment factors using value differences developed from capitalizing differences in the per-bed *NOI* suggest that values will vary between $500 and $1,000 for every 1% difference in quality mix. An analysis of the comparable sales suggests the same. The following analysis shows the sale prices for all three sales after all other adjustments have been applied (see subsequent quantitative adjustment grid). The difference between the adjusted prices for Sales 1 and 3, representing the lowest and highest prices and quality mix levels, is $22,160. The difference in quality mix for these two sales is 29.0%. Based on these coordinates, the bed value changes $764 for each 1% difference in quality mix.

Sale	Quality Mix	Adjusted Price
Sale 1	20.0%	$62,840
Sale 3	49.0%	$85,000
Differences	29.0%	$22,160
	Result	
$22,160 / 29.0 = $764/bed for each 1.0% difference in quality mix		

The regression analysis in Figure 16.5 shows the three adjusted sale prices before the quality mix adjustment is applied, which confirms the factor calculated.

Figure 16.5 **Linear Regression Analysis With Trend Line for Comparable Sales, Prices Adjusted for All Other Elements of Comparison**

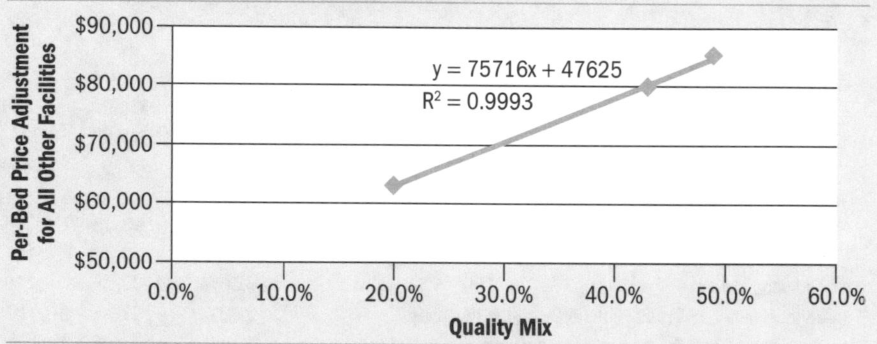

Using an adjustment factor equal to $750.00 for each 1% difference in quality mix produces the following per-bed price adjustments for the sale comparables.

Quality Mix Adjustment Calculations

	Sale 1	Sale 2	Sale 3
Subject quality mix	42.4%	42.4%	42.4%
Less quality mix of the sales	20.0%	43.0%	49.0%
Quality mix difference	22.4%	-0.6%	-6.6%
Adjustment factor ($750/1.0%)	$750	$750	$750
Net price adjustment	$16,763	-$487	-$4,987

Note: Figures are rounded.

- **Use (zoning).** No adjustment is necessary.
- **Non-realty components of value.** No adjustment is necessary.

Conclusion of the Quantitative Sales Comparison Analysis

The analyses described above present comparisons and specific, isolated calculations made to the sale prices for the elements of comparison. The summary grid shown in Table 16.7 draws together all of the price adjustments and provides a range of value indications. Given the tight spread in adjusted prices and rounding to a significant factor, a value of $80,000 per bed is concluded in the quantitative adjustment process in the sales comparison approach.

Table 16.7 Sales Comparison Summary and Adjustment Grid—Applying Quantitative Adjustments

	Subject	1	2	3
Facts of the sale				
Sale date		- 6 months	- 12 months	- 3 months
Total sale price	N/A	$3,120,000	$10,080,000	$9,000,000
Number of beds	120	78	140	90
Gross building area	48,000	26,158	57,846	41,520
Effective building age after immediate repairs	14	28	22	8
Overall building condition	Average	Average	Average	Good
Land area	5.00	8.90	8.80	5.00
Economic data				
Occupancy rate	89.3%	89.0%	87.0%	92.0%
Medicare/managed care mix	11.0%	8.0%	15.0%	15.0%
Private-pay mix	31.3%	12.0%	28.0%	34.0%
Medicaid capital cost rate	$9.20	$6.00	$10.00	$14.00
Effective gross revenue	$7,106,587	$4,190,955	$8,024,489	$6,021,734
NOI or *EBITDAR*	$1,127,881	$384,345	$1,423,391	$1,146,826
Elements of comparison & quantitative adjustments				
Property rights and assets conveyed		100.0%	98.0%	100.0%
Financing terms		100.0%	100.0%	100.0%
Conditions of sale		105.0%	100.0%	100.0%
Capital expenditures made immediately after purchase		100.0%	105.1%	100.0%
Net adjusted price before time and market conditions		$3,276,000	$10,378,400	$9,000,000
Time and market conditions		102.0%	105.0%	100.0%
Net adjusted price		$3,341,520	$10,897,320	$9,000,000
Adjusted price per bed		$42,840	$77,838	$100,000
Adjusted effective gross revenue multiplier		0.80	1.36	1.49
Adjusted price per square foot		$127.74	$188.39	$216.76
Other quantitative adjustments				
Location		$5,000	$0	$0
Physical (age, condition & quality)		7,000	4,000	-3,000
Economic				
Medicaid capital cost rate		8,000	-2,000	-12,000
Occupancy rate		0	0	0
Quality mix (private & Medicare)		16,763	-487	-4,987
Net adjustment		$36,763	$1,513	-$19,987
Adjusted price–value indication	$80,000	$79,603	$79,351	$80,013

Case Study—Qualitative Sales Analysis

The same three sales studied in the quantitative analysis are used to demonstrate the qualitative analysis. In both applications, the adjustments for property rights, financing, conditions of sale, capital expenditures made immediately after purchase, and time and market conditions are the same. The differences in location, physical characteristics, and economic characteristics are treated using several qualitative techniques. The summary grid presented in Table 16.8 presents some of the same information shown in Table 16.7, which profiled the quantitative adjustments.

Qualitative adjustments are applied to the sales to account for differences in location, the physical plant, Medicaid capital reimbursement, occupancy rate, and quality mix. A discussion of the qualitative analysis applied is presented as follows.

- **Location.** Sale 1 has an inferior location, as evidenced by demographic trends and general economic conditions within the primary market. The inferior location is also evident in the lower quality mix of the sale. The location characteristics of Sales 2 and 3 are similar to the subject. Like the subject, they are situated in stable suburban settings surrounded with similar use, household income, and property value levels.
- **Physical characteristics.** The physical characteristics of Sales 1 and 2 are inferior to the subject. These two buildings are older than the subject and have greater levels of physical deterioration and functional obsolescence. As a result, the remaining economic lives of these two facilities are measurably less than the subject's. Sale 3 is a newer, more functional building than the subject. It has more private patient rooms and a larger and more prominent therapy center than the subject, which allows it to achieve a higher Medicare census.
- **Economic characteristics**

  Medicaid capital reimbursement. The Medicaid capital reimbursement rate for Sale 1 is inferior to the subject's rate and the capital rate for Sale 3 is superior. The slight difference in the capital rate for Sale 2 is considered insignificant to the qualitative adjustment process.

  Occupancy rate. The market does not perceive any price difference attributable to the slight variations in occupancy rate between the subject and the comparables.

  Quality mix. Sale 1 has a significantly inferior quality mix. Sale 2 has a slightly superior, or higher, quality mix. The combined Medicare and private-pay mix for Sale 3 is clearly superior.
- **Use (zoning).** No adjustment is necessary.
- **Non-realty components of value.** No adjustment is necessary.

The comparable sales are arrayed relative to the qualities of the subject. From this array, a single value, or value range, emerges.

Sale Number	Overall Comparability	Adjusted Price*
1	Highly inferior	$42,840
2	Roughly equal	$80,590
3	Superior	$100,000

* The adjusted price equals the per-bed price of each sale after adjustments are applied for property rights, financing, conditions of sale, capital expenditures made immediately after purchase, and time and market conditions.

Table 16.8 Sales Comparison Summary and Adjustment Grid—Applying Qualitative Adjustments

	Subject	1	2	3
Facts of the sale				
Sale date		- 6 months	- 12 months	- 3 months
Total sale price	N/A	$3,120,000	$10,080,000	$9,000,000
Number of beds	120	78	140	90
Economic data				
Occupancy rate	89.3%	89.0%	87.0%	92.0%
Medicare/managed care mix	11.0%	8.0%	15.0%	15.0%
Private-pay mix	31.3%	12.0%	28.0%	34.0%
Medicaid capital cost rate	$9.20	$6.00	$10.00	$14.00
Effective gross revenue	$7,106,587	$4,190,955	$8,024,489	$6,021,734
NOI or *EBITDAR*	$1,127,881	$384,345	$1,423,391	$1,146,826
Elements of comparison & quantitative adjustments				
Property rights and assets conveyed		100.0%	100.0%	100.0%
Financing terms		100.0%	100.0%	100.0%
Conditions of sale		105.0%	100.0%	100.0%
Capital expenditures made immediately after purchase		100.0%	106.6%	100.0%
Net adjusted price before time and market conditions		$3,276,000	$10,745,280	$9,000,000
Time and market conditions		102.0%	105.0%	100.0%
Net adjusted price		$3,341,520	$11,282,544	$9,000,000
Adjusted price per bed		$42,840	$80,590	$100,000
Adjusted effective gross revenue multiplier		0.80	1.41	1.49
Adjusted price per square foot		$127.74	$188.39	$216.76
Other adjustments–qualitative				
Location		–	=	=
Physical (age, condition & quality)		–	–	+
Economic				
Medicaid capital cost rate		–	=	+
Occupancy rate		=	=	=
Quality mix (private & Medicare)		–	+	+
Overall comparability		– – – –	=	+++
		Highly inferior	Similar	Superior

Inferior = –
Substantially inferior = – –
Superior = +
Substantially superior = + +

Sale 2 emerges as the most comparable property and produced an adjusted price of $80,590 per bed. It is not uncommon to see a large spread in the unadjusted sale prices of nursing facilities simply because of the limited volume of transactions. Further refinement of the qualitative process can narrow the range of adjusted prices.

Reconciliation of the Sales Comparison Approach

If more than one technique is applied in the sales comparison approach, then a reconciliation of the techniques is performed to resolve differences and conclude a single value or value range for the subject. Reconciliation involves consideration of the strengths and weaknesses of each technique relative to the quality and quantity of the data, the reasonableness of the analysis, and the available support for price adjustments.

While a per-bed value is typically the primary unit of comparison, the value developed from this comparison can be expressed in other units of comparison, such as the price per square foot, net revenue multiplier, and overall capitalization rate. The value conclusion developed for the subject can also be compared to salient facts and to the averages of various value drivers for the sales. Value drivers may include effective building age, occupancy rates, quality mixes, *NOI/EBITDAR* margins, and *NOI/EBITDAR* per bed. Should the value conclusion of the subject fall outside the range indicated by other units of comparison, then many of the value drivers can also be expected to fall outside the range in a corresponding direction.

Case Study—Sales Comparison Reconciliation

The quantitative analysis produces a value indication of $80,000 per bed. The qualitative analysis supports the $80,000-per-bed value. Table 16.9 shows value drivers for the subject and compares the subject's characteristics with the average implied square foot value, effective net revenue multiplier, and implied overall capitalization rate of the sales.

Table 16.9 Reconciliation and Test of Reasonableness of the Sales Comparison Approach

	Subject	Sale Average	Comment
Effective building age after immediate repairs	14	19	Subject is superior
Gross building area per bed	400	403	Comparable
NOI/EBITDAR per bed	$9,399	$9,279	Subject is superior
NOI/EBITDAR margin	15.9%	15.3%	Subject is superior
Occupancy rate	89.3%	89.3%	Comparable
Medicare/managed care mix	11.0%	12.7%	Subject is inferior
Private-pay mix	31.3%	24.7%	Subject is superior
Medicaid capital cost rate	$9.20	$10.00	Subject is inferior
Overall comparability			
Indicated value per bed (adjusted price)	$80,000	$73,559	
Adjusted price per square foot	$200.00	$177.63	
Effective net revenue multiplier	1.35	1.22	
Overall capitalization rate	11.7%	12.7%	

The average time-adjusted sale price for the comparable sales is $73,559 per bed. The concluded value of the subject exceeds the average per-square-foot price and the net revenue multiplier of the comparables. The overall capitalization rate of the subject is slightly lower than the average of the sales. Using a qualitative analysis, the subject is compared to the sale average in terms of several value drivers. The subject is a newer building, with a slightly higher *NOI* per bed, a higher *NOI* margin, and a higher private-pay census mix. These relationships suggest that the subject is superior to the average of the sales. However, the subject has a slightly lower Medicare mix and Medicaid capital rate when compared to the average of the sales. Overall, the principal value drivers of the subject are superior to the sale average. Therefore it is reasonable that the value of the subject, measured on a per-bed, per-square-foot, and net revenue multiplier basis, will exceed those of the comparables. It is also reasonable that the overall capitalization of the subject may be less than the sales, given that the subject is a newer building and has a greater *NOI/EBITDAR* margin.

Summary

In the development and application of the sales comparison approach to a nursing facility, the appraiser considers a myriad of issues. The process involves collecting and analyzing sales data, applying appropriate price adjustment techniques, adjusting sale prices for differences in elements of comparison, and reconciling a final value conclusion. Appraisers can review changes of ownership filed at state departments of health, which may provide considerable insight into the transaction. A review of the buyer's first Medicaid cost report will provide considerable information on census, revenue, expenses, and capital costs. Armed with this research and other publicly available information, the appraiser is prepared to successfully interview a party to the sale.

The market typically frames nursing facility values on a per-bed basis. However, use of net revenue multipliers, prices per square foot, and earnings multipliers (implied overall capitalization rates) offer a test of reasonableness. The price adjustment process for nursing facilities is very similar to the adjustment process for other types of real estate. However, nursing facilities have unique elements of comparison, which include conveyances of property rights, payor mix, and Medicaid capital reimbursement. Using per-bed *NOI* adjustments as a primary adjustment technique in the sales comparison approach is tantamount to an income approach and the results may be misleading if the *NOI* forecast is flawed.

The sales comparison approach is most persuasive in the valuation of nursing facilities when there is a sufficient number of recent sale transactions that are comparable to the subject in as many ways as possible: location, physical plant age, quality, size, and economic factors such as occupancy, census mix, reimbursement levels, and earnings. Same-state data best reflects the influence of Medicaid and CON policies. In the absence of recent sales data from within the state, the appraiser may need to use sales from other states and recognize the differences in CON policies and reimbursements in the adjustment process. The sales comparison approach is essential to the valuation process even in the absence of ideal sales data. Properties under contract, offers, refusals, options, and listings may be better market indicators than actual sales of nursing facilities if the only sales available are exceedingly dissimilar to the subject.

Chapter 17

Cost Approach

The cost approach involves estimating separate values for the land, real estate improvements, tangible personal property, and intangible assets. Like the sales comparison and income capitalization approaches, the cost approach is based on comparison. Land valuation is typically developed by comparing the sale prices and relevant characteristics of comparable vacant sites to the subject site as if it were vacant and available for development to its highest and best use. The improvement value is based on the replacement or reproduction cost of the improvements less depreciation. The value of the tangible personal property, or furniture, fixtures, and equipment (FF&E), is also developed by estimating replacement cost less depreciation. The value of the intangible assets can be developed with a number of less precise techniques, which are described in Chapter 18. The summation of these values provides an indication of property value.

The principle of substitution has great relevance to the cost approach. A prudent buyer of a nursing facility will not pay more for the assets of the property than the cost to acquire a similar site, erect an equivalent set of improvements, equip the facility, and expend the financial and entrepreneurial resources needed to create the business without undue delay. The principle of supply and demand is relevant too as buyers of nursing facilities may opt to develop new facilities when the value of existing facilities exceeds the full cost of new development.

The cost approach is the least applicable technique in the valuation of the total assets of a nursing facility. Its underlying assumptions do not reflect the rationale of the market. The cost approach is generally considered more appropriate for newer properties that have not been affected by the three forms of depreciation: physical deterioration, functional obsolescence, and external obsolescence.

The greatest usefulness of the cost approach could be in allocating the total assets of the business to real estate, tangible personal property, and intangible personal property assets, under the theory that the value of an asset cannot exceed the cost to replace it in a timely manner, less reasonable amounts of depreciation. The cost approach can be very useful in determining the feasibility of a proposed nursing facility. If the prospective value of a proposed nursing facility exceeds the value of the land, the replacement cost of the improvements, and the tangible personal property value, plus the estimated cost to receive certifications and permits, recruit staff, absorb beds, reach stabilization, and set the business up in a profitable position, then the development project is usually considered economically feasible.

Procedural Steps

The procedural steps in the cost approach are summarized as follows.

1. Estimate the market value of the land as though vacant and available to be developed to its highest and best use.
2. Determine the appropriate cost basis for the improvements–replacement cost or reproduction cost.
3. Estimate the hard (direct) and soft (indirect) costs of the improvements
4. Estimate a market-appropriate profit or incentive for the developer or entrepreneur.
5. Add the hard and soft costs and the profit or incentive together to arrive at the total improvement cost.
6. Estimate the amount of depreciation caused by physical deterioration, functional obsolescence, and external obsolescence.
7. Deduct the total estimated depreciation from the total cost new of the improvements to arrive at the indicated value of the improvements.
8. Add the value of the land to the depreciated improvement value to arrive at the estimated real estate value.
9. Repeat Steps 2 through 7, focusing on the facility's personal property, to arrive at the value of the tangible personal property assets.
10. Add the value of the intangible personal property assets to the value of the real estate and tangible personal property assets to arrive at the market value of the total assets of the business. This step may be performed to allocate the value of the total assets, after the final value of the property is reconciled from the various approaches to value.

Land and Site Valuation

The valuation of the land may be presented as a stand-alone section of the appraisal or folded into the cost approach. The land is valued in accordance with its highest and best use as though vacant and available for development to its most economic use.

In estimating land value, sales comparison is generally the preferred methodology. To apply the sales comparison technique, the appraiser analyzes, compares, and adjusts sales of similar, vacant sites with highest and best use and value characteristics similar to those of the subject site. Other land valuation techniques include market extraction, allocation, and land residual methods. Only a cursory treatment of these alternative techniques is presented here since most nursing facility sites are valued based on comparable sales. It should be noted that these other techniques may be more practical in some urban markets, where land is fully developed and land sales are scarce.

Market extraction is applied by deducting the depreciated cost of the improvements, the depreciated cost of the tangible personal property assets, and the value of the intangible assets from the sale price. Land residual techniques hinge on a more complicated extraction technique, which requires that individual asset values, income, and capitalization rates be developed to arrive at an income and capitalization rate attributable to the land. The difficulty of evaluating the intangible assets, coupled with the market's general disregard of the cost approach in the valuation of nursing facilities, eliminates these techniques from practical application in nearly every instance.

The application of the sales comparison technique to derive land value is very similar to the procedure described in Chapter 16. The research of comparable land sales, listings, offers, and options for properties with a similar highest and best use is typically performed on a local level. However, land sales in other market areas are often considered if these areas have property values and rental levels that are similar to the subject market and the sales involve sites purchased for nursing facility or senior housing developments. Many developers of nursing facilities consider the affordability of land relative to their operating expectations, and those expectations are set by regional and national economic factors that are specific to the industry.

The comparable land sales are typically reduced to a common unit of comparison, such as price per square foot, price per acre, or price per bed. The local market and sales data will often dictate the appropriate unit of measurement. The elements of comparison and adjustment techniques applied in land valuation are very similar to the techniques applied to compare improved sales in Chapter 16. *The Appraisal of Real Estate* and other books and articles published by the Appraisal Institute can be used as references in the development of land value.[1]

Replacement Versus Reproduction Cost

The cost to construct the nursing facility improvements on the effective appraisal date may be developed using the reproduction or replacement cost. These costs are defined as follows.

> *Reproduction cost* is the estimated cost to construct, as of the effective appraisal date, an exact duplicate or replica of the building being appraised, insofar as possible, using the same materials, construction standards, design, layout, and quality of workmanship and embodying all the deficiencies, superadequacies, and obsolescence of the subject improvements.[2]
>
> *Replacement cost* is the estimated cost to construct, as of the effective appraisal date, a substitute for the building being appraised using contemporary materials, standards, design, and layout. When this cost basis is used, some existing obsolescence in the property may be cured. Replacement cost may be the only alternative if reproduction cost cannot be estimated.[3]

Replacement cost is generally preferred in appraising nursing facilities since costs are easier to obtain and some forms of obsolescence are eliminated. However, many existing nursing home buildings have deficiencies that would be included in the replacement cost. The materials, standards, design, layout, and quality of nursing facilities have evolved dramatically over the past several decades to meet changing regulatory, market, and reimbursement standards. The first wave of nursing facilities were developed within 10 years of the creation of the Medicaid and Medicare programs and their designs often included three- and four-bed patient rooms, shared semi-private toilets that do not meet current accessibility standards, and less than 300 square feet of total building area per licensed bed. Increased emphasis on therapy services beginning in the early 1990s caused a shift towards designs that include spacious areas for therapy services and eliminate the use of ward rooms. Facilities developed in this era often contain more than 400 square feet per bed. Current standards call for more private patient rooms, more common areas, and more square footage per bed.

---

1. See also James H. Boykin, *Land Valuation Adjustment Procedures and Assignments* (Chicago: Appraisal Institute, 2001).
2. *The Appraisal of Real Estate*, 13th ed., (Chicago: Appraisal Institute, 2008), 385.
3. Ibid.

The current replacement cost for the building improvements of a nursing facility may easily exceed $100,000 per bed, but the reproduction cost for a 30-year-old facility with similar materials and quality of construction in the same community may be $60,000 per bed. These older facilities will have smaller patient rooms, fewer toilets, and fewer and smaller common areas for patients and support services. While the cost per square foot of the two buildings may be similar, the per-bed cost will vary substantially.

If the replacement cost estimate treats the superadequacies or inadequacies of the subject building inappropriately, the reproduction cost may prove to be more reliable. However, if the building is older and contains elevated levels of physical, functional, and/or external obsolescence, the cost approach may have little or no relevance in deriving a final value estimate, regardless of the type of cost developed. Therefore, the appraiser may opt to economize his or her efforts and eliminate the cost approach.

Cost Estimates

Cost estimation involves the development of direct (hard) and indirect (soft) costs. Both types of costs are significant and must be included in any reliable cost estimate. Direct costs essentially include the costs incurred at the building site, and indirect costs generally include expenses that are incurred from activities conducted off the construction site.

Direct costs include the cost of:

- Building permits
- Installation of and connections to utilities
- Construction materials, products, and mechanical and other equipment
- Labor for the construction
- Use of construction equipment
- Security, temporary buildings, and storage
- Contractors' overhead and profits
- Performance bonds

Soft costs include costs for:

- Regulatory approvals (CON, etc.)
- Architect and engineering fees
- Legal, accounting, consulting, and appraisal fees
- Carrying cost of the land and construction interest and loan fees during construction
- Insurance and property taxes during construction

- Funding operating deficits during initial absorption
- Pre-opening marketing and recruiting expenses

To develop replacement and reproduction cost estimates, the appraiser compares construction costs for comparable buildings. Construction costs can be obtained from contract-reporting services, cost-estimating services, the appraiser's own collection of construction cost information obtained from prior assignments involving new developments, a review of costs filed in Medicaid cost reports and certificate of need applications, and contractor bids.

The importance of the cost approach to the valuation might guide the selection of cost source(s). For practical purposes, most appraisers primarily rely upon cost-estimating services such as Marshall and Swift , F.W. Dodge Corporation, and R.S. Means Company, Inc. The published cost manuals will typically include all direct costs and varying amounts of indirect, or soft, costs.

There are three cost-estimating methods:

- Comparative-unit
- Unit-in-place
- Quantity survey

The comparative-unit method is the most economical approach to estimating the construction cost of a nursing facility. It is also the most frequently applied method since the cost approach is generally the least applicable approach to value for nursing facilities. It involves comparing the overall construction costs of similar buildings, usually on a square-foot basis, and making adjustments for physical differences and construction cost trends. Published costs from cost-estimating services are generally relied upon in the development of the comparative-unit method, but costs from comparable buildings known to the appraiser can also be used. The publishers of cost manuals offer comprehensive training in the use of their services.

To apply the unit-in-place, or segregated-cost, method, the appraiser estimates individual unit costs for the various building components and subcomponents. The per-unit costs are applied to the appropriate unit of measurement for the component–e.g., square foot, linear foot, number of units (for elevator cabs), packaged terminal air conditioners (PTAC) units, ton of air conditioning, etc. This method requires more details on construction quantities, which may prove difficult for older buildings when no building plans are available. The unit-in-place method provides a combined materials and labor cost for the complete installation of a particular building component.

As an example, the cost of the roof cover will include the underlayment, shingles, nails, and other materials and supplies plus labor and subcontractor profit. Again, the appraiser must determine if it is practical to develop a cost approach with this level of detail.

The quantity survey method is similar in some respects to the unit-in-place method in that separate cost estimates are made relative to the construction trade, rather than the building component. The costs reflect the quantity and quality of all materials used, plus all categories of labor employed to complete the construction. For instance, in the quantity survey method, the cost of carpentry includes all materials and labor associated with that contractor or subcontractor agreement. In the unit-in-place, however, the carpentry costs are allocated to the exterior wall construction, interior construction, and structural roof construction.

Whichever cost method or methods are used to develop the replacement or reproduction cost estimate, the appraiser should carefully avoid counting the same cost twice or excluding costs. *Marshall Valuation Services*, published by Marshall and Swift/Boeckh, LLC, is a popular cost-estimating guide that provides comparative-unit (calculator) and unit-in-place (segregated) costs. The guide's cost figures include the following:[4]

- Nearly all direct costs
- Architect and engineering fees (separately calculated in the segregated cost, or unit-in-place, method)
- Interest on the building construction cost during the period of construction
- All appropriate local, state, and federal taxes for all material and labor costs
- Normal site preparation costs, including grading, foundation excavation, and finish (for the structure only)
- Utility lines and connections to the lot line, with normal setbacks
- Contractors' overhead and profit, including job supervision
- Worker's compensation and unemployment insurance
- Casualty and liability insurance during construction
- Construction equipment expenses
- Temporary facilities
- Construction site security

4. *Marshal Valuation Services*, Marshall and Swift/Boeckh, LLC, January 2008, Section 1, page 3.

The comparative-unit and unit-in-place cost figures in *Marshall Valuation Service* exclude a number of indirect costs, including the following:[5]

- All cost associated with acquiring the site and making the site ready for construction (legal, zoning, escrow fees, right-of-way expenses, demolition, storm drainage, and rough grading)
- Extraordinary foundation costs, including hillside foundations and pilings
- Land planning, preliminary concept plans for land use approvals, feasibility studies, certificates of need, environmental and other impact reports, appraisals, and consulting fees
- Discounts paid for financing, startup operating funds, negative cash flows during construction, project bond issuance, permanent financing fees, and the purchase of personal property (FF&E)
- Site improvements, including driveway and parking pavement, sidewalks, signage, fencing, landscaping and driveway lighting, septic systems, wells, lawn irrigation, and landscaping
- Off-site fees, impact and entitlement fees, off-site roads, and utilities
- All costs associated with pre-opening advertising and marketing as well as costs for occupancy and staff recruiting
- Furniture, fixtures, and equipment
- All expenses incurred immediately after construction is completed and accepted until stabilization occurs

While not specifically mentioned, all expenses incurred immediately after construction is completed and accepted, the cost to achieve economic or operational stability (operating deficits), and developer or entrepreneurial profit and incentive are not included in the cost figures provided in *Marshall Valuation Service* or other cost-estimating manuals.

Cost to Achieve Economic or Operational Stability

The nursing facility will experience negative cash flows from operations during the initial absorption process. Operating expenses are typically incurred even before the facility opens, as the operator recruits staff and advertises. Once opened, the facility begins the initial absorption process, which may take six months to well over a year. The operating cash flows during this initial period are typically insufficient to cover all or some of the debt service and a market level of return to the equity. The difference between the initial cash flow and the stabilized

5. Ibid.

NOI or *EBITDAR* during this period represents another soft development cost that is not measured elsewhere.

An example of the operating deficits experienced during the initial absorption of the case study property is presented in Table 17.2 . Typically, initial operating deficits for skilled nursing facilities approximate 10% to 20% of the improvement cost, prior to developer incentive and profit.

Developer or Entrepreneurial Profit and Incentive

Entrepreneurial incentive refers to the amount that the market would recognize the developer is entitled to receive as compensation for providing coordination and expertise and for assuming development risks. *Entrepreneurial profit* is the difference between the stabilized market value (or realized value) and the total, all-in cost, including the developer's incentive and operating deficits during the initial absorption. Because nursing facilities can have significant intangible value, much of the entrepreneurial profit may be interpreted as being intangible value. The estimation of profit is a fundamental component of total cost.

Entrepreneurial incentive and profit should be derived through market analysis and interviews with developers of nursing facilities. Entrepreneurial incentive and profit are typically expressed as a percentage of direct cost; direct and indirect costs; direct, indirect, and land costs; or the total cost of the completed project.

Case Study—Estimating Improvement Cost

Table 17.1 illustrates the development of a cost estimate using the comparative-unit method. The costs shown represent the costs of the improvements on the case study property. In this example, the building materials and mechanical systems of the subject improvements are consistent with current standards in the market, but the building lacks adequate storage and therapy space. While a replacement cost estimate would eliminate these functional deficiencies, the case study application will use the reproduction cost with the imbedded obsolescence. The base improvement cost is derived from *Marshall Valuation Service* and assumes good-quality, Class "D" (wood frame) construction as is typical for convalescence hospitals. The multipliers reflect a hypothetical *building and location*.

Note that contractor's overhead and profit and some indirect costs are included in the base cost and adjustments. *Marshall Valuation Service* should be studied for a full understanding of the costs included in the published base amount and adjustments. The replacement cost can be developed in the same steps and sequence.

Table 17.1 Cost New Improvement—Comparative-Unit Method (Reproduction Cost Basis)

Development of direct costs		
Building improvements		
Base unit cost from cost-estimating service, per square foot		$152.41
HVAC and other adjustments	+	0.00
Subtotal		$152.41
Fire sprinklers	+	1.80
Subtotal		$154.21
Number of stories multiplier (if applicable)	×	1.00
Subtotal		$154.21
Height per story	×	0.98
Subtotal		$151.13
Floor area perimeter multiplier	×	1.02
Subtotal		$154.15
Local cost multiplier	×	$0.98
Subtotal		$151.07
Current cost multiplier	×	1.0500
Refined cost per square foot		$158.62
Building area (square feet)		48,000
Base building improvement RCN		$7,613,694
Site improvements, total	+	386,306
Total direct construction cost		$8,000,000
Indirect costs not included in manual	+	550,000
Subtotal–direct and indirect costs		$8,550,000
Initital operating deficits - absorption expense	+	1,140,000
Subtotal		$9,690,000
Entrepreneurial Incentive (not profit)	+	484,500
Total cost for the nursing facility improvements		$10,174,500
Allocation of total cost		
Building improvements		$9,683,191
Site Improvements		$491,309

Source: *Marshall Valuation Service*

Case Study—Estimating the Cost of Initial Absorption—Operating Deficits

Table 17.2 shows likely absorption for the subject property if it were new and had to experience initial absorption. The analysis is performed on a quarterly basis. The census grows each quarter as the "new" facility competes for admissions that originate from the market. (An example of absorption using a turnover technique is presented at the end of Chapter 10.) Initially, the census for a new facility will have higher ratios of Medicare and private-pay patients because patients often must spend down their resources to get Medicaid, which takes some time to work into the census. The rates applied for the different payor classes and the other per-diem revenues are the same as those used in the stabilized forecast. The operating expenses represent a mix of fixed and variable expenses. The fixed expenses are equal to the specific total stabilized expense multiplied by the fixed percentage proportion. The variable expense equates to the stabilized per-patient-day expense, multiplied by the total patient days, multiplied by the variable percentage proportion. The operating deficit is the difference between the *EBITDAR* during that quarter and the anticipated stabilized quarterly *EBITDAR*. The total operating deficit has not been discounted to a present value.

The estimated initial operating deficit equates to $1,140,000, which equals 13.3% of the building cost, before developer incentive and profit.

Table 17.2 Operating Deficit During Initial Absorption

	Q1	Q2	Q3	Q4	Stabilized
Patient days					
Private, VA & other	1,000	1,650	2,200	2,800	3,066
Medicare Part A	400	650	850	1,000	1,077
Medicaid	1,200	2,600	3,900	5,000	5,639
Totals	2,600	4,900	6,950	8,800	9,782
Occupancy rate for the quarter	23.7%	44.7%	63.5%	80.4%	89.3%
Occupancy rate at end of quarter	30.0%	54.0%	72.0%	89.3%	
Routine revenues, per patient day					
Private, VA & other	$184.28	$184.28	$184.28	$184.28	$184.28
Medicare Part A	338.82	338.82	338.82	338.82	338.82
Medicaid	147.13	147.13	147.13	147.13	147.13
Ancillary (Medicare Part B and other)	1.75	1.75	1.75	1.75	1.75
Other revenues	0.50	0.50	0.50	0.50	0.50
Bad debt	(0.50)	(0.50)	(0.50)	(0.50)	(0.50)
Routine revenues					
Private, VA & other	$184,285	$304,070	$405,427	$515,998	$565,018
Medicare Part A	135,528	220,234	287,998	338,821	364,825
Medicaid	176,552	382,530	573,795	735,634	829,685
Ancillary (Medicare Part B and other)	4,550	8,575	12,163	15,400	17,119
Other revenues	1,300	2,450	3,475	4,400	4,891
Bad debt	-1,300	-2,450	-3,475	-4,400	-4,891
Total net revenue	$500,916	$915,409	$1,279,382	$1,605,853	$1,776,647
Operating expenses					
Direct care expenses	$383,000	$557,600	$713,200	$853,600	$928,166
Support costs	165,300	207,000	244,100	277,600	295,416
Property cost	38,500	38,500	38,500	38,500	38,542
Administrative, liability insurance and management	132,000	156,500	178,400	198,100	208,552
Provider tax ($800.00/bed)	24,000	24,000	24,000	24,000	24,000
Total operating expenses	$742,800	$983,600	$1,198,200	$1,391,800	$1,494,676
Net operating income or *EBITDAR*	-$241,884	-$68,191	$81,182	$214,053	$281,970
Operating deficit	-$523,855	-$350,162	-$200,788	-$67,917	$0
Total operating deficit, rounded	-$1,140,000				

Expense Assumptions:

- Direct care expenses are 20% fixed and 80% variable (fixed equals $185,633/quarter, variable equals $75.91/PD
- Support cost expenses are 40% fixed ($118,166) and 60% variable ($18.12/PD)
- Property cost are 100% fixed
- Administrative, liability insurance and management are 50% fixed ($104,276) and 50% variable ($10.66/PD)
- Provider tax ($200.00/bed/quarter)

Depreciation

Depreciation is the difference between the cost of an improvement and its contributory value as of the appraisal date. In the purest form, depreciation can be estimated by comparing the costs of comparable assets (buildings) and their sale prices. However, from a practical perspective, this procedure is difficult to apply to nursing facilities since non-real estate assets are involved. Depreciation emanates from one or more of three sources.

- Physical deterioration
- Functional obsolescence
- External obsolescence

Physical Deterioration

Physical deterioration can be curable or incurable. Curable deterioration, which is also called *deferred maintenance*, refers to components in need of repair on the date of the appraisal. This category is measured as the cost of restoring an item to new or reasonably new condition. To be curable, two tests must be satisfied. First, the cost to cure the item should result in a value increment equal to or greater than the expenditure. Second, if the expenditure produces an incremental value that is equal to or less than the cost, but it will preserve the value of the other improvements, then it is generally considered curable.

Incurable physical deterioration reflects items of deterioration that cannot be practically or economically corrected as of the effective date of the appraisal. Incurable items are classified as short-lived and long-lived.

Short-lived building components have useful life expectancies that are less than the remaining useful life of the structure. The deterioration of these components is measured individually. The depreciation is typically measured separately for each item using an age-life ratio. The age used may be the actual or effective age of the item. Professionally prepared property inspection reports are often required by lenders and investors for financing and acquisition transactions. These reports, which identify short-lived items, their age, their expected lives, and replacement costs, may be useful to appraisers.

Because nursing facilities are licensed healthcare centers, they must meet higher standards for maintenance and the replacement of short-lived building components and mechanical systems. A nursing facility will typically receive more wear and tear than most commercial buildings because the buildings are intensely used every hour of every day and do not close at night or on weekends. Moreover, the buildings have higher-than-normal occupancy, often with less than 150 square feet for each occupant, considering patients, staff, and visitors. These extraordinary factors add to the demands placed on the mechanical systems and interior finishes and may shorten the time frame for the replacement of short-lived items.

Some items that will probably require replacement prior to the end of the economic or useful life of the building include:

- Roof cover and insulation
- Interior construction items such as cabinetry, nurses' stations, hand railings, interior wall finishes in high-traffic areas, interior doors and frames, and decorative features
- Plumbing items such as water heaters, sinks, and toilets and some supply and drain piping in high-use areas such as the kitchen, laundry, and tub rooms.
- HVAC items such as in-room PTACs, furnaces, heat-pump units, A/C units, fans, climate controls, and air treatment items
- Electrical components, including lighting fixtures, emergency generators, and life-safety systems
- Exterior items such as various siding materials, windows, and doors
- Site improvements, including parking surfaces, fencing, exterior lighting fixtures, landscaping features, and major components of on-site sewage treatment systems

Long-lived components are expected to have remaining economic lives that are equal to or exceed the remaining economic life of the entire structure. All items not treated as deferred maintenance or short-lived must be treated in the estimate of long-lived depreciation. Similarly, all costs not covered under short-lived items or deferred maintenance are long-lived items. Among the items that are expected to remain valuable throughout the economic and useful life of the building are:

- Foundation
- Structural floor(s)
- Framing
- Exterior and some interior wall systems
- Roof systems
- Certain portions of the mechanical systems (wiring, piping, and ducts)
- Some finishes (exterior siding, windows, partitions, ceilings, and floor coverings)

Functional Obsolescence

Functional obsolescence is a loss in value resulting from defects in design or materials or from changes in standards. The obsolescence can be curable or incurable. Defects are curable if the replacement cost is the same as or less than the anticipated increase in value. Curable functional obsolescence is measured as the cost to correct the condition through addition, substitution, or modernization. In some instances, the obsolescence may be attributable to excessive or overly adequate designs or materials. Chapter 8 identifies a number of items of obsolescence frequently found in nursing facility buildings.

Many facility-specific, cost-based Medicaid reimbursement systems will allow the costs of renovations, replacements, and additions to be covered in the capital reimbursements in some fashion.

External Obsolescence

External obsolescence is a loss in value resulting from forces outside to the property, and it is often incurable. The conditions that cause external obsolescence can be temporary (e.g., a reduction in Medicaid reimbursements to balance a state's budget) or permanent. Permanent conditions would include long-term shortfalls in Medicaid reimbursement caused by tying capital reimbursement to the original cost basis set many years ago at levels that are substantially lower than the current physically depreciated cost.

Methods of Estimating Depreciation

Three methods are used to estimate depreciation.

1. Market extraction method
2. Economic age-life method
3. Breakdown method

The economic age-life method of estimating depreciation is most frequently used in the appraisal of nursing facility improvements since the concepts are easier to apply and understand. Central to all methods of estimating depreciation is the age-life relationship. In theory, an improvement loses value as it ages.

Actual or Effective Age

To set the stage for the calculation of depreciation, the actual or effective age is measured against the total economic or expected life of the improvement. Actual age, often referred to as *chronological age*, is the number of years that have elapsed since the building was constructed or the existing component was installed. Effective age considers the condition and utility of the total structure or the component and requires the appraiser to make judgments and interpret the market. Because levels of maintenance, capital replacement, and functional obsolescence vary, the effective age may be less or greater than the actual age.

Total Economic and Useful Life

Total economic life is the time between when the building is constructed and when it no longer contributes value to the underlying land. The useful life is the expected period of time the improvement will perform the function for which it was designed. The economic life may exceed the useful life since the building may cease to provide utility for the intended original use, but it may be economically feasible to renovate and/or convert the building to a different use. Since nursing facilities are special-use structures, economically feasible alternative uses of the building are limited. The physical life expectancy of a nursing facility should substantially exceed the economic or useful life, as functional and external obsolescence reduce the life expectancy.

For many nursing facilities, the market may not currently recognize some forms of functional and external obsolescence; however, these issues may arise later. As an example, assume that the subject facility and a number of the competitors in the market have a considerable number of three- and four-bed wards. Currently, the market and subject have high occupancy levels, which are attributable to the chronic bed shortage caused by certificate of need or new bed moratorium regulations. The market, especially the Medicaid market, has no alternative but to accept these accommodations. Gradually, as demographic and economic changes occur in the market, or suddenly, when new and or replacement beds enter the competitive mix, the facilities with ward beds will experience the first losses, all else being equal.

The life expectancy of nursing home buildings is affected by many of the same factors that influence most commercial and residential real estate. However, extensive regulatory and government reimbursement policies add a further dimension to the estimation of economic life.

Estimating the economic life of a nursing facility involves considerable judgment. The appraiser must consider population trends, the presence or absences of bed supply regulations in the form of certificates of need or moratoriums for Medicaid certification, and the potential expansion of alternatives to nursing facilities (if Medicaid waivers can be used for assisted living and home health care). Other considerations that can affect economic life include the underlying land value, highest and best use, and the physical and functional quality of the subject's design and construction. In many cases, the economic life of nursing facilities may be extended by bed shortages created by tight certificate of need policies or by inadequate reimbursements for new buildings that undermine the economic feasibility of new construction. Management and financial strength of the ownership can affect the useful life of similar nursing facilities differently.

Remaining Economic Life and Remaining Useful Life

Remaining economic life is the estimated time over which the existing improvements are expected to continue to contribute economically to property value–i.e., make a positive economic contribution to the property.[6] The total economic life minus the effective age will approximate the remaining economic life. Of course, the remaining economic life can be extended through timely and strategic capital replacements and improvements that reduce the effective age.

Market Extraction Depreciation Method

In its simplest form, the market extraction method involves comparing the replacement cost of the improvements to the sale price of the property, less land value. The percentage difference between the value and cost of the improvements is an expression of overall depreciation. That percentage may then be divided by the effective age of the improvements to arrive at an annual rate of overall depreciation. This technique simplifies the possibly complex interplay of physical, functional, and external causes of depreciation. For the extraction method to produce reliable results, the appraiser should analyze several comparable improved sales with buildings of similar age, functional utility, and physical condition. Because nursing facilities are typically sold as going concerns and the sale prices typically include tangible and intangible personal property, the extraction process quickly becomes convoluted.

Table 17.3 illustrates the principles of the extraction technique. The big assumption being made in this example is that the values of the tangible and intangible assets have been clearly identified and supported. This example goes so far as to provide an indication of the total life expectancy of the building.

The market extraction method for estimating building depreciation is most reliable when there are a number of comparable nursing home sales and the estimates of the tangible and intangible personal property assets are well substantiated. The method is limited since intangible asset value can be extremely difficult to segregate. The comparable properties should have similar building qualities and ages and comparable levels of

6. *The Appraisal of Real Estate*, 13th ed. (Chicago: Appraisal Institute, 2008), 415.

Table 17.3 Example of Market Extraction Method of Depreciation

	Sale 1	Sale 2	Sale 3
Sale price	$7,200,000	$9,000,000	$10,800,000
Less land value	500,000	600,000	1,200,000
Less value of tangible personal property	225,000	250,000	400,000
Less value of intangible personal property	1,350,000	1,800,000	1,800,000
Indicated depreciated cost of improvements (value)	$5,125,000	$6,350,000	$7,400,000
Cost of improvements new	$7,650,000	$9,000,000	$11,400,000
Less depreciated cost of improvements	5,125,000	6,350,000	7,400,000
Total depreciation	$2,525,000	$2,650,000	$4,000,000
Total depreciation as a percentage of cost	33.0%	29.4%	35.1%
Effective age of comparable property	15	12	20
Average annual depreciation rate	2.20%	2.45%	1.75%
Total economic life expectancy	100% / 2.20%	100% / 2.45%	100% / 1.75%
	45.5 years	40.8 years	57.0 years

physical, functional, and external obsolescence. Given the complexities of estimating the intangible asset values of comparable sales and the general dearth of comparable data, the market extraction method is difficult to apply to nursing facilities.

Economic Age-Life Depreciation Method

To apply the economic age-life method, the appraiser simply divides the effective age of the facility by the total economic life and multiplies that product by the total cost to arrive at an estimate of depreciation. This technique covers all forms of physical deterioration and functional and external obsolescence. The formula is

$$(\text{Effective Age} / \text{Total Economic Life}) \times \text{Total Cost} = \text{Depreciation}$$

This method has limitations. First, the technique assumes straight-line depreciation, yet there is often evidence that suggests that the rate of depreciation varies over the lifespan of a building. Also, this method does not separately treat the various physical, functional, and external causes of depreciation or differentiate between short- and long-lived items of physical deterioration. To improve on this method, the total cost can be modified to reflect a deduction for immediately curable physical deterioration and functional obsolescence.

Breakdown Depreciation Method

The breakdown method segregates depreciation according to its physical, functional, and external causes and, as such, this method offers more precision. For a comprehensive discussion of this multi-step depreciation procedure, refer to *The Appraisal of Real Estate*, 13th edition, published by the Appraisal

Institute. This method may require the application of several techniques to calculate the different types of depreciation. The techniques include:

- The *cost to cure* physical deterioration (deferred maintenance) and functional obsolescence–usually the depreciation deduction is expressed as a whole dollar amount
- An *economic age-life ratio*, which is used to estimate curable and incurable short-lived and long-lived physical deterioration
- The *capitalized loss in earnings* (*NOI* or *EBITDAR*) caused by the lost revenue or excessive operating expenses stemming from incurable functional obsolescence and external obsolescence
- *Market data analyses* (paired sales, extractions, or other techniques), which reveal and measure functional and external obsolescence
- The *functional obsolescence procedure*, which provides comprehensive treatment of all forms of loss due to functional issues

The breakdown method is a sequential process in which physical deterioration is estimated first, followed by estimation of functional and then external obsolescence. For physical deterioration, deferred maintenance is treated first, then deterioration in short-lived components, and finally deterioration in long-lived components.

A case study is presented in this section to illustrate and tie together the salient principles and techniques applied in the breakdown method.

Procedures for Calculating Physical Deterioration

In the breakdown method, deferred maintenance, or immediately curable physical deterioration, is treated first. Deferred maintenance is estimated as the cost to replace or restore the item(s) to new or reasonably new condition. The cost of deferred maintenance is deducted from the total cost new, and the remainder is then treated for other forms of deterioration.

Short-lived physical deterioration is typically measured for each short-lived component separately. First, the costs of the short-lived items are estimated. Then, the effective age and expected life of each item are developed. From this information, a straight-line, age-life depreciation calculation is made for each item, and the sum of the depreciation amounts represents the estimated incurable, short-lived deterioration.

The estimation of long-lived deterioration is the final step in the calculation. The cost new of the long-lived building components equals the total building cost minus the cost new of the short-lived building components (curable and incurable). Typically, the age-life method is applied to calculate long-lived physical deterioration. First, the ratio or percentage of effective age to the total economic or useful life of the building is calculated. That percentage is multiplied by the cost of the long-lived components to produce the estimate of long-lived deterioration.

Procedure for Calculating Functional Obsolescence

Regardless of the type of functional obsolescence, whether it is curable or incurable, caused by a deficiency or superadequacy, use of the method shown in Table 17.4 ensures that all components of functional obsolescence are treated consistently, without any omission or duplication of costs or deductions.

Table 17.4 **Procedure for Calculating All Forms of Functional Obsolescence**

Step 1	Cost of existing item		$xxx,xxx
Step 2	Less depreciation previously charged	–	xxx,xxx
	plus		
Step 3	Cost to cure (all cost)	+	xxx,xxx
	or		or
	Value of the loss	+	xxx,xxx
Step 4	Less cost if installed new	–	xxx,xxx
Step 5	Equals depreciation from functional obsolescence		$xxx,xxx

Procedure for Calculating External Obsolescence

There are two methods for measuring external obsolescence. The net income loss attributable to the negative influence can be capitalized at an appropriate rate to quantify the amount of obsolescence. The other method is to compare sales of similar properties that are subject to the negative influence with other properties that are not. This comparison indicates the amount of obsolescence.

One major source of external obsolescence for nursing facilities is inadequate Medicaid reimbursement. This inadequacy may apply only to capital reimbursement, or other specific components of the rate or the overall rate may be inadequate. The rate inadequacy may be capitalized into a value loss indication. If a calculation for the rate inadequacy is being applied, the appraiser should consider the potential duration of the condition. It is likely that states will amend their systems from time to time and, as a result, eliminate or shift such inadequacies. Typically, the market will not specifically consider this issue in the development of depreciation, even if the cost approach is actually used as a pricing factor. However, Medicaid reimbursement rates are often inadequate and this causes substantial loss in value.

The breakdown method will be applied to the case study property, using the improvement costs estimated earlier in this chapter.

The subject building has been well maintained and has an actual age of 14 years. Since few building components have been replaced, or needed to be replaced, the effective age is also 14 years. The total economic life is estimated to be 50 years and that estimate is largely based on the expected life tables found in various cost-estimating services, the current stage in the life cycle of the neighborhood, and market expectations.

Physical Deterioration

Curable physical deterioration—deferred maintenance. Many of the PTAC units in the patient rooms are original and will require replacement very soon. In addition, the rooftop A/C units serving the common areas are also original and require immediate replacement The cost for these immediately curable items is $40,000.

Incurable physical deterioration—short-lived Items. The short-lived items that are not ready to be replaced as of the appraisal date, but will probably require replacement prior to the end of the economic or useful life of the building, are listed in Table 17.5 along with their current estimated replacement costs, effective ages, and expected lives.

Table 17.5 Incurable Physical Deterioration—Short-Lived Components

	Cost for Short-Lived Components	Curable Physical	Net Cost Curable Physical	Age	Life	% Depr.	Incurable Depreciation
Roof cover	$125,000	$0	$125,000	14	20	70.0%	$87,500
Interior construction	160,000	0	160,000	14	20	70.0%	112,000
Ceilings	75,000	0	75,000	14	20	70.0%	52,500
Plumbing	72,000	0	72,000	14	20	70.0%	50,400
HVAC	60,000	40,000	20,000	8	12	66.7%	13,333
Electrical	75,000	0	75,000	14	25	56.0%	42,000
Exterior walls and windows	120,000	-	120,000	14	25	56.0%	67,200
Totals	$687,000	$40,000	$647,000			65.7%	$424,933

Note. The replacement cost new (RCN) of the various components only includes the costs for the individual short-lived items and excludes items such as ductwork, interior walls, and partitions. These items will most likely never be replaced, making them long-lived components.

Incurable physical deterioration—long-lived items. The long-lived items include everything not treated as deferred maintenance or short-lived items. The long-lived deterioration is based on an age-life method using the effective age of 14 years. In this case, the economic life and useful life of the building is the same, 50 years. Straight-line depreciation is applied to the long-lived cost. The calculations are shown in Table 17.6.

Functional Obsolescence

From a competitive market perspective, the subject improvements are functional, given their design, age, and condition. From an operational perspective, the building lacks adequate storage space and needs a larger employee break room with a locker area. In this case, the obsolescence is caused by deficiencies that are curable through an addition and substitution. Presently, the building's maintenance department is very cramped

Table 17.6	Incurable Physical Deterioration—Long-Lived Components	
Total cost new of the building		$9,683,191
Cost of curable & incurable short-lived components		– 687,000
Cost of long-lived components		$8,996,191
Effective age	14	
Expected economic or useful life (same)	50	
Depreciation percentage	28.0%	
Long-lived depreciation		$2,518,933

and the area is shared with general storage; neither is very functional and the problems are likely to be exacerbated over time as scavenged parts from replaced mechanical systems and FF&E pile up, along with medical records and other stored items.

The solution is to erect a 3,000-sq.-ft., freestanding, pre-engineered metal building on a rear corner of the site to house the maintenance department, some of the unsightly, loosely stored outdoor items found around the rear of the building, and other less critical materials. The total cost of the new maintenance shop building is $150,000—a cost to cure. The space in the nursing facility vacated by the maintenance shop will be reconfigured into a larger employee break room with a locker area and a separate, secured room for medical records. Note that these improvements will have no discernible impact on Medicaid capital reimbursement for the purposes of this case study problem. One bonus from this expansion and renovation is that the existing employee break room, which is adjacent to the therapy unit, will be reconfigured into a home-like kitchen and dining area for occupational therapy use. The expanded therapy area is not expected to have any measurable immediate benefit in terms of additional census from patients requiring these therapies; however, the new therapy area will allow the facility to remain competitive.

The partition separating the two rooms will be removed and many of the cabinets, plumbing, and appliances in these areas will be used for the occupational therapy program. The cost of the items that will be removed in the maintenance, storage and break room is $50,000. Because the existing items are mostly shorter-lived components, the estimated depreciation that has been previously charged is 50%, or $25,000. The cost for the building renovations (cost to cure), covering approximately 1,000 square feet of floor area, is $70,000. All of the work will be performed by an independent contractor and will be treated as a capital expense. If the building had been originally designed to include the retrofitted space, that cost would have been $40,000 (cost if installed new). Depreciation from functional obsolescence is calculated in Table 17.7.

Table 17.7	Functional Obsolescence Caused by a Deficiency Requiring an Addition and Substitution	
Step 1	Cost of existing item	$50,000
Step 2	Less depreciation previously charged (50%)	– 25,000
	plus	
Step 3	Cost to cure ($150,000 + $70,000)	+ 220,000
	or	
	Value of the loss	0
Step 4	Less cost if installed new	– 40,000
Step 5	Equals depreciation from functional obsolescence	$205,000

Note: This example is presented to illustrate the procedures for calculating functional obsolescence. However, many market participants may not actually recognize or be concerned with obsolescence initially, and only become aware of the problem years after the purchase. The appraiser will need to determine whether market participants will actually recognize and treat the obsolescence in establishing prices.

External Obsolescence

Overall, the subject facility enjoys a favorable competitive location and is able to compete effectively for patients and staff. There are no social, economic, or environmental influences in the area surrounding the subject that are expected to adversely impact its desirability or expected useful life.

As shown in earlier portions of the case study, the subject is expected to be adequately reimbursed for all of the allowable operating expenses associated with delivering services to the Medicaid census. However, based on the current cost to develop the subject, minus all physical and functional depreciation, the interest and depreciation costs substantially exceed the Medicaid capital reimbursement for the building. The difference between the appropriate capital reimbursement amount to satisfy a market rate of return on the physically and functionally depreciated cost of the tangible assets and the actual capital reimbursement amount is capitalized into a value indication (see Table 17.8).

Remember that the total Medicaid capital reimbursement includes interest and depreciation payments for the building, site improvements, and FF&E, based on original, historical costs, and these costs are not trended for inflation. Therefore, only that portion of the reimbursement rate that represents the building is used in this calculation. The reimbursement shortfalls for the site improvements and FF&E should be treated similarly

Table 17.8 **External Obsolescence—Inadequate Medicaid Capital Reimbursement**

Total building cost	$9,683,191
Less physical and function depreciation	
Physical, deferred maintenance	40,000
Physical, short-lived, incurable	424,933
Physical, long-lived, incurable	2,518,933
Functional obsolescence, total	205,000
Total depreciated cost of the building, before external obsolescence	$6,494,324
Combined market-level interest rate and recapture rate (sinking fund factor) for the building	9.0%
Combined market-level interest and recapture for the building	$584,489
Total patient days used in development of Medicaid rate	39,420
Appropriate Medicaid capital reimbursement for the building, at current cost levels	$14.83
Less actual Medicaid capital rate, minus amounts for site improvements and FF&E	– $8.41
Amount of Medicaid capital reimbursement inadequacy	$6.42
Number of annually forecasted Medicaid patients days	22,557
Total annual inadequacy of Medicaid capital reimbursement	$144,753
Capitalized value of the Medicaid capital reimbursement inadequacy (20%)	$723,765

in their respective depreciation calculations. The reimbursement inadequacy is only applied to the forecasted Medicaid patient days. The capitalization rate applied to the inadequate reimbursement is greater than the overall rate and considers the prospects that the capital reimbursement system may eventually be modified or corrected.

Site Improvements

To estimate depreciation in the site improvements, a modified economic age-life method is applied since the site improvements represent a relatively minor portion of the total cost new. The modification is used to account for any deferred maintenance that requires immediate treatment. The calculation of the site improvement depreciation is shown in Table 17.9.

Table 17.9 Depreciation of Site Improvements

Total cost of the site improvements		$491,309
Curable physical depreciation (deferred maintenance)		0
Cost net of curable physical depreciation		$491,309
Weighted average effective age	10	
Average economic life	25	
Depreciation percentage	40.0%	
Total depreciation of the site improvements		$196,524

Summation of the Real Estate Value

The cost approach represents one of the primary techniques for developing an allocation of the going-concern value of a nursing facility and the real estate assets. To arrive at the estimated value of the real estate assets, the land value and the depreciated cost of the building and other improvements must be calculated. Valuing the personal property assets, tangible and intangible, using the cost approach is discussed shortly.

Case Study—Cost Approach
Summation of the Real Estate Assets

The depreciated cost of the subject building and site improvements are added to the land value. For purposes of the case study, the land value is estimated to be $1,000,000. This amount is consistent with the principles of balance and contribution. A valuation of the land has not been presented in this material because this topic is treated extensively in other Appraisal Institute literature. The summation of the real estate assets is shown in Table 17.10.

Table 17.10 Summation of the Real Estate Value

Valuation of the building		
Total building cost	$9,683,191	
Less physical depreciation		
Deferred maintenance	– 40,000	
Short-lived, incurable	– 424,933	
Long-lived, incurable	– 2,518,933	
Physically depreciated building value	$6,699,324	
Less functional obsolescence from all causes	– 205,000	
Less extrenal obsolescence from all causes	– 723,765	
Deprecaited building value		$5,770,559
Valuation of the site improvements		
Total cost of the site improvements	$491,309	
Less depreciation from all causes	– 196,524	
Depreciated site improvements value		294,786
Total improvement value, rounded		$6,070,000
Plus land value		1,000,000
Total real estate value		$7,070,000

Note: Figures are rounded.

Valuation of the Tangible Personal Property—Furniture, Fixtures, and Equipment

Nearly all sale and lease transactions of nursing facilities include the tangible personal property or furniture, fixtures, and equipment (FF&E) in the conveyance of property rights. In fact, most buyers and prospective tenants will make only a cursory inspection and inventory of the FF&E when setting a bid. An inventory may be conducted later as part of the sale or lease process. For accounting and reimbursement purposes, most buyers will simply assume the prior owners' asset basis. In new construction, the total cost of all FF&E is often less than 10% of the total development cost.

USPAP requires the appraiser to analyze the effect on value of such non-real property items.[7] USPAP Standards Rule 1-2e(iii) does not specifically state that personal property must be valued separately, but it should be identified and appropriately treated for the intended use and value definition of the appraisal.[8] Title

7. *Uniform Standards of Professional Appraisal Practice, 2008-2009 Edition*, Appraisal Standards Board, The Appraisal Foundation, Standards Rule 1-4(g), Page U-19.

8. USPAP Standard Rule 1-2e(iii) pertains to the consideration of FF&E. It states "In developing a real property appraisal, an appraiser must identify the characteristics of the property that are relevant to the type and definition of value and intended use of the appraisal, including… (iii) any personal property, trade fixtures, or intangible items that are not real property but are included in the appraisal."

XI of the Financial Institutions Reform, Recovery and Enforcement Act of 1989 (FIRREA) requires that the value of personal property must be separated from the real estate. Condemnation and real estate tax appraisal assignments typically seek the value of the real estate alone.

Through inspection of the property, an interview with the administrator and maintenance director of the facility, and a review of the asset records, the appraiser should be able to gain enough knowledge to determine the quality and quantity of the FF&E. If the building is relatively new, the asset records may provide a solid basis for valuation. For older buildings that have experienced multiple cycles of FF&E replacement, the asset records may be incomplete or too disorganized to be useful.

Generally, the valuation of the equipment is based on replacement cost less depreciation. The replacement cost can be developed in several ways. The appraiser can:

- Review the asset records of the facility and use the actual cost of the equipment, trended for inflation
- Perform an inventory of all the personal property assets and individually estimate the replacement cost (and depreciation) of each (Valuations are typically provided by an equipment appraiser.)
- Review and compare the actual costs for recently developed comparable nursing facilities using information obtained from developers, lenders, investors, operators, CON applications, or Medicaid cost reports
- Survey developers and operators
- Use cost-estimating services

Since the furniture, fixtures, and equipment are an integral part of the nursing facility operation, they are more valuable under continued use than they would be if removed and sold separately. Thus, the value is considered the "contributory value in use," which is consistent with the premise of going-concern value.

The depreciation of FF&E is typically estimated with an age-life method. The cost new and depreciation may be calculated as aggregate amounts or for individual items. If the scope of the appraisal assignment requires a detailed valuation of each item of FF&E, it may be necessary to secure the services of an equipment appraiser and incorporate his or her opinions in the report. In practice, most appraisal assignments will not require itemized equipment details and the appraiser can treat the cost and depreciation of FF&E as a single line item.

Few, if any, sales of recently assembled and intact FF&E are available for comparison purposes. Such sales might reflect a landlord purchasing the FF&E of the tenant at a lease termination or a wholesaling or liquidation of the FF&E of a closed facility. In these cases, the buyer would need to move and transport the items to a new location. These types of sales are probably not indicative of market value. Changes of ownership may include a report on the value or price of the FF&E, but these figures are often allocations that suit a particular accounting need and are not necessarily representative of market value.

Case Study—Valuation of Tangible Personal Property and Total Tangible Assets

The following example illustrates a typical valuation of the FF&E of a nursing facility. In the case of the subject property, the cost is developed from trending the historical total FF&E cost per bed from several newly developed facilities. Based on the comparables, the estimated cost new for the FF&E at the subject is $8,000 per bed, or $960,000. Since the subject facility leases the dishwasher and photocopier and expenses those payments, the replacement costs of those items are deducted from the estimated total cost new; the adjusted cost is $950,000. Nursing facilities will often lease equipment that requires considerable maintenance that cannot be performed by in-house personnel.

Although the subject is only 14 years old, approximately one-third of the equipment items, measured by cost, have been replaced at least once. Management expects to increase the pace of FF&E replacement in the foreseeable future. Most of the original equipment has been fully depreciated. Based on these considerations, and on inspection of the property, the estimated aggregate depreciation is 75%. Therefore, the estimated value of the total FF&E is $240,000, after rounding.

Table 17.11 Summation of the Real Estate & FF&E (Tangible Asset) Values

Depreciated cost of the building	$5,770,559
Depreciated cost of the site improvements	294,786
Total depreciated improvement cost, rounded	$6,070,000
Land value	1,000,000
Total real estate value	$7,070,000
FF&E or tangible personal property valuation	
FF&E cost new	$950,000
Less depreciation from all causes (age-life method)–75%	– 712,500
Depreciated FF&E, or tangible personal property, rounded	$240,000
Total value of the tangible assets (real estate and FF&E)	$7,310,000

Valuation of the Intangible Personal Property

The valuation of the intangible assets of the going concern is treated in Chapter 18. This discussion also covers the treatment of profit and entrepreneurial incentive.

Summary

Separate values for the land, real estate improvements, and tangible personal property are developed in the cost approach. The value of intangible assets can be developed after reconciliation of the final going-concern value and the value of the total assets of the business. The land is typically valued by comparing the sale prices and the relevant elements of comparison of comparable vacant sites to the subject. The valuation of the subject site should be considered as vacant and available for development to its highest and best use.

The improvement value is based on the replacement or reproduction cost of the improvements, less depreciation. Reproduction cost is the cost to construct an exact duplicate or replica, which includes existing obsolescence. Replacement cost is the cost to construct a substitute using current materials, standards, design, and layout, which may eliminate some existing obsolescence. Construction costs can be obtained from published sources, actual construction contracts, cost estimators, and costs for comparable buildings as reported by various services and through certificate of need approvals, cost reports, or local government permit applications. Cost may be developed on a per-square-foot or a per-bed basis. Cost estimates may be based on a total per-unit basis (comparative unit), on the costs of individual building components (unit-in-place), or on costs separated by construction trade (quantity survey).The cost should include all reasonable hard and soft costs. In addition to the soft costs normally incurred in the development of commercial real estate, a nursing facility may include the costs of obtaining a CON, operating deficits during the initial absorption, and pre-opening marketing and recruiting expenses. Entrepreneurial incentives and profit should also be considered in the cost estimate.

Depreciation is the difference between the cost of the improvement and its contributory value as of the appraisal date. Depreciation emanates from physical deterioration, functional obsolescence, and/or external obsolescence. On the most basic level, depreciation can be estimated by comparing the cost of comparable assets (buildings) and their sale prices. However, from a practical perspective, this exercise is difficult to apply to nursing facilities since non-real estate assets are involved. The most commonly applied depreciation techniques have been explored in this chapter including the extraction of depreciation from market data, the application of age-life methods, and the breakdown method, which treats physical, functional, and external obsolescence separately.

Tangible personal property, or furniture, fixtures and equipment, value is also developed by estimating replacement cost and depreciation. The valuation of intangible assets is addressed in Chapter 18, where several techniques are presented.

The cost approach can be very useful in determining the feasibility of a proposed nursing facility. The approach can be used in allocating the total assets of the business to real estate, tangible personal property, and intangible personal property assets under the theory that the value of an asset cannot exceed the cost to replace it in a timely manner, less reasonable amounts of depreciation.

Chapter 18

Reconciliation of Value Indications and Allocation of Going-Concern Value

Reconciliation

Typically, the appraisal of a nursing facility will involve the application of more than one approach, and the valuation indications developed from the approaches applied often differ. Resolving the differences in the value indications is known as *reconciliation*. Several values may be indicated by application of the income capitalization and sales comparison approaches. In the income approach, use of direct capitalization and discounted cash flow analysis will produce different value indications. Similarly, an appraiser using the sales comparison approach may apply several different types of analyses and techniques to the same or different groups of sale data and units of comparison. While the various methods applied produce different results that may be resolved to arrive at a conclusion to the particular approach, at least one value from each approach utilized is carried through to the final reconciliation.

The reconciliation process allows the appraiser to assess and compare the relevancy of each approach, given the quality and quantity of the data analyzed and the accuracy and appropriateness of the data and methods applied. Most appraisals set forth a single point value estimate. That amount is regarded as the most probable figure, not the only possible figure. Some clients may seek a value between a certain high and low amount or a probability range. It is highly unusual for the final value conclusion to lie outside the value spread indicated by the applied approaches.

The reconciliation process should include a quality-control assessment to determine that the data and conclusions drawn from one portion of the appraisal are applied consistently throughout. For instance, the effective age estimated for the property should be consistently applied in the development of depreciation, sale price adjustments, and the capitalization rate. Another example of consistency may pertain to the Medicaid capital rate that is used in the development of the income, as a factor of external obsolescence, and as an element of comparison in the sales comparison approach. Any inconsistencies should be corrected or noted and considered in the reconciliation process.

Generally, income capitalization is considered the most important valuation approach as most nursing facilities are controlled by for-profit ownerships seeking competitive investment returns. Since most nursing facilities are encumbered with debt, the lenders are not only interested in knowing loan-to-value ratios; the mortgages and bonds are also evaluated based on debt service coverage ratios. When the various components and critical parts of the income approach are developed with well-verified, comprehensive data and well-reasoned analysis, the income approach may warrant substantial weight in reaching a value conclusion. The credibility of the income approach is lessened when there is considerable variation in *EBITDAR* or *NOI* between the trailing periods and the forecast, even though the forecast may prove accurate in time. A well-researched competitive market analysis that establishes occupancy and payor mix levels and reflects a thorough understanding and analysis of Medicare, Medicaid, and market levels of private-pay revenue may be undermined if the operating expenses and capitalization conclusions are developed from limited comparable market data. However, if all four cylinders of the income approach (census, rates, operating expenses, and capitalization rates) are well-tuned to the market, this approach may easily possess the greatest strength.

The sales comparison approach is often used as a general guide to set valuation parameters for market participants. The fine tuning is often conducted in the income capitalization approach. The sales comparison approach is most meaningful when there are a number of recent comparable sales available for comparison and price adjustments are kept to a minimum. In the appraisal of nursing facilities, the number of sale comparables may be few and those sales that are available often require considerable adjustment for differences in the locational, physical, and economic elements of comparison. Even with well-supported adjustments, confidence in the sales comparison approach declines as the size of the price adjustments increases.

The cost approach is generally the least regarded approach because the economic actions of the market are not measured well using this approach, and the value of intangible assets may not be considered. Should the value conclusion developed in the cost approach exceed the value indications from the other approaches, it is likely that the full amount of external obsolescence has not been considered, or the improvements may not be the highest and best use of the property. The cost approach is generally considered more reliable when the improvements are newer and do not suffer much depreciation. As the next section will show, the cost approach is important to the allocation of the going-concern value.

Case Study—Reconciliation of the Final Value

The reconciliation process begins with the value indications developed for the subject property in previous case study applications. The values are:

Income capitalization approach	$9,325,000
Sales comparison approach	$9,600,000
Cost approach	$7,310,000

The cost approach is afforded no weight in the conclusion of the going-concern value since this approach has not considered intangible values. If the cost approach is representative of the tangible assets, then considerable value is attributable to the intangible assets.

The sales comparison approach was developed by analyzing three sales. Sale 1 sold for $40,000 per bed and required substantial upward adjustments. The concluded value was twice the sale price and, even though the adjustments are well-reasoned and well-supported, the approach is weakened somewhat by the substantial adjustments. Sale 2 sold for $72,000 per bed and, based on the limited amount of adjustment, it is fairly comparable to the subject. Sale 3 is a superior property and sold for $100,000 per bed; it required several downward adjustments, but the adjusted price is well-supported and the value indication is meaningful. The conclusion of the sales comparison approach supports the income capitalization approach, and both approaches were developed fairly independently from one another.

The income capitalization approach is generally the preferred approach since most buyers in the market are for-profit entities seeking to profit from operating nursing facilities. In the case study applications, the census, revenues, operating expenses, and capitalization rate conclusions were all developed from extensive, well-confirmed data. This allowed for efficient and comprehensive analysis and resulted in a meaningful value indication. The direct capitalization approach is given greater weight than the DCF analysis. In this case, the value indication from the DCF analysis is less than the value estimated by direct capitalization and the value indications from the sales comparison approach.

In the final analysis, the sales comparison and income capitalization approaches are well- researched and considerable analysis was performed in both approaches. Slightly more weight is placed on the income capitalization approach because this approach more closely reflects the economic motivations of the market.

Concluded value of the going concern: $9,450,000

Allocation of the Going-Concern Value

Most appraisal assignments will require the appraiser to perform an allocation of the concluded value of the going concern or the total assets of the business between the real estate and the personal property. While not specifically required under USPAP, Title XI of FIRREA requires an allocation. Appraisals for property tax assessment certainly require the separation of the real estate value. There are other instances in which an allocation is necessary.

The assets in the going-concern value of a nursing facility include:

- Real estate–fee simple, leased fee, or leasehold
- Tangible personal property–furniture, fixtures, and equipment
- Intangible personal property–including the assembled work force, licenses, certifications, approvals (certificates of need, or CON), patient records, goodwill, and management

The methods for allocating the going concern of a health care facility seem to be a subject of on-going debate. Generally, appraisers will apply a top-down approach to allocation, whereby the going-concern value is developed first. Developing a total value can be well supported by direct market evidence–i.e., sale comparables and the capitalization of unallocated *NOI* or *EBITDAR*; however, sales of just the real estate or just the business assets, without the real estate, occur less frequently. Buyers and sellers of nursing facilities do not contemplate the going-concern value by adding the value of the real estate to the separate values of the tangible and intangible personal property; they focus on the overall value.

The bottom-up approach essentially implies that the value of the intangible assets, FF&E, and real estate can be developed in some independent manner and then added together to arrive at the total value of the business or going concern. The difficulty with this approach is that there is little market evidence to support the value of any single asset component. Moreover, the value of the whole may be different from the sum of the individual values. The concept of highest and best use demands that the assets be evaluated at their most profitable, sustainable level.

HUD has wrestled with this problem in administering the Multifamily Accelerated Processing (MAP) program, which insures mortgages on existing and proposed nursing and assisted living facilities. Under the MAP program, HUD may only insure loans backed by real estate and tangible personal property (e.g., major movable equipment). The MAP appraisal guidelines require the appraiser to develop an opinion of the going-concern value first, and then determine the value of the real estate as a subset.[1]

The allocation of value is critical in ad valorem tax assessment and condemnation assignments. Most jurisdictions prohibit the inclusion of non-realty assets for real estate taxes and in condemnation actions. On rare occasions, a real-estate-only value may be required to satisfy the terms of a purchase option during or at the termination of a lease or a long-term management agreement. In real estate tax assessment appeals, taxpayers often try to minimize taxes on viable nursing facilities by making an erroneous argument that the real estate should be evaluated without the positive contribution of the intangible assets.

There is no single, correct approach for performing an allocation of the going-concern value of a nursing facility. Several techniques are available and, when the allocation is a critical component of the appraisal, using several techniques, just like using more than one valuation approach, will produce a more convincing allocation.

Cost Approach

When the depreciated cost of the tangible assets and the land are less than the overall business enterprise value, the cost approach can be a proxy for real estate value. After all, the old adage that the cost approach sets the upper limit of value does have some truth. This is a top-down, residual technique that begins with the best known and supported values and works back to the unknown.

Under most circumstances, a profitable nursing or senior housing facility will have value greater than the depreciated replacement cost of the tangible assets, suggesting that there is intangible value. However, there are cases in which the going-concern value, meeting the definition of highest and best use, will be less than the land value plus the physically and functionally depreciated cost of the improvements and FF&E. In these cases, the difference between the concluded going-concern value and the depreciated cost represent a portion of the yet-to-be determined external obsolescence. In cases in which the going-concern value is less than the tangible asset value, prior to full treatment of external obsolescence, the appraiser will need to revise the estimated obsolescence downward enough so that the final concluded cost approach

1. *Multifamily Accelerated Processing Guide*, Revised March 15, 2002, Office of the Assistant Secretary for Housing, FHA Commissioner, Chapter 7, page 22. "The appraiser must first identify the overall 'Business Value' a.k.a. 'Going Concern Value' prior to establishing a proprietary income adjustment and 'Real Estate Only' value."

value is equal to, or less than, the going-concern value. Then the question remains, will the external obsolescence be great enough so that there is still some positive difference between the going-concern value and the fully depreciated cost, which could be considered intangible value?

Entrepreneurial or Proprietary Profit Capitalization

Some appraisers consider deducting an entrepreneurial profit from the *NOI* or *EBITDAR* and capitalizing that portion to arrive at an indication of the intangible value. Other techniques frequently relied on in the allocation process include some method of striping or parsing off a piece of the gross revenue or *NOI* to satisfy the intangible component.

FHA-insured mortgages, offered through the Multifamily Accelerated Processing (MAP) program at HUD, have been the largest single source of financing for skilled nursing and assisted living facilities in the past decade. The MAP program is value-based and limits loan amounts for existing facilities to no more than 85% of the market value of the real estate and major movable equipment. MAP appraisal guidelines require that a minimum of 15% of the net operating income be excluded from the valuation of the tangible property through a "proprietary earnings" deduction. That 15+% represents a return to the intangible assets.

The allocated *NOI* or *EBITDAR* to the intangible assets may be capitalized into an indication of the intangible asset value. The capitalization rate for the intangibles can be developed by residual techniques, using sales of nursing facilities; deduced from sales of nursing facility leasehold interests; or based on capitalization rates developed from sales of health care service providers such as therapy and pharmacy companies, which have no real estate assets when operated out of leased property. Normally, capitalization rates for health care service companies are greater than overall capitalization rates for nursing facilities, reflecting their perceived additional risks. While commercial real estate capitalization rates often fall below 10.0%, capitalization rates for therapy, home health care, and pharmacy companies frequently exceed 20%. Business brokers and trade journals can be sources of comparable data on "business" capitalization rates. A capitalization rate for intangible assets can be calculated as follows:

Overall rate		12.5%
Less real estate & FF&E capitalization rate	10.0%	
Real estate portion of overall value	75.0%	
Deduct the real estate component of the overall rate (10% × 75%)		– 7.5%
Portion of overall rate relating to intangible personal property		5.0%
Indicated overall capitalization rate for intangible assets (5.0% / 25%)		20.0%

An example of an allocation technique using the HUD "proprietary earnings" deduction is shown below.

Net operating income		$1,000,000
Proprietary earnings	15.0%	150,000
Capitalized proprietary earnings ($150,000 / 20.0%)		$750,000
Overall going-concern value ($1,000,000 / 12.5%)		$8,000,000
Less intangible value	–	750,000
Less FF&E tangible personal property–via depreciated cost)	–	250,000
Indicated real estate value		$7,000,000

Lease Income Versus Operational Earnings

Some market participants make the argument that long-term, absolute net leases are based largely on real estate value and, therefore, recently leased properties with rents and other conditions set at market levels are proxies for real estate value. Conversely, the difference between the business *EBITDAR* and market rent represents the market return to the tenant or proprietary position. The tenant's capitalized anticipated earnings from a recently set, market rate lease represents intangible value rather than leasehold value in the real estate. This argument assumes that if market rent and contract rent are the same, then the tenant has no leasehold value in the real estate. Therefore, the capitalized value of the tenant's earnings is intangible value. Additional intangible value may be attributable to the landlord's interest since the landlord possesses many of the intangible assets prior to the commencement and after the termination of the lease, and the value of these assets are built into the rent payments. As a result, the capitalized value of the tenant's earnings in a market-rate lease represents a minimal value for the intangible assets–the tenant's portion, not the landlord's portion.

Historically, absolute-net, skilled nursing facility market rents have typically ranged from 70% to 85% of *EBITDAR*. This does not mean that rents set at percentages outside this range are not market rent. Thus, 15% to 30% of *EBITDAR* is available for the operator or tenant. The appraiser can research lease data in much the same way improved sales are researched to confirm this. Obtaining market capitalization rates for the tenant's interest from comparable sales is problematic. Sales of leasehold interests in nursing facilities occur from time to time, but the price may include value attributable to 1) a real estate leasehold interest–where contract rent is less than market rent and 2) the value of the "tenant's profit" or difference between market rent and *EBITDAR*. The appraiser must realize that any capitalization rate developed from leasehold sales may include both and the indicated rate may be indicative of both interests. The appraiser may also rely on capitalization rates derived from sales of allied businesses such as outpatient therapy companies, pharmacies, and nursing home management companies. Because the purchase of leasehold interests or nursing facility management companies are difficult to finance, greater use of equity is required and market equity rates typically achieve a substantial premium over mortgage rates.

The following formula and example illustrates the concepts just discussed.

$$V_I = (EBITDAR \times (1 - (1 / ErRR)))/R_I$$

Where:

EBITDAR = Earnings before interest, taxes, depreciation, amortization, and rent

EtRR = Market EBITDAR-to-rent ratio

R_I = Overall capitalization for the intangible interest

V_I = Intangible value

EBITDAR		$1,000,000
Market EBITDAR-to-rent ratio (*EtRR*)	1.25	
Market rent ($1,000,000 divided by 1.25)		– 800,000
Tenant "profit"		$200,000
Capitalized value of tenant's interest (16.67%)		$1,200,000

Start-up and Operating Deficits Prior to Stabilization and CON and License Value Segregated from the Going-Concern Value

In some states, it is possible to segregate the value of the license or certificate of need since these rights may be sold and transferred to a different location. There is evidence that much of the intangible value can accrue to the certificate of need in some states. Ohio allows bed licenses to be transferred to other facilities within the same county, and an active market exists for the purchase and sale of licenses in some of the state's more populated counties. Missouri has a similar policy, and even allows beds to be moved into adjacent counties, with some distance restrictions. In these states, the licenses often command prices in excess of $5,000 per bed; there have been instances in Ohio where beds have sold for more than $20,000. Where there is an active and legal market for the sale of licenses (or CONs), it is possible to identify this value and include that figure in the intangible value.

Some argue that the value of the license or the CON is a component of the land or real estate value since the license is property-specific and represents another type of zoning or use permit. If including the value of the CON with the real estate, or treating it as a non-realty asset, becomes a critical aspect of an appraisal assignment, resolving the issue may require a judicial opinion. The appraiser needs to exercise caution and use extraordinary assumptions when valuing the CON as part of the real estate rights.

In addition, a portion of the start-up cost, or the operating deficits that occur prior to opening and through stabilization, may be considered part of the intangible value. The difficulty with this approach is that there is little market evidence to support the value of licenses in most states. Moreover, the operating deficits are speculative and other intangible assets are not included.

Medicaid Implied Rental/Value

The tangible asset value could be tied to the allowable property cost basis of the facility recognized in the Medicaid reimbursement rules of the particular state. Any profit derived from a facility-specific, cost-based reimbursement system beyond the capital reimbursement is achieved through cost-savings incentives, or it is simply a single-occurrence profit that will vanish after the next cost re-basing. For facilities with very high proportions of Medicaid, the only sustainable EBITDAR or NOI may be achieved through the capital reimbursement. In these cases, an argument can be made that the allowable capital cost basis, or the capitalized value of the Medicaid capital reimbursement, is tantamount to the value of the tangible assets. This technique is less reliable as the Medicaid mix is reduced. The following example illustrates the Medicaid capital approach.

Medicaid capital rate	$10.00
Occupied days per bed, per year	330
Annual total Medicaid capital reimbursement	$3,300
Medicaid capital reimbursement capitalization rate	10.0%
Indicated tangible asset value per Medicaid bed	$33,000

This approach is most effective when the census is primarily Medicaid, the private-pay rate approximates the Medicaid rate, there is little or no Medicare or private insurance census, and the operating expenses and the reimbursement for all other expenses are nearly equal. The value could be broken down further, according to the reimbursement amounts for the real estate and the tangible personal property assets.

Under most Medicaid reimbursement systems, the capital payment is based on a historical cost and does not reflect current market costs and values. Essentially, the capital rate is legislated and the payment is analogous to rent-controlled housing.

Using Sales of Similarly Constructed Real Estate as a Proxy for SNF Realty Value

Residential and medical office buildings often have similar location and construction qualities as nursing facilities. Some appraisers will use such sales to demonstrate the value of the real estate of a nursing facility. Comparing the per-square-foot prices of buildings in similar locations with comparable building ages and construction qualities to the subject can set a general parameter for real estate value. In addition to the adjustment process and elements of comparison discussed in Chapter 17, adjustments may be applied to the "real estate comparable" sales to reflect differences in construction and other costs. This technique can be used to indicate real estate value if appropriate adjustments are applied for differences in the characteristics of the real estate and if the highest and best use of the subject and the sales represent the original, intended uses. The application of this technique should be subordinate to the techniques discussed earlier. This approach is not recommended when the value of the going-concern or total assets of the business appears to be less than the real estate value indicated by "proxy" or similarly constructed property sales.

Summary of Allocation Techniques

Most appraisal assignments require that the appraiser provide a separately stated value for the real estate or an allocation of the total assets of the business or going concern to the real estate, the tangible personal property, and the intangible property assets. There are no standard techniques generally applied for the allocation, and the various approaches described here are only a sampling of a number of common techniques that are used by appraisers. Market participants are generally less concerned about the allocation of the assets of the nursing facility than the total value. The cost approach is often considered the best approach for developing the real estate value when the going-concern value exceeds the fully treated depreciated cost of the tangible assets plus the land value. Generally, the cost approach is more effective when the improvements are newer and suffer from little or no functional or external obsolescence.

The capitalization of entrepreneurial or proprietary profit is commonly used when the cost approach is believed to be less reliable and when the appraisal assignment involves an FHA-insured mortgage through HUD's Multifamily Accelerated Processing program. This technique can be applied without the development of a cost approach analysis, and it can be presented simplistically. However, the technique is difficult to apply since segregating and parsing the income between tangibles and intangibles is problematic and capitalization rates must be deduced from various data, because sales of stand-alone proprietary interests seldom occur.

Recent, absolute net leases and *EBITDAR*-to-rent coverage ratios can provide the basis for developing a value for the real estate or the intangibles. The allocation assumes that a substantial portion of the rent is attributable to the real estate and tangible personal property assets and that a substantial portion of the tenant's *EBITDA* is associated with the intangible assets. The value of the leased fee interest, while largely tangible, may also include the value of the licenses, certifications, and other intangible assets, which may effectively be leased as well and returned to the landlord when the lease expires or terminates. Therefore, this technique may not fully distinguish the value of the intangible assets.

The Medicaid capital cost basis or the capitalized value of the Medicaid capital reimbursement can represent the tangible asset value when a facility has a census that is nearly all Medicaid and all of the operating expenses are being covered, dollar-for-dollar, under a facility-specific, cost-based reimbursement system. The usefulness of this technique quickly disintegrates when increasing proportions of non-Medicaid census are introduced, or the reimbursements for the operating expenses fail to cover the actual expenses over the long run.

Sales of similarly constructed real estate in similar locations may reflect real estate-only value in limited situations. However, the highest and best use of the subject and sale buildings should match their initial intended uses and designs. This approach fails to measure any effects caused by different levels of demand for the various property types.

Developing an opinion of the market value of the going concern or total assets of the business often involves the application of two or three valuation methods. Similarly, the allocation process can certainly employ multiple techniques. The importance of using multiple techniques becomes more critical if the primary purpose of the appraisal is to develop an opinion of just the real estate value.

Case Study—Allocation of Value

Using the data from the ongoing case study, the various allocation techniques are demonstrated.

Allocation Based on Cost Approach

Going concern value	$9,450,000
Less depreciated cost of the improvement and land value	– 7,070,000
Less depreciated cost of the tangible personal property (FF&E)	– 240,000
Indicated value of the intangible assets	$2,140,000

Allocation Based on Capitalized Value of the Proprietary Earnings

Net operating income	$1,127,881
Proprietary earnings (22.5%)	$253,773
Proprietary earnings capitalization rate	20.0%
Indicated value of the intangible assets (rounded)	$1,270,000
Overall going-concern value	$9,450,000
Less intangible value	– 1,270,000
Less FF&E tangible personal property (depreciated cost)	– 240,000
Indicated real estate value	$7,940,000

Lease Income Versus Operational Earnings

EBITDAR or *NOI*	$1,127,881
Market *EBITDAR*-to-rent ratio	1.30
Market rent	– $867,601
Tenant "profit"	260,280
Capitalized value of tenant's interest (20.0%), rounded	$1,300,000
Overall going-concern value	$9,450,000
Less intangible value	– 1,300,000
Less FF&E tangible personal property (depreciated cost)	– 240,000
Indicated real estate value	$7,910,000

Start-up and Operating Deficits Prior to Stabilization and CON and License Value from the Going-Concern Value

Value of identifiable intangible assets:	
Value of the CON ($10,000 per bed)	$1,200,000
25% of initial operating deficits and stabilization cost	285,000
Indicated value of the intangible assets	$1,485,000
Overall going-concern value	$9,450,000
Less intangible value	– 1,485,000
Less FF&E tangible personal property–via depreciated cost	– 240,000
Indicated real estate value	$7,725,000

Medicaid Implied Value

Because the subject has more than 40% non-Medicaid census, this technique is not applicable.

Sales of Similarly Constructed Real Estate as a Proxy for SNF Realty Value

Sale	1	2	3	4
Property type	Apartment	Apartment	Medical office	Medical office
Adjusted sale price*	$10,000,000	$9,000,000	$12,000,000	$7,500,000
Less land value	– 1,250,000	– 1,000,000	– 2,000,000	– 1,250,000
Improvement value	$8,750,000	$8,000,000	$10,000,000	$6,250,000
Building area	102,500	95,800	72,000	48,000
Price per square foot, building only	$85.37	$83.51	$138.89	$130.21
Sales - direct cost new per square foot	$110.00	$110.00	$165.00	$165.00
Subject direct cost per square foot	$166.67	$166.67	$166.67	$166.67
Cost differential	151.52%	151.52%	101.01%	101.01%
Cost-differential adjusted price	$129.34	$126.53	$140.29	$131.52
Concluded building value, per square foot				$130.00
Building area				48,000
Indicated improvement value				$6,240,000
Plus land value				1,000,000
Total real estate value				$7,240,000
Tangible personal property (FF&E) value				240,000
Intangible asset value				1,970,000
Going concern or total value of the business				$9,450,000

* The sale prices have been adjusted for all elements of comparison except for the physical and economic qualities that may be reflected in cost differentials. None of the sale improvements suffer from any significant obsolescence. Their locations are similar to the subject and any differences in value because of location are considered in the land value.

Summary of the Allocations Using the Various Techniques

	Real Estate	FF&E	Intangibles	Total Assets
Cost approach	$7,070,000	$240,000	$2,140,000	$9,450,000
Entrepreneurial profit capitalization	7,940,000	240,000	1,270,000	9,450,000
Lease versus EBITDAR	7,910,000	240,000	1,300,000	9,450,000
License value and operating deficits	7,725,000	240,000	1,485,000	9,450,000
Proxy real estate sale comparison	7,240,000	240,000	1,970,000	9,450,000
Averages	$7,577,000	$240,000	$1,633,000	$9,450,000

A reconciliation of the various allocation techniques will consider the strengths and weaknesses of each technique applied and a single, final allocation will be concluded.

Summary

Reconciliation of the differences in the value indications involves assessing the quality, quantity, and accuracy of the data and the appropriateness of each approach. Generally, the income capitalization approach is favored over the sales comparison approach, and the cost approach is least indicative of the market value of a nursing facility.

The cost approach does not consider the value of the intangible assets or that value is developed through relative abstractions that cannot be measured through analysis of market evidence. Simply put, participants in the nursing facility market give little emphasis to the cost approach and do not generally contemplate the value of the assets separately.

The sales comparison approach is most applicable when several comparable sales that required few or minor price adjustments are analyzed and the adjusted prices are within a tight range. The absence of recent sales that reasonably match the physical, locational, and economic characteristics of the subject nursing facility reduces the reliability of the value indication.

The income capitalization approach is typically favored when the revenue and operating expense forecasts are supported by the historical results of the subject property and by well-documented results from comparable facilities. Analyzing facilities that have experienced a history of irregular earnings or will face the prospects of census, reimbursement, and operating instability reduces the effectiveness of the income capitalization approach. The reconciliation considers the quality of the data used to develop the capitalization rate and the internal rate of return or discount rates, and the degree of consistency between the subject and the comparables in the development of earnings estimates and risk assessments. The final value conclusion must be reasonable in light of all the approaches applied.

Most nursing facility appraisal assignments will require an opinion of the market value of the going concern (total assets of the business) or the value of only the real estate. The real-estate-only value is generally sought in property tax assessment engagements or to satisfy a specific need defined in a contract. Most sale transactions and appraisal engagements are concerned with the value of the going concern.

The methods for allocating the going concern value are the subject of on-going debate. Generally, appraisers will apply a top-down approach to allocation, whereby the going-concern value is developed first and then an allocation is made between the real estate and the tangible and intangible personal property assets. The allocation process should start with the "best" known value(s). This chapter has explored several allocation techniques, including

- Use of the cost approach
- Capitalization of entrepreneurial or proprietary profits
- Use of ratios of market rent to operational earnings
- The cost of obtaining initial operating stability plus the value of the license or certificate of need
- Implied value from Medicaid capital reimbursements
- The proxy value of pure real estate asset sales such as office or apartment properties that have locations and building qualities similar to the subject.

Other allocation techniques should not be ruled out. The key to using an allocation method is its reasonableness.

Chapter 19

Valuation of Partial Interests

Partial interests are estates in real property that represent less than the whole, or fee simple, interest. Typically, appraisers will encounter partial interest assignments involving leased fee and leasehold estates. The leased fee interest belongs to the landlord while the leasehold interest belongs to the tenant.

Most nursing facility leases involve absolute net terms and extend from five to more than 20 years. Typically, the entire facility is leased to a single tenant. In fact, many leases will involve multiple properties, with a single master lease covering them all. In exchange for rent, a typical lease conveys the rights of use and occupancy of the real estate, equipment, certificate of need, and other permits and governmental approvals from the applicable licensing and certification agencies regarding the ownership and operations of the facility. The assembled work force and responsibilities for providing care to the patients are typically conveyed through a transfer operating agreement. Together, the agreements comprise many of the assets associated with the business or going concern. Upon termination, most leases require the cooperation of the terminating tenant in conveying licenses, certifications, work forces, patient records, and other operational assets and obligations to a succeeding operator. Occasionally, the tenant may bring the certification of need to a real estate developer and offer to lease a building (and FF&E) for a particular term that allows the real estate investors to recapture their investment and receive a market rate of return, while the tenant continues to own the certificate of need. At the termination of the lease, the tenant could vacate the property, take the certificate of need elsewhere, and leave the real estate investors with an unlicensed property.

Some leases are vague as to which party controls the rights to these intangible assets at lease termination or when the tenant wants to exercise a purchase option. Legal and valuation disputes often arise from confusing nursing facility leases and operating contracts. Leased fee and leasehold valuations can be adversely affected if the lease is vague on critical issues such as the ownership of intangible assets at the termination of the lease or purchase option.

The typical nursing facility lease is absolute net, meaning the tenant is responsible for all operating expenses and capital replacement. Also, the tenant is typically required to carry a fairly significant amount of general and professional liability insurance. The tenant must maintain all licenses and certifications during the lease term. Most contemporary leases will require the tenant to provide the landlord with financial and operating statements regularly. Moreover, many leases require minimum *EBITDAR*-to-rent-coverage ratios and may provide specific definitions for revenue and expense items.

For conventional real estate, the values of the leased fee and leasehold interests are typically subsets of the fee simple value. While this is not necessarily true in all cases, the sum of the leased fee and leasehold values often approximates the hypothetical fee simple value of the property.

Nursing facility leases are often created between related parties for various business reasons and, while the terms and rents identified in related-party leases may be consistent with the market, the valuation of one or both partial interests may be a moot point. In these cases, lenders may require the leasehold interest to be subordinated to a mortgage. The appraiser should seek direction from the client regarding the property interest to be evaluated and determine if a hypothetical condition is necessary to appraise an interest that in fact does not exist, i.e. a fee simple interest when a long-term lease is in place.

Leased Fee Valuation

The income approach is usually applied in the valuation of a leased fee interest. Direct capitalization and discounted cash flow analysis techniques are typically applied. Both techniques measure the anticipated rent over the expected term of the lease, plus the residual value of the property at lease termination. The direct capitalization approach will typically be applied to capitalize the current rent using an overall capitalization rate derived from market evidence. In discounted cash flow analysis, the expected rents over the anticipated term of the lease, or the holding period, and the value of the property at the termination of the lease or holding period are discounted to present value using a market-derived discount or yield rate.

When either technique is applied, the quality and durability of the rental income is paramount. Comparing the estimated net operating income or *EBITDAR* to contract rent provides insight into the potential duration of the lease, the ability of the lessee to pay rent (and thus the risk to the leased fee position), and the residual value.

Rental rates for newly constructed nursing facilities are typically based on a rate of return for the development costs. These development costs may exclude the cost of assets that the tenant brings to the property and operating deficits during the initial absorption. Rents for existing nursing facilities are often based on a formula of *EBITDAR* to rent. Some leases specifically spell out this formula when rents are to be reset to market rent during the term or an extension of the lease. Typical market levels of *EBITDAR*-to-rent produce coverage ratios ranging from 1.15:1 to 1.40:1. As the lease term goes on, the coverage ratios often change because annual rental increases and earnings change at varying rates. A portion of the *EBITDAR* is saved for the tenant as an economic incentive for the operational risks. The tenant may also achieve profits and other benefits through a management fee.

An *EBITDAR*-to-rent coverage ratio that equals or exceeds initial market ratios provides the landlord with greater certainty that the tenant will perform under the terms of the lease because the tenant has sufficient economic incentive to comply with the lease. If the *EBITDAR* is less than market, then there is a greater risk that the tenant will not adhere to the terms of the lease. The selection of the leased fee capitalization rate and internal rate of return places substantial emphasis on the *EBITDAR*-to-rent coverage ratios during the anticipated lease term. Other factors influencing the rate selection include property and competitive market qualities, guarantees, and the creditworthiness of the lessee.

Most nursing facility leases extend over many years to allow the tenants time to establish a business and recover their investments in personal property assets, including FF&E, working capital, the assembled work force, and management skill. Most leases will grant one or more multiple-year lease extensions or renewal options, provided all terms and conditions are being met to the satisfaction of the landlord. Typically, rents are increased using some type of formula that considers a common price index, an *EBITDAR*-to-rent formula, or an adjustment based on market rent.[1] Leases often include a definition of

1. Market rent, as defined by *The Dictionary of Real Estate Appraisal*, 4th ed., is " the rental income that a property would most probably command in the open market; indicated by current rents paid and asked for comparable space as of the date of the appraisal."

market value for rental resets, and the appraiser is obligated to follow the definition in the lease contract when engaged by a party to the lease for the rent determination. The estimated *EBITDAR*-to-rent coverage ratio at the time of a renewal is very useful in determining the probability that the tenant will renew or extend the lease. Note that if the tenant does not find the lease profitable, the tenant has little incentive to make capital investments in the building beyond the minimum during the waning years of the lease. In this case, the landlord is likely to face the prospect of finding a new tenant and making substantial capital improvements to the facility for the next operator.

Market rent is typically estimated using income and rent comparison techniques, processes very similar to those applied in the income capitalization and sales comparison approaches. Using the income approach, the net operating income or *EBITDAR* is converted into market rent through an *EBITDAR*-to-rent coverage ratio or its reciprocal, rent as a percentage of *EBITDAR*. Like the development of an overall capitalization rate, the ratio or percentage is developed by analyzing comparable lease transactions, market surveys, and other market relationships. Alternatively, rental value can be developed by comparing rental rates from comparable properties and adjusting the rent, usually measured on a per-bed basis, for many of the same elements of comparison considered in the sales comparison approach. For existing nursing facilities, the cost approach has limited relevance in determining market rent, unless only the real estate and tangible personal property assets are to be included in the rent.

To develop market support for a leased fee capitalization rate or an internal rate of return, the appraiser first looks to the market for sales of the leased fee interest in nursing facilities. Such sales are fairly scarce and the search may necessitate casting a wide geographic net to gather a meaningful number of comparables. Healthcare REITs are a good source for comparable rental and leased fee sales data. Most sales data will show that leased fee capitalization rates are typically a few hundred basis points lower than capitalization rates for the going concern or business enterprise of a similar property. The lower rate is generally appropriate when the rent is at or below market levels since the landlord does not anticipate assuming the operational risks of conducting the business. The following issues warrant consideration in the selection of an appropriate leased fee capitalization rate or internal rate of return:

- Amount and frequency of scheduled rental increases
- *EBITDAR*-to-rent coverage ratio–high rent coverage reduces risks and rates

- Minimum *EBITDAR*-to-rent coverage requirements and provisions to ensure that positive coverage is achieved, such as cross-defaulting and multiple property leases between the same tenant and landlord
- Remaining term of the lease and prospects and cost of transitioning the property to the next operator
- Building condition, remaining economic life, and location
- Credit quality of the tenant and guarantees
- Atypical lease terms or unconventional leases
- Anticipated reversion value, relative to the current value
- Tenant's ability or inability to compete with the existing leased facility after the termination of the lease–assuming the tenant might develop a replacement facility in the same market area
- Landlord's contribution to property expenses

In the development of a discounted cash flow analysis, the appraiser must estimate future rents, a reversion value, and possibly a lease expiration date. The reversion value may be based on 1) a leased fee value, assuming a continuation of the existing lease or a new lease at market rent, or 2) a going-concern value, including an unencumbered fee simple interest after the lease terminates and ownership is transferred. The internal rate of return (*IRR*) is developed from market evidence, typically from sales in which the internal rate of return is apparent or from investor surveys. In the absence of comparable leased fee data for nursing facilities, market capitalization rates and IRRs can be inferred through analysis of rates from other net leased property types, provided appropriate consideration is given to the differences. Extracting *IRR*s from absolute net leases can be fairly simple when the rental increases are clearly defined. For example, an *IRR* of approximately 12.0% is indicated from the sale of a leased property that has a going-in overall capitalization rate of 10.0% and 2.0% annual rental increases for each of the remaining 15 years of the lease. The rate depends on the anticipated percentage change in the value of the property over the lease term. The rate may be lower, if the annual value increase is less than 2.0%, or higher, if the property value is believed to increase more than 2.0% per year.

Most valuations of the leased fee interests with long-term, absolute net structures assume no vacancy or operating expenses in the *NOI* or cash flow because the market incorporates these factors into the capitalization and discount rates. It is important to treat the market data used to derive these rates in a manner that is consistent to the treatment of the *NOI* of the subject. If the subject property and the comparable sales involve absolute net leases, then deducting for vacancies and operating expenses from the rent of one property but not from the rent of the other will produce an inaccurate value. Most REITs will report capitalization rates based on full rent when the lease is absolute net, without deductions for vacancy risk, management fees, or other potential expenses. For absolute net leases, the possibility of vacancy and expenses associated with the property in a premature tenant transition can be incorporated into the capitalization rate.

Using a residual approach to estimate the leased fee value, by deducting the leasehold value from the hypothetical fee simple value, is not recommended. The sales comparison and cost approaches are not practical for the valuation of the leasehold interest and may have only limited significance at best in the valuation of a leased fee interest.

Leasehold Interest Valuation

A leasehold interest may exist when the contract rent is less than market rent and the lease has provisions that permit the tenant to transfer its interest to another. Additional value to the leasehold interest may be realized when the expected *EBITDAR* exceeds market rent. Allocating these values (i.e., the difference between market rent and contract rent and between *EBITDAR* and market rent) to the real estate and the tangible and intangible personal property assets is problematic. In most leasehold sales, the two are combined into a single consideration (see Figure 19.1).

Generally, the risk to the leasehold interest is greater than the risk to the leased fee interest since the rent must be paid prior to recognizing earnings to the leasehold. Moreover, the leasehold earnings have greater volatility and the interest is usually not entitled to the reversion. Developing capitalization rates and internal rates of return for leasehold interests is very difficult since leasehold transactions are infrequent and the earnings are volatile. Like fee simple and leased fee capitalization rates, the leasehold capitalization rate equals income divided by value. Is this case, the income is the difference

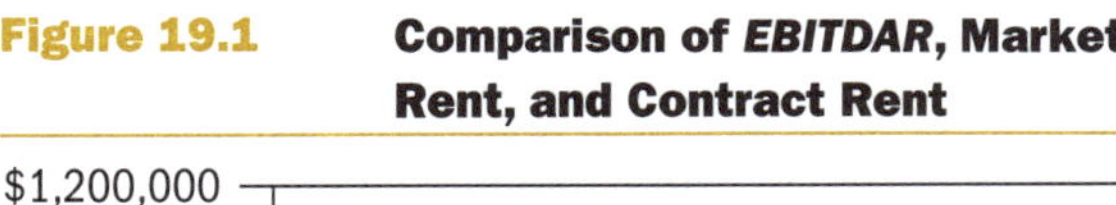
Figure 19.1 **Comparison of *EBITDAR*, Market Rent, and Contract Rent**

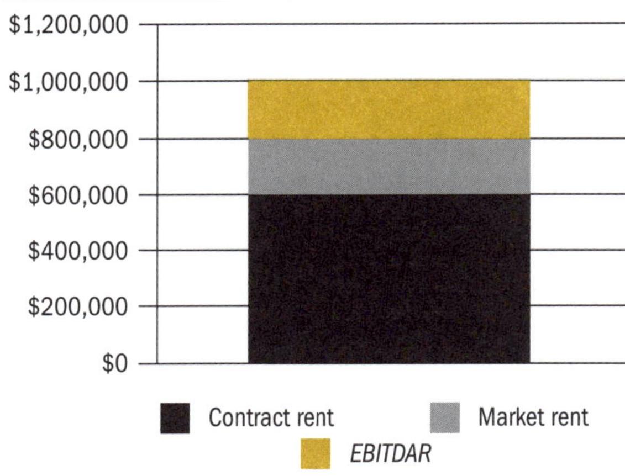

between either the market rent and the contract rent, or between *EBITDAR* and contract rent. For the most part, leasehold valuations capitalize the positive difference between *EBITDAR* and contract rent. Depending on the stability and predictability of the leasehold earnings, a direct capitalization and/or a discounted cash flow analysis may be employed to value this interest. Unless demonstrated by the market, the leasehold interest is not necessarily equal to the difference between the hypothetical fee simple and the leased fee interest. The difference between the fee simple and leased fee interests can be used as a test of reasonableness when reconciling the capitalized value of the leasehold interest.

Allocation of Leased Fee and Leasehold Value

Even though the leased fee interest is receiving rent for the facility, it has effectively leased and is receiving payment for its interests in the tangible and some of the intangible assets of the nursing facility. Therefore, it may be improper to claim that the entire rent is attributable to the value of the real estate and FF&E. Likewise, it is possible that the leasehold value possesses both tangible and intangible value.

It is extremely unlikely that the market will provide any meaningful evidence regarding the allocation of value to these partial interests. The cost approach may provide some insight into the real estate and FF&E value for the leased fee interest, provided the leased fee value exceeds the land value and the depreciated costs of the improvements and FF&E. If the leasehold value is represented as the capitalized difference between *EBITDAR* and market rent, then an argument can be made that this value has a significant intangible component. The capitalized difference between the market rent and contract rent may have a greater proportion of value allocated to real estate and FF&E. In fact, as the tenant continues to add and replace FF&E over the term of the lease, this asset group could represent increasing proportions of the leasehold value.

Summary

The ownership of many nursing facilities is fragmented, with the real estate owned by a "property entity" that leases the assets to a tenant that is the licensed operator. It is imperative to consider the relationship between the landlord and tenant and determine if the parties are related or unrelated. If the parties are related and the intended use of the appraisal is to consider a fee simple interest, then there may be no reason to evaluate the separate leasehold and leased fee interests. Many nursing facilities have fragmented ownership involving third-party property leases. In either case, the appraiser must identify the interest or interests being appraised and state any necessary hypothetical conditions that are contrary to the facts of ownership.

Most nursing facilities operated under third-party leases involve long-term, absolute net leases that require the tenant to assist the landlord in transferring the operating rights to the next operator upon termination of the lease. The leased fee value is generally estimated through income capitalization and/or discounted cash flow analysis. The quality and durability of the cash flow largely hinges on the *EBITDAR*-to-rent coverage ratio. Positive coverage provides the tenant with economic incentives to remain faithful to the terms and conditions of the lease. Negative coverage increases the risk to the landlord, as the tenant may be unable to continue the lease under the current rent, if at all.

The terminal or residual value of the property at the termination of a long-term lease should consider the likelihood that the building will suffer higher-than-normal levels of deterioration since the tenant has had little incentive to make capital improvements, beyond necessary replacements, in the later periods of the lease. Valuations of leasehold interests deal with marginal earnings or incomes that have considerable volatility. Market support for capitalization rates and *IRR*s is difficult to obtain. Unless this is demonstrated by the market, the leasehold interest is not necessarily the difference between the fee simple and leased fee interest.